SMOKING UNDER THE TSARS

SMOKING UNDER THE TSARS

A History of Tobacco in Imperial Russia

TRICIA STARKS

Cornell University Press *Ithaca and London*

First published 2018 by Cornell University Press

Printed in the United States of America

Library of Congress Cataloging-in-Publication Data

Names: Starks, Tricia, 1969– author.
Title: Smoking under the tsars : a history of tobacco in imperial Russia / Tricia
  Starks.
Description: Ithaca [New York] : Cornell University Press, 2018. | Includes
  bibliographical references and index.
Identifiers: LCCN 2018006952 (print) | LCCN 2018008823 (ebook) | ISBN
  9781501722066 (pdf) | ISBN 9781501722073 (ret) | ISBN 9781501722059 |
  ISBN 9781501722059 (cloth ; alk. paper)
Subjects: LCSH: Smoking—Russia—History—19th century. | Russians—Tobacco
  use—History. | Tobacco—Social aspects—Russia—History. | Russia—Social
  conditions—1801–1917.
Classification: LCC GT3021.R8 (ebook) | LCC GT3021.R8 S73 2018 (print) | DDC
  394.1/4094709034—dc23
LC record available at https://lccn.loc.gov/2018006952

To Mike

I do not know which taste or what pleasure they find in it . . . the taste of tobacco can be appreciated fully only by smokers. No language can express this pleasure; this feeling will never be completely defined.

—S. B. *Torzhestvo tabaku: Fiziologiia tabaku, trubki, sigar, papiros, pakhitos i tabakerki*, 1863

Contents

Tables and Maps

Tables

Maps

Acknowledgments

I have been working on tobacco since 2002, and in that time, the one planned monograph has turned into two, and two edited volumes hopped on for the ride. Needless to say, I have accumulated enormous debts. Research for this project was funded by grants from the National Institutes of Health and the National Library of Medicine; the National Council for East European and Eurasian Research and the National Endowment for the Humanities; and the Kennan Institute at the Wilson Center and the Slavic Research Lab at the University of Illinois. At the University of Arkansas, the Office of the Provost, the Fulbright College of Arts and Sciences, and the Department of History all provided assistance. Renee Vendetti was extremely patient with all my questions about application processes, and Jeanne Short, Brenda Foster, and Melinda Adams continue to be the hardest working administrative team in Fulbright College. Deans from the college, including Don Bobbitt, Robin Roberts, and Todd Shields, provided additional support, as did the chairs of the department, Jeannie Whayne, Lynda Coon, Kathryn Sloan, and Calvin White. I have imposed on many others during the application process, and I am indebted to Bryan DeBusk, Ellen Leen-Feldner, Eve Levin, Julie Stenken, Beth Schweiger, Robert Finlay, Judyth Twigg, Paula Michaels, Elizabeth A. Wood, Gwen Walker, and David L. Hoffmann for their help during the hunt. David took me in years ago when I was a student adrift, and his consummate professionalism, good humor, and unfailing generosity continue to serve as my model.

In workshops and conferences I tried out different pieces of the project, and it is all the stronger for the many useful suggestions I received and the enriching conversations I enjoyed. Thank you to the organizers of these events—Lynda Park, Natalia Lvovna Pushkareva, David L. Hoffmann, Fran Bernstein, Chris Burton, Dan Healey, Susan Gross Solomon, Gregory Dufaud, Matthew P. Romaniello, Cynthia Buckley, Christopher J. Gerry, and Dora Vargha. Readers for essays and chapters that appeared along the way—Barbara Alpern Engel, Aaron Retish, Sally West, and anonymous readers—provided much needed guidance. The formidable Pushkarevy historians—Natalia Lvovna and Irina Mikhailovna—continued to show me the way forward, as did the amazing archivists of the University of Illinois, National Library of Medicine, and State Archive of the Russian Federation. The women of the Leninka stoically served up the stacks of books I requested, and S. N. Artamonova supplied help and access to the stunning graphics. At the University of Arkansas, the divine Beth Juhl and the indefatigable staff of our Inter-Library Loan department made the impossible available. My collaborator on the NEH/NCEEER grant, Iurii P. Bokarev, provided valuable insight into the economic story of Russian tobacco, and for the NIH/NLM grant, Kenneth A. Perkins reached across the humanities-STEM divide to introduce me to the latest research on cigarette dependence. He opened a new way for me to look at Russia's tobacco history. At Cornell, Roger Malcolm Haydon and Meagan Dermody guided the manuscript through the process with skill and humor; Sara R. Ferguson (the guardian of all that is good) and Julia Cook edited with great care. Kate Transchel and Alison K. Smith read and critiqued the manuscript for the press, providing extremely helpful ideas on structure, content, and interpretation. I appreciate the perspectives that all of these scholars imparted and apologize for any continued pigheadedness on my part that they see in the book.

A few poor souls have suffered through even more. Lynda Coon has been not only a brilliant critic, reading every stitch, but also a great colleague and friend, always ready with enthusiasm, empathy, or humor. She inspires me with her generosity as a scholar, kindness as a mentor, keen mind as a theorist, and acumen as an administrator. Matthew P. Romaniello has been my partner in tobacco, plowing through hundreds of emails, at points obsessive, at others picayune, and yet always his breadth and depth of knowledge about everything—theory, history, profession, or pop culture—stuns me and embiggens this work. I have been fortunate that he has tolerated me through dozens of conferences, including one at the University of Hawaii, and through not one but two edited volumes. He read every part of this book, sometimes multiple times, the poor dear.

Mike Pierce edited, encouraged, and suggested while pursuing his own career of researching, writing, editing, and teaching—and then taking care of kids and house when the "work day" was done. When I left the country, he did it all. People ask us how we work together, but I do not know how it could be otherwise. I just know every day how lucky I am that he is my friend, my colleague, and my partner. We are both extremely fortunate to have Don and Pat Pierce and Dick and Sharon Starks, who came in at a moment's notice to care for the kids and us. And Ben and Sam made it all easier by being patient and helpful when needed and funny and distracting when necessary. Thanks, guys—you make me happy, every day.

A Note on Translation

Although Russians called tobacco processing plants "fabriki," the term "factory" has been used here, rather than "mill," to conform to western terminology. Transliteration of the Russian conforms to Library of Congress style except in cases where clarity or style are hampered; thus concluding hard signs have been eliminated, and with such names as "Tolstoy" established forms are observed. Unless indicated in the notes, all translations, and their errors, are my own.

SMOKING UNDER THE TSARS

INTRODUCTION

Papirosy and Dependence

A cigarette does not taste as it smells. A freshly opened pack releases an earthy, sweet scent, but the initial inhalation delivers flavors of metal. Nicotine's odor and taste is of burning rubber.[1] Tobacco smells like nature but tastes of industry. A swirl of sensations accompanies the drag as it fills the palate and tickles the throat, while a chemical cocktail of nicotine, tars, and toxins infuses the lungs to pass into the blood and circulate around the body. The burning inhalation pulls through the mouth and nose—felt, smelled, tasted, and heard—and the embers that bring it all to life smolder close to the face while the crackling and popping of the leaves and paper intrude on the ear and dazzle the eye.[2] Language attests to this muddle of mind, body, and cigarette. For Russians, the scent of tobacco could be audible (*slyshno*) or felt (*chuvstvenno*).[3] Despite the sensory banquet, smokers do not speak of savoring their first cigarette. More often new users report nausea, headache, and dizziness.[4] To become a regular smoker takes an endurance to move beyond that initial revulsion for other reasons: for addiction, for comfort, for prestige, or for pleasure. It is these "other reasons" that dominate this analysis, but I begin with the sensory appeal of the cigarette.

There are many ways to consume tobacco—snuff, chaw, pipes, water pipes, poultices, teas, and even fumigating enemas—but the focus here is on the point of mass use of tobacco that developed in Russia in the late nineteenth and early twentieth century with the rise of a unique form of Russian cigarette called a papirosa (singular –a; plural –y), a smoke composed of two parts—a hollow, cardboard mouthpiece and a tissue-paper cartridge stuffed with domestic tobacco (figure I.1).[5]

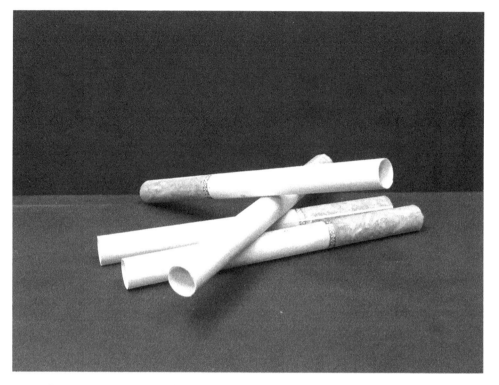

Figure I.1   Papirosy: Modern manufacture made according to the tsarist-era style. Note the tissue-wrapped leaf (the *kurka*) and the hollow, cardboard mouthpiece (the *gil'za*). Author's collection.

Papirosy enjoyed sharply rising popularity in Russia in part because they delivered nicotine quickly, intensely, and smoothly.[6] Unlike the half-hour languor of a pipe or cigar, the smoke of a papirosa could be bolted down on the go in a few short minutes, making for a habit in keeping with the pace of the modern city.[7] Pipes could break. Cigars were expensive and could spoil. The easy availability of cheap papirosy from street sellers and their porta-bility made for a more mobile, modern, and convenient habit. Further, the inhalation of cigarette smoke carries a more intense, faster-acting dose of nicotine since the acidic smoke can be brought into the lungs, while alka-line cigar and pipe smoke absorbs in smaller doses more slowly through the mouth lining. Inhaled smoke rapidly spreads from the lungs to the blood delivering over 90 percent of the nicotine in less than half a minute.[8] The intensity of the experience is hard to duplicate with other tobacco products or even nicotine in patches.[9] In addition to its likely being more addictive, smoother, acidic smoke may have enticed new, adult, male consumers but also perhaps lured women and children to the habit.[10]

More efficient in delivery and easier to use, papirosy exploded in production and consumption.[11] Russian tobacco excise tax receipts showed the precipitous increase. In 1889 the tax generated about twenty-two million rubles and by 1913 it was almost seventy million, an increase of nearly 250 percent, due almost entirely to expanded production rather than higher tax rates. Tobacco was on the rise as a percentage of taxed products. In 1913, tobacco was second only to sugar for taxes and ahead of petroleum and matches.[12] Yet taxed tobacco was only a fraction, and an unknown one, of the total tobacco consumed in Russia, as the excise system did not include locally grown and consumed tobacco. Contemporaries observed that much Russian tobacco production and use escaped count.[13]

Perhaps even more astonishing than the growth in tax revenue was the climbing percentage of tobacco produced as papirosy out of all tobacco worked. By 1914, 49.5 percent of all tobacco processed in Russia came out as papirosy. The war years only accelerated the change so that by 1922/23 that reached 83.2 percent.[14] As comparison, the cigarette only reached half of total production in Britain in 1920, in the United States in 1941, and in France in 1943.[15] Contemporaries estimated that almost every urban Russian male consumed about a pack a day at the turn of the century.[16] A report in Russia's journal *Vrach* (Doctor) in 1887 noted "among men a nonsmoker is, unfortunately, already almost impossible to find."[17] And while commentators lingered on the ubiquity of smoking among men, the large number of women that openly smoked astonished them.

The early transfer of the tobacco market to papirosy may hold profound significance for health outcomes as the easy access to a convenient means of inhaling smoke creates circumstances that may make for more addictive use and therefore more dangerous outcomes than consumption with pipes or cigars.[18] The addictive nature of the papirosy also poised the product for steady demand despite economic downturns or changes of fashion.[19] The large community of smokers, male and female of all classes, likely led to increased pressure for nonsmokers and for those who might wish to quit. Russia arguably became a society of smokers earlier and more fully than any other market in the world.

Well into the twentieth century, large numbers of Russians smoked factory-produced, hand-rolled papirosy stuffed with either Turkish leaf varieties or increasingly the Ukrainian/Russian tobacco—makhorka (*nicotiana rustica*). Makhorka, one of about one hundred known tobacco species and one of two domesticated types, was the nicotine-heavy variety brought by Sir Walter Raleigh from the New World.[20] Nicotine, the alkaloid identified in the nineteenth century as a component of tobacco and a powerful poison in isolation, is recognized as the primary chemical cause of dependency, though other elements in smoke might enhance this effect.[21] When inhaled through smoke, nicotine binds with receptors in the brain, which then release dopamine, creating a pleasurable effect.[22] Nicotine does not produce the same results for every user and in every method of delivery.[23] Age, genetics, gender, and environment all contribute to the experience. Adolescents may be more susceptible than adults, women more than men, and children of smokers more than those of people who never used tobacco.[24] Systematic engineering by tobacco companies has changed the amount of nicotine delivered and the speed with which it enters the body, assuring that the cigarette of today also differs substantially from the smoke of a century ago. American manufacturers worked over their tobacco for nicotine content, but Russian makhorka started at a point of higher nicotine than others.[25]

Even though tobacco species are very similar genetically, their flavor can vary widely because of disparities in soil, climate, and curing.[26] In most markets, the "harsh and sour" and at times hallucinogenic makhorka fell to the wayside in preference for the "mild, sweet" *nicotiana tabacum* of Virginia, but throughout Russia and Ukraine, makhorka, with its shorter growing season and tolerance for cooler climates, maintained primacy, becoming an emblem of Russian difference and imparting an exceptional smoking experience.[27] In 1899, of the 60,000 *desiatin* (almost 162,000 acres) of land sown with tobacco in the empire, 35,000 was makhorka, another 5,000 simple Russian sorts, and only 6,000 allotted to American and 14,000 to Turkish leaf.[28] The share of makhorka in tobacco production grew with time. From 1900 to 1908 the production of cheaper papirosy utilizing rough tobacco increased by an average of 10.1 percent each year while the average yearly growth in general makhorka production was 5.7 percent.[29]

Makhorka carried a distinctive smell, taste, and effect to Russian papirosy. Virginia "bright tobacco" is flu-cured in barns with charcoal fires and has a light taste and scent, though it is deceptively high in sugar and nicotine and therefore considered very addictive. Burleys of South America and the Mediterranean, cured in open-air barns, impart a buttery flavor and have a nicotine content of around 5.2 percent.[30] Turkish tobacco, also called "Oriental" leaf, was the second most produced tobacco in imperial Russia; it is sun-cured in the open air, is more acidic and easily inhaled than Virginia tobacco, and contains less sugar and nicotine (.86 percent or so), yet has a powerful taste because of the highly aromatic yet tiny leaves.[31] In addition to leaf differences, behaviors of individual smokers or tobacco additives, such as ammonia, as used in Russia, can cause variations in nicotine content and bioavailability from 3 to 40 percent.[32] Still, Russian papirosy, made from either higher-nicotine makhorka (up to 16 percent) or more acidic and therefore more easily inhaled Turkish, may have had greater potential for dependency than smokes made from other types of leaf or those of Western manufacturers.[33]

The prevalent use of low-grade makhorka tobacco—fragrant, harsh, high in nicotine, yet still inhaled deeply—makes the Russian smoking experience remarkable, and the unique sensory markers of Russian smoking occupied many a memoirist and foreign traveler, indicating that at least the broad distinctions between Western and Russian cigarettes were easily visible in the nineteenth century.[34] Memoirists noted the peculiar scent, taste, style, and potency of Russian papirosy. Consumers and bystanders readily contrasted the odor of Russian tobacco with the lighter aromas and more delicate flavor of Virginia leaf. It would seem that nineteenth-century Russian papirosy must have had a quite heady, if not overwhelming, effect, according to the testimony of contemporaries.

Despite the pervasive consumption of tobacco in Russia, recognized as comparatively high even in the late nineteenth century, the details of Russia's smoking history remain obscured.[35] This is not because the problem has disappeared. Despite recent progress, Russians remain some of the heaviest smokers in the world. According to the World Health Organization in 2014, over 60 percent of men and 20 percent of women in Russia smoke. Such high consumption reveals itself in disastrous health consequences. About 400,000 Russians—parents, spouses, siblings, and friends—die every year from smoking-related illnesses, the rough equivalent of yearly tobacco mortality in the United States, which has about double the population of Russia.[36]

The extent of the contemporary problem underscores the need for a scholarly account of Russia's tobacco history. This volume investigates how tobacco went from a product of occasional use to become a mainstay of Russian identity by the eve of World War I, detailing how papirosy became part of nearly every aspect of Russian culture, politics, and society, as well as infiltrating individual Russian bodies and all their tissues. Papirosy were not just everywhere; they were important to nearly everything—from revolutionary activity to empire building, from male power to female emancipation, from moral concern to professional focus, and from individual pleasure to societal danger. As smoking became embedded in Russian identity, it sent down roots into the culture and society that would be as difficult to eradicate as those of the addictive chemicals of tobacco itself. So universal is the experience of tobacco to Russia, and so deeply entrenched, that for Russians to give up smoking they must induce a type of cultural amnesia, giving up what they thought they had always been.

Central to this story is not just the production and style of Russian tobacco, but also its reception on an individual level as both embodied behaviors and physical reactions. Tobacco provokes visceral responses, as smoking engages the entire body in tasting, smelling, feeling, seeing, and hearing. These are more than just fleeting sensations. While chemical dependency is often seen as the primary motivation for continued tobacco use, the sensory stimuli tied to smoking can trigger cravings and the symptoms of withdrawal. These same cues can at times alleviate the desire to smoke.[37] The importance of the sensory experience explains why patches and nicotine replacement therapies today, disconnected from the physical act of smoking, are sometimes not successful cessation treatments, as well as the proposed change in 2012 of testing for "Cigarette Dependence" rather than simply "Nicotine Dependence."[38] The sensory experience of tobacco use, in the Russian case the primacy of the papirosy, is central to understanding the history of Russian tobacco dependence.

Papirosy have changed with time, and taste and scent, arguably the most important senses to tobacco use, are not the same today as they were a century ago. Taste can vary from person to person and by age.[39] Sweets are alluring to the young, and the aged often crave bitter, strong flavors. Experience and associations can influence what is considered sweet, savory, or desirable; for instance, over the course of the eighteenth and nineteenth centuries, as sugar became more available, tastes changed and thresholds for "sweetness" shifted.[40] Discussion of scent has been largely absent in global tobacco histories. Perhaps this lacuna can be attributed to the fact that scent is difficult to discuss; plagued by the ephemeral and contingent nature of odor, language seems inadequate to its description in the present moment let alone in the historical. But while the ability to smell is a constant, how one smells is not a cultural monolith.[41] Sensory historians argue for massive changes in the intellectual contexts of perception over the course of the eighteenth and nineteenth century as the Enlightenment changed the hierarchy of what senses were considered civilized and refined as opposed to those termed backwards and bestial.[42] At the same time, the line between stench and perfume relocated, influenced by new medical concepts, urban relationships, political expectations, social fears, and gendered assumptions.[43] Taste and scent played across concepts of class, order, and respectability, and issues of nation, modernization, and health.[44] In the case of tobacco, as Russians became acquainted with foreign blends and internal industry advanced, tobacco once thought of as smooth became harsh in comparison, and society viewed those who smoked low-grade tobacco with increasing condescension for their coarse tastes, which were connected to a perception of their unrefined manners and low intellect.

The body, its perceptions, and its surroundings spur the desire to smoke through symptoms of withdrawal or conditioned stimuli that cue the desire for tobacco—like smelling smoke, seeing an ashtray, watching another smoke, engaging in work, or gathering with friends.[45] A biopsychosocial web of hungers ensnares the smoker in continued use; these spaces, situations, ideas, people, and senses are not static, but rather framed by culture and history. These influences play out throughout the life of the smoker. They change as smoking spreads and becomes more socially visible, accepted, and normative, and as ideas about class and status develop. They adjust as marketers and producers suggest tobacco's attractions, and as authorities in science and medicine debate tobacco's effects. Yet some things remain surprisingly constant. In Russia of over a hundred years ago, as today, social groups fostered onset of tobacco use, usually in adolescence, efforts to quit were deterred by mingling with other smokers, and low education and socioeconomic status predicted use of higher nicotine, more addictive products.[46]

While the chemistry of nicotine produces certain physical responses, the interpretation of these reactions by individuals, and whether they should be conceived of as good or bad, is tempered by context. "Addiction" itself is a term dependent on historical context—alternatively termed "dependency," "habit," or "weakness" and seen as disease or individual failing. The perception of addiction, like the experience of use and withdrawal, is subject to its surroundings. Specialists now know that physical withdrawal from tobacco reveals itself in cravings, irritability, anxiety, depression, restlessness, cramping, nervous ticks, or increased appetite, but a cigarette alleviates these symptoms. Thus smoking becomes associated with calming anxiety, easing depression, satisfying hunger, and reducing tedium. To avoid the unpleasant experience of withdrawal, which usually is not noticed for some time but can return after only an hour, smokers light up again and again. It is this compulsion to continue using tobacco, even in the face of overwhelming evidence of its hazards, that is a hallmark of contemporary definitions of addiction.[47] Yet, there was not a widespread appreciation of the connection between tobacco use and danger, nor between withdrawal symptoms and use, in the past. Most Russian cessationists argued that tobacco, unlike opium or alcohol, had no withdrawal symptoms.[48] Because there was no agreement about withdrawal and a conflicted case regarding tobacco's dangers, today's definition of addiction—continued use despite knowledge of harm—cannot be imposed on the user of the past. For the Russian smoker of the past, chemically induced physical reactions to tobacco were interpreted alternately, assigned to other causes, or perhaps not noted at all.

Tobacco's impact stretches beyond biology and social context. Cigarettes, like all commodities, are more than just items for consumption by individuals; they serve as ways for people to display, manipulate, and communicate identity, as well as to express ideas and negotiate social relationships.[49] Tobacco circulates itself more readily through communities and more equally than most other products because it is easily distributed and can be differentiated greatly in terms of price and quality, which allow it to spread to lower and upper classes, rural and urban consumers.[50] Smokers connect to others through consumption, signaling their relationship to groups by displaying their brand choice, their style of smoking, and their accessories for the habit. These messages are more than just a language of status or belonging. Marketers as well as smokers can manipulate them. Russia's radical feminists or hardened revolutionaries might signal to others their pure politics through taking up the habit, offering a smoke, or showing a preference for a certain brand. For instance, papirosy were primarily associated with the urban population, with higher grade tobacco as a point of class distinction, while rural inhabitants more often used rough, mercerized makhorka in pipes or self-rolled smokes in scrap paper called "dog legs" (*koz'ia nozhka*).[51]

Things are not always, or maybe ever, passive objects that we manipulate and display to others in a language of "stuff." Cigarettes can influence conduct in ways that come from the biological dependency tobacco creates, the dictates of the physical act, or the social and cultural connections of the habit, and in a circular manner they can, in turn, trigger physical cravings for tobacco for the user and for others.[52] Things influence behaviors in ways both subtle and constant even as users insist they are in control and onlookers swear they are beyond the sway of the material.[53] For example, papirosy did not always burn well. Windy, damp weather and the need to keep the embers of sometimes poorly-made products smoldering forced users to cup the palm and fingers around the burning end of the papirosa while holding the mouthpiece with forefinger and thumb. This pinched, furtive posture would have obscured the light of the papirosa in military situations or hidden it in spaces that might have discouraged smoking. Thus a way of smoking associated with a lower-quality smoke became also a bodily-style indicative of class, war experience, means, and nation. The choosing, lighting, holding, and inhalation of a cigarette are actions that are at once chemically altering, pregnant with significance, and habitually transformative, yet bound to their historical context for interpretation.

The signals sent by the smoker do not always come from gestural cues or special accessories. The provocation of the cigarette for body and bystander continues after the butt is stubbed out, as tobacco marks the flesh in ways easily identifiable to observers, lingering for hours or even days after consumption. Smoke bathes the skin, hair, and clothing, anointing the user with a sign of their habit for all to discern. Tobacco perfumes the body from the inside out as tissue absorbs then slowly diffuses the scent. Stale odor betrays heavier smokers through the rancid-tobacco scent of their sweat and their metallic, musty breath even as the smell cleaves to clothes and hair. Smokers become like censers for the habit—slowly releasing their devotion to the weed over the course of their day. Still other somatic inscriptions divulge the habituate. The smoker's hack or husky voice attends tobacco consumption, and even the absence of use has its signifiers. The cravings of addiction can produce jitteriness, irritability, and attention problems when abstinence from tobacco continues beyond a few hours.

Smoking's signs stand outside the control of the user, serving as clues to others of their habit, and perhaps even cues for bystanders' own compulsions. In imperial Russia, they also occasioned revulsion. For instance the habit of snuff created many memorable impressions as a particularly vile form of tobacco use. As one observer of military men remarked, "The majority of snuffers had an unclean visage. The aftermath of tobacco stood on mustache and beard. From the nose coursed a brown slime."[54] In smokers, other signs became sources of disgust and markers of their poor habit. The stained fingers, blackened teeth, dingy facial hair, and yellowed nails remained well after the smoke had dissipated. For women, the signs of tobacco held particular power and danger, some considering them an attractive addition to a woman's charms and others arguing that they so spoiled a woman as to make her repellent.

The biological, cultural, social, and psychological experience of tobacco use has changed according to time and place. To be a smoker carried different meanings before smoking was connected to cancer, before nicotine was understood to be addictive, in places where cigarettes were made from exotic materials with other stories of production, when odor and smoke carried other meanings, when social stigma did not cling to smokers, and before citizenship carried the weighty obligations of continued health as well as obedience. For example, smoke in the nineteenth century indicated productivity and progress; in the twenty-first it suggests pollution.

Knowledge of the horror of tobacco-related death, and of the menace drifting in cigarette smoke, has changed the relationship of smokers and nonsmokers noticeably in the last half century. According to current surveys of smokers in the United States, most want to quit, but this was not the case over a century ago, and it is not the case even today elsewhere in the world.[55] Addiction research has affected attitudes toward smokers as well as the therapies offered. Knowing that one in three who try tobacco will become daily users, and that of these less than 5 percent will be successful in any one attempt to quit, brings a different attitude toward the dependency created for tobacco, the support needed for cessation, and the relationship to smokers by nonusers.[56] Perceptions from outsiders have changed as secondhand smoke has arisen as a threat from the individual to society as a whole.

We now know that tobacco smoking is addictive and deadly and we can see the contrary sensory story of agonizing smoking-related health complications. The cardio-pulmonary effects of smoking—emphysema, asthma, or COPD (Chronic Obstructive Pulmonary Disease)—leave the smoker gasping for breath, wracked with pain, and physically exhausted. But these diagnoses are modern, and while certain researchers suspected smoking caused weakness of the heart and lungs in the late nineteenth century, most of the public would be decades later in recognizing these problems as smoking related. We now know many cancers result from smoking—lip, esophagus, stomach, and lung among others—and bring their own narratives of fatigue, nausea, physical pain, and emotional trauma from the disease itself, the harrowing treatments of chemotherapy, tumor extraction, and organ removal, and the emotional and financial toll on families, friends, and the sufferer. Such knowledge is also, however, modern. At the turn of the century, only lip cancer from cigar use was accepted as a problem directly attributed to smoking, appearing in literature as early as the 1880s.[57] But generally no lingering, painful illnesses were attributed to smoking. When so many of the manifestations of smoking took so long to develop, blame did not always go to the responsible killer, and conceptions of smoking took on a different tenor.

This book is an exploration of the papirosy experience in all of its social, cultural, and as much as possible, sensory and physical manifestations, at a certain time and place. In describing the historical papirosa—from its extreme intoxicating effects to its unique, non-mechanized production; from its pungent, intense taste to its ubiquitous use—this book reveals the exceptional tobacco experience of one of the countries most threatened by the practice today. It also contributes to global histories by examining the sensory experience of tobacco alongside the cultural and social contexts, and complements studies of consumption and material culture by making the papirosa an active player in the story of tobacco rather than a passive receptor of consumer behavior. There are many scholarly histories of tobacco that detail its cultivation, production, and marketing, but none for Russia.[58] No Russian medical history has approached tobacco, and general public health studies of tobacco's rise often portray addiction as an ahistorical constant, downplay medical contention, neglect industrial advances that changed the addictive quality of cigarettes, or overemphasize the influence of antismoking advocates at the expense of contemporary reveries on the joys of smoking.[59] Cultural histories of tobacco tend to concentrate on the art and miss out on the social, economic, industrial, and medical understandings of the habit.[60] In isolation, each approach provides only a narrow view of tobacco use and users and neglects the many ways in which each aspect—physical experience, medical understanding, cultural construction, social context, and business practice—played off the other.

This volume is not, however, just a tobacco history. The emergence of the papirosa in the 1830s, its rise in visibility in the 1860s, and its introduction into mass use and marketing from the 1890s on to 1914 coincided with a vibrant period of political, economic, societal, and cultural change in tsarist Russia. Stung by the humiliating defeat of the Crimean War (1853–56), Tsar Alexander II (r. 1855–81) embarked on an ambitious series of reforms for Russia in the 1860s and '70s, emancipating the serfs, establishing local governance, creating new educational structures, amending judicial systems, and modernizing the military.[61] While far less revolutionary than many of the politically and socially forward elite might have wished, the era ushered in a period of rapid change, and Russia's military fortunes turned with the successful conclusion of the Russo-Turkish War of 1877–78. Alexander II's life came to an end with the regicide of 1881, and Alexander III (r. 1881–94) attempted to dissuade social and cultural changes, pushing instead for economic modernization and industrial development through projects like the Trans-Siberian Railway, begun in the 1890s under his Finance Minister, Sergei Witte (1849–1915).[62] Tobacco factories, spurred by the rising entrepreneurial interests of the day, the ready market, and the expansion of tobacco cultivation, became party to the economic, military, and industrial fortunes of the times.

The rapid urbanization of the last decades of the nineteenth century created conditions for the spread of tobacco cultivation and production, but also for tobacco's place in the negotiation of identity for swiftly-rising social groups—newly emancipated peasants, urbanizing workers, emerging bourgeoisie, and professionalizing bureaucrats—and the reconstruction of social roles for old estate groups—nobility, clergy, townspeople, and peasantry—against the fractured background of Russian regional variation, ethnic diversity, and rapidly devolving estate structures.[63]

Although Russian collectivism is often touted, the search for the self had its place in these tumultuous years, for workers and others as well as for aristocrats and intelligentsia.[64] These various groups encountered a city that allowed fresh ways of participation by becoming part of consumer culture, displaying novel commodities, and discovering original places to consume.[65] Commercial culture—be it consumption of leisure activities, purchasing art prints, reading pulp literature, or following high fashion—created space for people urban and rural, middle- and lower-class, owner and worker, conservative and radical, male and female to explore divisions between them as well as identify points of agreement.[66] Russian women, constrained by patriarchal authority in their choice of living arrangement, education, and employment, found in consumer culture a space to express new identities, aided in part by the fact that Russian women legally retained their property rights after marriage, unlike in much of the West.[67]

Problems from the rapid pace of industrialization and urbanization emerged alongside opportunities. New workers found employment neither steady nor well remunerated. Those that could find jobs worked long hours and returned to housing that was cramped and plagued by sanitary shortfalls. Medical and legal professionals, a rising educated bureaucratic stratum, representatives from the local governments, and increasing numbers of radicals of various political stripes voiced concerns about the pace and direction of modernization and mediated an entire set of discussions revolving around rights, responsibilities, and freedoms for men and women from peasant to aristocrat.[68] Even as they brought up problems for the state to address, they defined norms of acceptable behavior for the people, thereby singling out some as deviant or antisocial. These professionals worked to secure their own positions even as they feared they might at any moment lose their newly won status in an environment of startling change.[69]

Papirosy, humble and mundane, became party to this massive project of Russian political, social, and cultural creation. Starting with, and then expanding beyond, cultivation and production statistics, the chapters that follow reconstruct historical tobacco use, utilizing sensory theory, gender studies, medical history, semiotics, and contemporary tobacco research. These chapters employ material mined from newspapers, journals, industry publications, etiquette manuals, propaganda images, popular literature, memoirs, cartoons, and advertising images. Concentrating on the period when papirosy were established as the primary form of tobacco use in Russia—roughly the last forty years of the autocracy—this study traces Russian smoking under tsarist power until the collapse of the autocracy in the revolutionary era, after which the new political, cultural, social, production, and medical contexts framed a very different smoking experience.

Each chapter—"Cultivated," "Produced," "Tasted," "Condemned," and "Contested"—follows one root that papirosy put down into Russian society and culture, moving thematically from the papirosa's foundation as a cultural and imperial concept and its emergence as a mass-use product of revolutionary potential, to its later construction as a liberating object for tsarist subjects, toward discussion as a moral and medical problem, and concluding as it became a point of conflict for reformers and purveyors as well as for therapists and moralizers. Together, the chapters recreate how smokers and the society around them experienced, understood, and presented their habit and trace the development of the deep, wide, and influential presence of tobacco in Russia.

Apart from this introduction, in which I employ modern medical concepts and contemporary experiences, I present the remainder of this book in the past tense, even when working with visual and literary sources. Though it is possible to think of these as living sources that interact with the modern viewer in a vital way, the messages they conveyed about tobacco are not ahistorical. The present tense does not serve these sources. These posters, appeals, and attacks all had a very different meaning before addiction became medicalized, before cancer became defined as a tobacco death sentence, and in different contexts of ethnicity, gender, consumption, and class. The interpretation of these sources does not transcend their time and context, or at least the argument here is that they do not, and throughout this manuscript they are situated firmly in the past.

As the chapter "Cultivated" argues, makhorka and Russian-grown Turkish seed served as a symbol of Russian difference, but also as a tool for imperial domination. Domestic tobacco production overwhelmingly favored these strong, highly aromatic tobaccos, thereby imparting a distinctive Russian smoking experience.[70] When Russians expanded their empire, they took tobacco with them, linking the sowing of the lands of Crimea and Central Asia to the expanding habit. The primary force in imperial conquest, the Russian military, was also the primary user of tobacco in its earliest incarnations, first in pipes, then increasingly over the course of the century in cigars, and finally in papirosy. Between the use by soldiers and the deployment of tobacco seed in newly conquered areas, an exceptionally militant association grew just as papirosy use spread to the general population. Advertisers later capitalized on this connection to sell tobacco as valorous, patriotic, and manly, using two main avatars for smoking—the manly Cossack and the sexually available odalisque—to tempt Russians to try a new means for invigorating and pleasuring the political and individual body. Marketing cemented an association of tobacco and militarism founded earlier in the soil of empire.

"Produced" details the singular form, content, and manufacture of Russian papirosy. Russian consumption predated tobacco trusts and vertical integration, making the story covered here extraordinary. Most tobacco histories concentrate on the development of the Bonsack machine in 1885, and the entrepreneurial acumen of manufacturers like James B. Duke, to tell a story of mechanized production, vertical integration, trust building, aggressive advertising, and expanding consumption.[71] But in Russia, even before the explosion of mechanically produced cheap smokes, and with less aggressive advertisement, papirosy had already hooked a vast number of urban males and females. Making papirosy affordable and everywhere was essential to expanding the market, but instead of mechanizing the industry, Russian tobacco factories kept adding females and child laborers working at lower wages to meet demand and keep down costs.[72] This led to one more idiosyncratic feature—the revolutionary workforce of radicalized women who would become flesh-and-blood symbols of Russia's exploitative industrial relationships. For workers, for radicals, and for bourgeois smokers, these relationships of the factory were highly visible, so that product choice held political implications that a user could be reminded of, on average, twenty times a day. The papirosa emerged as a mix of modern styles made with backward techniques in abusive shops by radicalized workers under cynically philanthropic owners.

The Russian smoking experience was distinctive because of the production peculiarities, the eccentric papirosy, the coarse makhorka, and the early, sizeable market. Additionally, the cultural, political, and gendered associations of smoking in Russia developed differently from those in other regions of the world.[73] The chapter "Tasted" notes how an unusual social context led to the curious construction of Russian tobacco connoisseurship as a realm open to both men and women and inclusive of all classes, yet pushing strongly hierarchical visions. Connoisseurship—educated consumption of a product that allows users to distinguish themselves in terms of knowledge, status, and taste—developed alongside tobacco. In Russia as in the West, users, nonusers, cultural authorities, advertisers, and etiquette manuals together constructed rules and accessories for cultured use, spaces for shared consumption, and philosophical justifications that underscored class division while promising social inclusion. Unusual was the presence of women in the realm of respectable smoking. Although statistics are not available for the period, according to outside observers, marketing indicators, and antitobacco activists, women smoked in greater numbers in Russia than in Western nations, placing Russian habits in line with the patterns of countries like China.[74]

The relation of the user to tobacco today is tempered by anxiety, but this is not a creation of the last few decades or even a result of the medical understanding of tobacco that emerged in the twentieth century. From its earliest days in Russia, tobacco occasioned alarm from the state, church, and society, and its move to mass, visible use brought forward only more apprehension. Russia's boom in tobacco cultivation, production, and use came as increasing worries about gender roles, national strength, and social problems proliferated around the globe in a general age of anxiety. The chapter "Condemned" focuses on the fears that rising tobacco use tapped into as new medical, national, and psychological concerns about popular health, morals, and decline emerged, both in the West and in Russia. Nineteenth-century fixations on odor, neurasthenia, and degeneracy greatly affected the antitobacco movement, as did the social and political instability of an urbanizing society, fears of autocratic overreach, and disquiet over a swiftly increasing number of radicalized workers. Smoking marked the body, social spaces, and the land in ways that users deemed transformative and opponents argued threatened morality, individual health, the family, the city, and, increasingly in the age of imperialism and social statistics, the economy, society, and the nation. The rise of etiquette, health, and improvement literature in tandem with a developing interest in public health as a state resource took an occasional habit and turned it into a discursive explosion of treatises denouncing tobacco.

Essential to the tobacco experience today are the concepts of addiction and danger, but as the chapter "Contested" shows, these were not constants. The arguments against tobacco, the concept of dependency, and the therapies proposed for cessation in the late nineteenth century developed in a society without medical or public consensus. Antismoking advocates waged their war against tobacco in an environment of increased political power for medical and health professionals, yet doctors did not unify in opposition to tobacco or in comprehension of its dangers—or even on whether or not it was addictive. Instead, approval for moderation emerged in scientific literature, and ridicule for the stridency of antitobacco messages came out in popular forums. This suspicion and derision of antitobacco arguments created space for connoisseurs, marketers, and producers to peddle their own image of tobacco as healthful and enjoyable and antismoking polemics as shrill and ridiculous.

Industries develop. Businesses innovate. Cigarettes evolve. People are diverse, and sensory input is felt differently according to the era, the age, or the area. The epilogue concludes the story of smoking's foundation in Russia by showing how the experience of tobacco changed with the collapse of old production relationships, the popular acceptance of smoking, the disavowal of tobacco prohibition, and the dawn of a new era for tobacco in terms of medical consensus. The onset of World War I brought prohibition of alcohol but an eruption of tobacco use on the front lines. Even as the Bolshevik Revolution caused the downfall of bourgeois producers and ushered into power a new state with its own conflicted relationship to tobacco, use of papirosy was booming. The triumph of public health as a major policy point with the Soviets did not mean the victory of antismoking ideas; rather, it closed one chapter on tobacco's connection to state and citizen and brought forth a new era for antitobacco advocacy even as tobacco use was firmly embedded in the daily life of the Soviet citizen. The image of tobacco created in the nineteenth century and the medical understandings developing during that same period would prove remarkably long-lived, influencing policy on smoking, cessation, and therapy for decades to come.

1 : CULTIVATED

Exotic Blends and Imperial Designs

In 1852, under fire and finding his pipe damaged, a Zouave from one of the famed Bedouin fighter battalions of the Crimean War dumped the gunpowder and bullet out of a paper-wrapped cartridge shell, replaced it with tobacco, and lit up the world's first cigarette.[1] Kindled in the heat of combat, the cigarette blazed into prominence among the ranks, supplanting the more cumbersome pipe and the now passé snuff. As soldiers returned from deployment and spread the habit, the association of cigarettes with the military changed this once diminutive smoke—an effete cigar—to a marker of vigor, valor, and virility.[2] While this charming vignette maintained a hold on the popular imagination for years to come, paper cartridges stuffed with tobacco appeared on the European market decades earlier than the apocryphal anecdote would allow. French documents from 1708 referenced cigarettes, and the Napoleonic Wars along with the development of lighter papers diffused the style throughout Europe well before the Crimean conflict.[3]

Russia's first cigarettes came via France in the 1830s, wrapped in corn-husk and called *pakhitosy*, soon to be replaced in the 1840s by the more familiar, delicate, paper-wrapped style, touted by another Frenchman. Like the cigarette of the French Bedouins, the Russian's unique papirosa was born of the barracks when an enterprising officer filled his cartridges with low-grade domestic makhorka tobacco rather than the more expensive, imported Maryland leaf and began selling them.[4] Russian troops, already primed by the pipe, found the papirosa convenient, and the smoke soon traveled to the rest of Russian society. An 1843 magazine article noted, "No more than thirty-five years ago, smoking tobacco was seen in the same level as drinking spirits. Seamen, old soldiers, and primarily cavaliers smoked." Now, the author said, smoking had invaded all of society.[5] The papirosa were not yet supreme, however. In his *Sevastopol Stories,* set during the Crimean conflict, Lev Nikolaevich Tolstoy (1828–1910) described smoking as so firmly rooted in the military and in such proliferation that a complex culture of tobacco use as signifier of rank and class emerged to distinguish grunts (pipes) from officers (papirosy) and high command (cigars).[6]

The longevity of the Zouave origin story indicated the strong connection of cigarettes to a romanticized image of the military in the nineteenth century and particularly to the conflicts in Crimea. The Zouave captured the imagination of the public for their fierce tactics, elaborate drills, and eccentric uniforms—vibrant, sapphire blue jackets paired with red harem pants or sashes, gold embroidered jackets festooned with shiny buttons, all topped with jaunty turbans or fezzes. Their unusual, if not tactical, attire inspired copycat styles among soldiers in the American Civil War, as well as in the Spanish and Polish militaries. The smoking soldier became an enduring and iconic figure, and the striking imagery of a man dressed as a tropical bird lent itself easily to the emerging field of color posters and cigarette packs. In the late nineteenth century, France's Job and Zig-Zag cigarette papers employed a Zouave in their advertising, as did the Russian firm A. Miller for their 1899 poster for their *Pushka* brand—an interesting choice as the Zouave's fought for Russia's enemies.[7]

Even before the papirosa, tobacco and soldier were united in the Russian imaginary. Nikolai Gogol (1809–52) twirled tobacco, soldiers, empire, and nation together in his 1835 story "Taras Bulba," in the love affair between the titular stalwart Cossack defender of faith and his tobacco pipe, *liul'ka,* which was his constant companion on all his campaigns. But the smoking soldier was more than just an imagined type in imperial Russia. The soldier and sailor, tied to tobacco use as early as the Thirty Years War (1618–48), provided an ideal vector for smoking, and their martial lives of tedium broken by terror proved "natural incubators for drug abuse," as one historian noted. Their mobility allowed for the easy transfer of their habit to all areas of the globe.[8] After the Crimean War, European consumption rose significantly as soldiers' love of tobacco on the front lines flowed back to the home front.[9] The British saw smoking take off.[10] So too would the Russians. The influence of the Russian military on the rest of society was heightened by the practice, beginning after the reforms of Alexander II, of military men returning to civilian life after a set time. Military units thus became perfect routes for tobacco use as soldiers went in, learned to smoke under pressure, and then returned home to spread the habit further.

While one author attributed the 1870 victory of the Germans over the French "to Germans smoking pipes, Frenchmen cigarettes," no such worry over the manliness of the papirosa appeared to bother the smoking Russian soldier or his adoring public.[11] According to Archibald Forbes, a war correspondent during the next Crimean conflict, the Russo-Turkish War of 1877–78, the zeal among the Russians for tobacco was matched only by the Turks. As he described from the front lines, "Cannon smoke and tobacco smoke hung over both camps like thunderclouds."[12] By 1897 the Military Medical Academy stated that smoking had so taken hold that soldiers were puffing away before they even got to war. According to the academy's own statistical analysis, 55.85 percent of its first-year students smoked, consuming an average of 18.35 to 25.29 papirosy per day. They started somewhere between ages sixteen and eighteen, not waiting for the fatigue of war to embrace the soldier's friend.[13]

The frequency of conflict with the Ottomans near the primary source of Russian tobacco and the experience of many smokers watching returning soldiers puffing away created an exceptionally masculine and militaristic smoking culture in imperial Russia strongly linked to imperial expansion and patriotic nationalism. Papirosy emerged as a product of empire, and in their imagery served as a producer of empire. In the early nineteenth century, gallant fighters like the dashing Denis Davydov (1784–1839) were nearly inseparable from pipes in their cultivated images.[14] The infamous Nadezhda Durova (1783–1866), who disguised herself as a man to serve in the Russian military, finished her soldier's ensemble not just with the look of a military man but also with his style of sitting and smoking.[15] In literature and in popular culture, connections between the military, tobacco, and nationalism started decades before advertising took hold, so that when later posters deployed an image of a Russian soldier, users connected these gallant puffers not just to manliness and vigor but also to national pride, historic Russian greatness, and imperialist dreams. In popular literature, visions of Russia's massive empire fired up nationalist sentiment, and tobacco advertisements fed into and off of such popular reveries.[16] Unlike the narrative of the western cigarette, where manufacturers created a consumer product through marketing, the story of Russian papirosy instead showed a market and image already well entrenched.

More than just the use of tobacco by soldiers and the use of the military by tobacco promoters connected smoking to the imperial project. Martial meaning infused papirosy from production and consumption to promotion and trade. The materials for smokes came from around the empire, while manufacturers enhanced the flavors of tobacco with essences from across the globe. Acquiring leaf, paper, and seasonings required engaging the peripheries of the world and securing the edges of empire. Crimean tobacco gained a reputation as being of exceptional quality, as did that from the Kuban region further to the east and from newly conquered areas of Central Asia. Every inhalation conveyed the importance of empire to the smoker and flavored his habit with patriotic feelings, manly posturing, and imperialist pretensions. Tobacco's military connections supported the cultural construction of empire as an essential part of being Russian.[17]

Imperial imagery need not take only the male form. The odalisque (harem woman) combined promises of pleasure and luxury with tobacco and became an inducement for visiting strange lands and tasting these pleasures more intimately. The image of the Muslim "other" was frequently featured in Russian popular literature, where the stereotype became a prop for contemplations of national identity, a foil for anxieties of disquiet from the masses, and an object for projecting thoughts barbarous and sensual.[18]

The experience of empire fed back into the perception of tobacco use. Soldiers became acquainted with smoking as partners in these imperial projects, and then these same men of uniform were transmuted into the symbol of the venture in popular culture. Returning to the metropole, the Russian imperial soldier was life imitating art. As he smoked on the streets, he became a walking billboard for tobacco use as manly, dominating, and gallant, reinforcing the connection of tobacco's taste to empire, the messages that advertisers crafted, and the primacy of smoking to a soldier's life. Society, advertising, culture, masculinity, and daily life intertwined to assure that some of the strongest associations for papirosy in their formative period of intense growth were the empire, the nation, and the soldier.

The connection of smoking to imperialism in Russia is particularly important to arguments regarding the creation of civil society in the late tsarist period.[19] The linking of mass consumption to the creation of national symbols, culture, and ideals occurred in other industrializing countries of the period, like the United States and Britain, but neither of these experienced a violent, revolutionary upheaval akin to the Russian revolutions of 1905 and 1917. Some have argued that the lack of unifying national symbols and the trumpeting of imperial ideals led to the downfall of the tsarist state during World War I. The images connected with papirosy, however, show a marked unity in their vision of smoking as part of Russian military tradition and the Russian imperial ethos, underscoring the ways in which Western models sometimes fall short in explaining the peculiarities of Russian culture.[20]

ACCORDING to the contribution by S. V. Lebedev and noted St. Petersburg tobacconist V. G. Shaposhnikov to the 1901 *Entsiklopedicheskii slovar* (Encyclopedic dictionary), subjects of the empire relied on imperial sources for their tobacco, utilizing leaf from Crimea, the Caucasus, Bessarabia, and the Kuban region in Ukraine, rather than foreign imports. Higher-quality tobacco products might utilize Turkish tobacco, but there was also Russian-grown tobacco cultivated from Turkish seed.[21] Imperial expansion enabled Russians to grow some excellent leaf, first with Catherine the Great's annexation of Crimea in 1783, then with imperial movement into Georgia and the Caucasus after 1801.[22] Russians had imported Virginia tobacco from the time of Peter the Great and tobacco from the Ottoman Empire and China since the eighteenth century.[23] An 1852 manufacturing manual indicated Russians had a sophisticated understanding of, and access to, the major global varieties of tobacco, including Hungarian, Ukrainian, and that from regions like Virginia, Louisiana, Ohio, and Santa Domingo. They also named their blends for tobacco's global greats, like Maryland, Puerto Rico, or the Maracaibo Basin of South America. Russians grew much tobacco that was lower quality than Turkish and American varieties. An 1852 Russian tobacco manual claimed, "Ukrainian tobacco, as with most Russian tobacco, is very strong and stupefying, but also has an unpleasant scent and a sharp taste."[24] This description of a highly potent and poor-tasting tobacco likely indicated use of *nicotiana rustica* or makhorka.[25] Makhorka remained the major tobacco crop, constituting 58 percent of cultivation in 1899. Turkish was 23 percent of the crop, and only 10 percent consisted of American sorts.[26] In 1911, makhorka continued to be over half the tobacco crop, though by this point higher-quality sorts of tobacco were on the rise, climbing much more quickly than lower-quality sorts.[27]

Botanists claimed that Russia had arable regions similar to those of Virginia, but cultivation of Virginia tobacco would have a slow start in Russia. The Shtaf brothers brought back Maryland and Virginia seed from Philadelphia in 1830 through a Moscow agrarian society, but it took two years of working with the seeds to get enough for a sufficient planting.[28] By 1845, Russians claimed growth of American, Turkish, and Crimean tobacco in Crimea. In Ekaterinskaia province (along the Azov Sea), they grew Havana, Virginia, Maryland, and Abako. Tobacco was cultivated in almost every area of the empire—from Finland to the Caucasus.[29] Turkish tobacco from Odessa, Kishenev, and Dubossarakh remained the prevalent leaf in most quality blends smoked in the mid-century.[30]

Foreigners noted and appreciated the difference of the Russian smokes. The papirosy of the Laferm factory of St. Petersburg and Leipzig had an international reputation from the nineteenth century onward. Robert Hart, who served from 1868 to 1907 as the inspector general of the Chinese Maritime Customs service, complained in a letter from China in 1884, "I find it difficult—in fact, so far it has been impossible to procure cigarettes exactly to my taste." He directed his friend to send him papirosy "from St. Petersburg—from the real Russia La Ferme (and not a German) there doing business." He rapturously noted that he had smoked some and "the tobacco was exquisite—and very expensive and the cigarette only gave five or six whiffs. I don't know whether you can manage to get me some of the *Russian La Ferme's* or not; if you could, it would oblige me immensely." He even drew a picture to help in their identification. The Russian papirosy were longer and thinner, but of course, because of the cardboard filter, only had a few inhalations of tobacco to recommend them.[31] Hart was not the only Brit to enjoy a Russian smoke. In his travelogue, *The Russians at Home*, Henry Sutherland Edwards commented that the Russian cigarettes were "far finer than any that can be produced in London."[32]

John Bain Jr., a prolific author of tobacciana in the United States, testified to the international reach of Russian cigarettes. In his 1906 *Cigarettes in Fact and Fancy,* Bain wrote, "The Turkish cigarette invaded the United States in the early seventies in at least four forms, the La Ferme, of Leipzig and St. Petersburg, the Nestor and Melachrino, of Egypt, the Monopol of New York, and the Dubec, of Richmond." The quality of the product was self-evident as "it is largely replacing the Virginia cigarette, especially in the large cities and summer resorts. At nearly all formal dinners and supper-parties, Turkish cigarettes are served with the coffee and at many banquets a small or ladies' cigarette of the same mark is served with the sherbet."[33] An American complimented Laferm in 1915 for producing one of "the best known grades of cigarettes made from genuine Turkish leaf" in the American import market.[34] This "genuine" Turkish leaf was not necessarily grown only in the Ottoman Empire, as by the turn of the century Russia's firms mixed foreign tobacco with leaf cultivated in Crimea, the Caucasus, Bessarabia, and Ukraine.[35] By this point, Laferm was one of the largest producers of tobacco products in Russia and the world.[36]

Not only leaf was an imperial project. Warsaw, St. Petersburg, and Berditchev supplied the fine paper needed for cartridges, and Vilnius, Riga, and St. Petersburg produced the heavier cardstock required for the mouthpieces.[37] "Sauce," used to restore moisture to dried tobacco, improve its flavor, or return sugars lost in the curing process, also engaged the edges of empire and the limits of trade, although Lebedev and Shaposhnikov maintained, "Very aromatic and exotic tobacco does not stand adjustment." They haughtily declared that Russians rarely used saucing, instead preferring to create complex leaf blends of up to ten different varieties. Laferm declared no additives of any kind.[38]

Despite such bravado, the amount of information on saucing in other sources indicated that it was a common practice of Russian manufacture. The 1852 volume *O razvedenii i fabrikatsii tabaka* (On the cultivation and fabrication of tobacco) argued, "One of the most important means for the improvement of tobacco is, without a doubt, fermentation. It destroys its harsh, sharp, and unpleasant taste for the most part and makes it fragrant and delicate."[39] The manual suggested flavorings that pulled together the world, including Russian standards like alcohol, sugar, dill, and tea; aromatics like ambergris, incense, lavender, amber, and flowers; and exotic spices such as nutmeg, cinnamon, clove, vanilla, cardamom, anise, bergamot, raisins, lemon peel, and licorice.[40] While other manufacturers might promote a national taste for unadulterated tobacco, the Zhukov factory did not hold to the "bare leaf" philosophy of Laferm and Shaposhnikov, including in their sauce at least sixteen ingredients, from sugar, berries, and orange to anise, carnation, and saffron.[41]

Imperial acquisitions in the late eighteenth and nineteenth century aided the Russian manufacturers' preference for oriental leaf. Although tobacco cultivation suited almost every district in the Russian Empire, in the eighteenth century Russian agriculture failed to fulfill demand. When Catherine the Great allowed free trade in tobacco after 1762, the next year saw leaf imported from China and Brazil.[42] Her annexation and overthrow of the khanate of Crimea in 1783 and the extension of Russian control of the region after the Russo-Turkish War of 1787–91, coupled with the signing of the Treaty of Jassy in 1792, extended the empire but also had great import for tobacco. The move, part of Catherine's plan to shift Russia's imperial gaze toward the south and the Ottoman Empire, opened up new, highly desirable land for cultivation.[43] The disruptions of the Napoleonic era gave strong incentives for the development of native Russian tobacco cultivation and production.[44] After 1815, the raw material base for Russian production widened, allowing for increased domestic manufacture.[45]

The supply of tobacco from Crimea remained uneven, however, as clashes with the Ottoman Empire disturbed cultivation and trade. Russian conflicts with the Turks occurred at four major points over the course of the nineteenth century: 1806–12, 1828–29, 1853–56, and 1877–78.[46] While the two most important of these conflicts, the Crimean War (1853–56) and the Russo-Turkish War (1877–78), did not entail major territorial loss, they did interrupt cultivation, preparation, and trade.[47] According to one account, the disruptions of the southern market hit tobacco hard, and only after Napoleon III's fall did things improve, though they rebounded strongly and even exceeded previous points.[48] Over the course of the nineteenth century, most smokers would have experienced price fluctuations, quality changes, shortages, or even the collapse of their preferred brands as the supply of raw materials wavered. Users probably would have seen the connection between the problems for their preferred brand and imperialist conflicts with the Turks.

Imperial areas fostered tobacco cultivation, military fortunes influenced supplies, and the terminology of papirosy connected even more forcefully the soldier to the smoke. The Russian word for the tobacco-filled shell at the end of a papirosa was *gil'za*—the same as for the shell of a gun. Sometimes they were called *patron*—the word for cartridge. The language carried over into the act of smoking. F. V. Greene, a lieutenant with the United States Army who observed the Russians during the Russo-Turkish War of 1877–78, indicated in his memoir the crossover between tobacco terminology and military orders. After a dinner with the tsar in August 1877 in the Village of Biella, Greene remembered,

> Just after the *compôte* . . . there seemed to be a silence, when the Emperor said something in Russian and the whole company responded with one loud simultaneous shout. I looked up startled and saw the Emperor staring at me and laughing very heartily at my confusion. He explained that it was the signal for smoking, and that I must learn to answer with the others. The words were *Vweenemai pah-h-h-* to which every one answered *tronn*; *vweenemai patron* being the Russian command "Take cartridges." After this little pleasantry every one produced from his pocket his silver cigarette case, lighted a cigarette, and smoked, and sipped his coffee.[49]

Although the company playfully performed the chant, the after-dinner smoke took on the character of a call to arms, flamboyantly performed in synchronous, obedient ranks. The ritual visualized the preparedness of the assembled to join in battle as well as the integral connection between tobacco and militarism. Fusing comradeship, fun, and combat, tobacco was not just the soldier's friend, but it made soldiers into friends.

Tobacco merchants had long promoted the idea that tobacco served military efforts as well as guns. In 1697, the British Board of Trade and Plantations petitioned Peter the Great in hopes of overturning his ban on tobacco by arguing that tobacco helped soldiers fighting fatigue in the cold Russian climate."[50] They found a ready audience in the tsar, who himself enjoyed a good pipe.[51] A saying from the French of the seventeenth century showed a similar understanding of tobacco's role in the military with the quip "pas de tabac, pas de soldat" (no tobacco, no soldier).[52] In the *Lancet* and the *British Medical Journal,* nineteenth-century British medical authorities went so far as to conclude that tobacco helped soldiers to deal with tedium, stress, and exertion in the Boer War.[53] Around the world, the cultural authority and prestige attached to a man in uniform rose through the middle of the century and graced the tobacco habit with the same debonair air the soldier brought back from the battlefront.[54] By the 1850s, papirosy were common at the Russian court and such a part of an officer's look as to be expected, like a saber or a dashing scar.[55]

Russians on the home front recognized the importance of tobacco to soldiers on the front lines early on, and such associations intensified as smoking became more common in Russia itself. In March of 1878, for instance, the Women's Committee of Iaroslavl sent almost twenty pounds of makhorka to the wounded and ill soldiers for solace.[56] After 1893, economic societies for Russian military officers provided tobacco as well as organizing cots, food, and boots.[57] An accounting of tobacco sent to the Far East in the period from February 20 to April 1 of 1904 displayed the increased importance of such giving by the time of the Russo-Japanese War, as it listed the nearly one million papirosy, almost four hundred pounds of Turkish tobacco, and over 2500 pounds of makhorka sent to the troops in that period from the cities' businesses and citizens. They also sent on papers, cartridges, three pipes, fourteen cigars, and papers for letters (which presumably might serve as smoking papers).[58]

Given the importance of conflicts with Turkey to tobacco cultivation and consumption and the already well-established connection of the military to tobacco use, the emergence of the imperial struggle in late-nineteenth-century tobacco branding and advertisements came as little surprise. Poster and newspaper advertising was in its early development in late-nineteenth-century Russia, without the barriers of education, class, or gender for entry to the marketing profession as with established occupations. This lent a more eccentric and less professional aspect to the industry. Before World War I, most manufacturers produced their own promotional materials. For instance, the owner of the Shaposhnikov and Co. firm was heavily involved in the conception of the stunning and inventive visuals used in advertising.[59] Although some still kept the work in house, a steady increase in the number of advertising firms attested to growing interest from many manufacturers in a professional group to handle marketing.[60] Many in the business community considered advertising a progressive business strategy, and the makeup of the industry backed this interpretation.[61]

Technical innovations in lithography and engraving, as well as inter-national examples, encouraged the development of Russian poster and newspaper advertising. The inspirations for Russian commercial art were evident in the terminology. The Russian word for poster (*plakat*) came from German and that for advertisement (*reklama)* from the French.⁶² The first showing of international posters in Russia in 1897, featuring works by Henri de Toulouse-Lautrec (1864–1901) and Alphonse Mucha (1860–1939), was a watershed for poster art in Russia, drawing the attention of Russia's World of Art group and encouraging the same cross pollination between high art and commercial art visible in Europe.⁶³ Despite the interest of the artis-tic community, most prerevolutionary posters were not signed.⁶⁴ Clothing, style, and themes pointed to in-house or at least native Russian artists in most cases. Often copy, however, was signed, and the inclusion of poetry and writing in advertisements made for a new era of advertising as more than just a listing of inventory.⁶⁵

No records show exactly where posters hung, how many eyes saw them, or whether they appealed to consumers. Even if an advertisement ran in a newspaper, it was not guaranteed that every subscriber read and believed its promises. But there can be little debate about the omnipresence of ad-vertising in the major urban areas. Newspaper, journal, and magazine pro-duction rose rapidly in the late nineteenth century.⁶⁶ Shop signs, fences, poster columns, theater curtains, streetcar placards, and window displays cloaked the nineteenth-century Russian city in calls to buy galoshes, cocoa, and powders. A 1909 critique of the city of Tashkent noted the ways in which advertisements for cigarettes and other products spoiled views and defaced facades.⁶⁷

Other appeals magnified the messages of signs and posters. Newspapers devoted a third to half of their pages to advertisements, and direct mail pleas and free items, like ashtrays, matchbooks, and calendars, became objects of daily use that further pushed products.⁶⁸ Certain tobacco brands gave out collectible cards to make the advertisement itself an item for acquisition. Packaging of tobacco products displayed and enticed even as it protected the wares. Store clerks piled packs of papirosy into elaborate displays to resemble a ship or perhaps a formidable pyramid.⁶⁹ Products showed brand marks on packaging so that advertising followed the purchaser home and even made it from the city to the countryside. All of these different avenues to the consumer assured that the marketed object was ubiquitous, that the images associated with brands could be seen daily if not hourly as part of an early manifestation of mass culture in Russia, and that they thus became part of the expected daily urban experience.⁷⁰

Venues for viewing advertisements dotted the city and lay around the home, but no market research firms surveyed focus groups for reactions in the nineteenth century. These advertisements may have reflected aspects of reality, or they may have represented something else or perhaps even something more. Advertising revealed the hopes of manufacturers for the reception of their product as well as their perceptions of their consumers and these consumers' desires. Marketers presented not life as it was, but the better life that one could have with purchase and consumption.[71] As they appealed to yearnings, they also revealed anxieties. Not surprisingly, manufacturers depicted the path to respectability as desirable and tended toward conservative, pro-business, procapitalism, pro-Russia, noncontroversial pitches. Advertisers probably did not try to offend with polemics, but rather encouraged potential users to see their product as life-transforming in the daily, if not politically revolutionary, sense.[72] Tea, tobacco, and cosmetic companies produced the most innovative advertisements because of market competition.[73]

The investment of Russian tobacco companies in advertising was low compared to contemporaries in other markets, most devoting only one-third to one-half a percent of their yearly sales to marketing.[74] In contrast, in the United States in 1889, Duke's American Tobacco laid out $800,000 on advertising—an investment of about 18 to 20 percent of their sales of around four to four and a half million.[75] The years before the onset of World War I were the most active in prerevolutionary Russian advertising, yet the number of tobacco advertisements appearing daily in newspapers averaged two and a half at most.[76] Still, the pack designs, name choices, and even limited posters and newspaper advertisements available would have held a deep resonance because of the extensive use of tobacco products and the high visibility of these items in daily life.

Tobacco brands, newspaper advertisements, and posters combined already-developed ideas about smoking and its associations with militarism, manliness, and empire and packaged them in the figure of the Cossack. Nikolai Gogol's Cossack hero Taras Bulba established the connection of tobacco and Cossack in Gogol's titular 1835 story. The nationalistic, anti-Semitic story of a father and his two sons took place in a hazy time a century past. If others termed tobacco the soldier's friend, in Gogol's story, Bulba's pipe *liul'ka* became a comrade for whom he was willing to sacrifice his life. Whereas Bulba shot his younger son for disloyalty, and slipped away as his older son was tortured and killed, when faced with the loss of his pipe, Bulba stopped his retreat, let fall his defenses, and got captured. In an ironic end to a man who lost sight of his own safety over his love for smoking, Bulba died by being burned alive. While Bulba smoked a pipe, the love of tobacco and soldier transcended means of smoking to embrace all products. The late-nineteenth-century papirosa brand *Taras Bulba* took its name from Gogol's story and featured a Cossack on horseback charging valiantly forward on its packs.[77]

The early connection of Cossack and tobacco penetrated down to the level of domestic organization. In the Nikolaevan era (1825–55), the well-to-do employed servant boys called "little Cossacks" (*kazachki*) just to offer care for pipes:

> The master of the house, laying on the divan or the Voltaire couch, from time to time yelled through the home: "Eh, Van'ka, Stepia, etc.—Pipe!" and the Little Cossacks would run like mad, rushing from one end of the home to the other with a burning splinter in their hand, lighting on the way an already primed pipe. Giving it to their master, the well trained little Cossack saw it as his duty to wipe the mouthpiece of spit onto the tail of his shirt. If the master was displeased then the little Cossack would get a smack on the head with the pipe.[78]

The "little Cossack" provided the aristocrat lounging on his couch easy access to the wild life of the steppe—one well-packed pipe at a time.

Like the papirosa and the military, the Cossack was an established figure who invoked powerful cultural, artistic, political, religious, homosocial, and imperial associations and reinforced an image of smoking as integral to manliness. Artistic representations, like those of Gogol, Ilya Repin (1844–1930), and Tolstoy, used the Cossack as a symbol of freedom, independence, bravery, steadfast faith, and excess. Political figures gave realistic expectations to cultural emblems. Alexander III praised the Cossacks as the embodiment of Russian values and hailed their defense of empire.[79] A guardian of Russia from the time of the Golden Horde, the Cossack fit perfectly into the imperial and tobacco agenda. The Cossack, defender of faith and opponent of the Turks, came just in time for a new period of hostility, and his embrace of tobacco made smoking into a political act connected to empire and, by the 1870s, Pan-Slavism. The union of all Slavic people became a more urgent political agenda after the massacre of thirty thousand Bulgarians by the Turks in 1876, which precipitated the Russian declaration of war on Turkey in 1877. The growing belief in creating a joined identity for Slavs across the Balkans, central Europe, and Russia only fanned the flame.[80]

Fueled by patriotic fervor and anti-Turk animosity, Nikolai Feodorovich Dunaev, a forty-nine-year-old peasant who moved into tobacco production in 1849, renamed his entire factory in the wake of the 1877–78 war. Dunaev's factory worked with makhorka brought from the Chernigov and Poltava districts of Ukraine. Because his tobacco was not southern sourced, he weathered smoothly the market fluctuations brought on by imperial conflict. Yet, even though his factory remained sheltered from the problems to the south, he did not stay apolitical. Somewhere around the period of the Russo-Turkish War, Dunaev renamed his firm "Balkan Star." With the new name came a new mark for the brand—a mounted Cossack with a lance in the uniform of the Russo-Turkish War under an exploding star. Although Dunaev left no record of his reasoning, the choice of uniform, timing, and name all point to a connection between tobacco, the imperial project, and military strength. Such a move would have been more than a symbolic change. For almost three decades, consumers had depended on the Dunaev name, making it one of the leading makhorka firms in the empire. Such a dramatic brand makeover might have conveyed a sense of innovation and change, but it would have been a risk, perhaps leaving many customers behind. Dunaev must have seen the project as worthwhile.[81]

"Balkan Star" immediately called to mind the Russian imperial interests in southeast Europe, but also specifically the Russo-Turkish War of 1877–78, when, with their ally Serbia, the Russians came to the aid of Bulgaria and Bosnia and Herzegovina. A second treaty concluded under pressure from Britain and Austria-Hungary chipped away at the initial victory of the Russians, but overall the Russians still saw substantial gains in their visibility in the larger Slavic world. The use of the mounted Cossack as the soldier connected to the Balkan Star image hinted at the religious conflict between the states as well as their military tensions. In the literary and popular imagery of the nineteenth century, the Cossack recalled the religious nature of this "Holy War" in defense of Russian Orthodoxy against Islam.[82] The profiled Cossack of the Balkan Star brand image held some resemblance in meaning and style to the mounted St. Michael, slaying the dragons and protecting the faith.

Other brands similarly pushed for a broader religious and imperial conflict. The papirosy brand Constantinople aspired to still more by backing Pan-Slavic ambitions of overturning Turkish control of the ancient city.[83] Their call was not alone. Ottoman, founded in 1882, was actually a Russian factory located in St. Petersburg.[84] The name borrowed from the good feelings engendered by the Russian victory, and used Cossack imagery in its advertising not as a celebration of Ottoman strength but of Russian triumph (figure 1.1). A poster for the brand appropriated the painting by Ilya Repin,

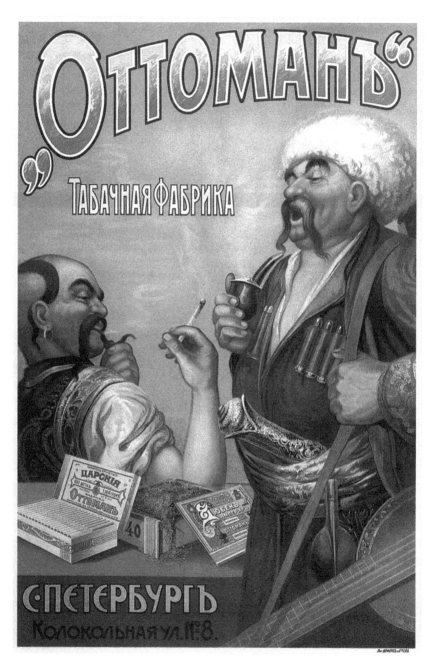

Figure 1.1   *Ottoman* poster. 1900s. Collection of Russian State Library, Moscow.

Reply of the Zaporozhian Cossacks to Sultan Mehmed IV of the Ottoman Empire. Here, a famous depiction of a notorious event for the Cossacks became a pitch for a brand named after the Ottomans. Repin took over a decade to finish the work, which Tsar Alexander III purchased in 1891 for the then-outlandish sum of 35,000 rubles. The painting depicted the seventeenth-century moment when the Zaporozhian Cossacks gathered to write an insulting reply to the demands of the Ottoman Sultan Mehmed IV (r. 1648–87) that they surrender. The painting was already soaked in tobacco as Repin depicted multiple Cossacks with pipes and one with an anachronistic papirosa. The marketers appropriated a close-up of two of the central figures, now reproduced as a pair of happy smokers. Instead of laughing over what greater insult they might hurl at the sultan, our happy Cossacks relax over "Ottoman" tobacco produced in St. Petersburg, a subtle hint that after centuries of effort the Ottoman Empire had been tamed and could now be consumed.

The 1904 poster for the *Kapriz* brand of papirosy of the St. Petersburg firm A. N. Bogdanov and Co. presented the empire of tobacco with its Cossack architect in its center (figure 1.2). A pantheon of five male smokers,

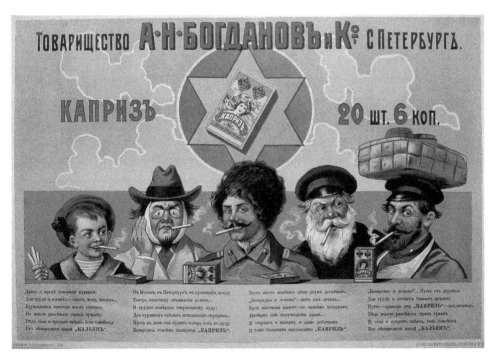

Figure 1.2   *Kapriz* poster. 1904. Collection of Russian State Library, Moscow.

all happily engaged in consuming their favored tobacco, drew the attention of the viewer. A boy, a bourgeois citizen, an old man, and a trader flanked a rakish Cossack in uniform with signature fur cap and a beguiling gleam in his eyes. Slightly taller than his compatriots, the Cossack held authority over his fellow smokers by his size, virility, and good health and commanded further attention by his central position in the composition and his straight-shouldered presentation, which took up more of the frame.

The young boy to the left looked on admiringly. The scamp, the only person in the composition without a designated pack, held a few loose papirosy and stared at our central figure, implying he had filched the smokes attempting to emulate the derring-do of his military idol. Only the Cossack and the boy visibly smiled, emphasizing the connection and the implication that smoking made men. The bandaged bourgeois man between the two was no match for the Cossack and fell to the background behind him and the boy as he depended on his papirosy to cure his debilitating toothache, a problem tobacco was believed to alleviate. On the right of the poster, an old man in a peaked cap, and a younger man who looked like his son, also in a cap but with apron and trader's basket, shared their own tableau of meaning. The artist communicated the unity of the figures by subtly stressing their common ethnic and familial backgrounds. Indeed, all five shared the same nose, coloring, and complexion, with four sporting rather distinctive red hair. The consumer society of *Kapriz* was not a diverse one but an ethnically-bonded one.

Behind the band of satisfied smokers, a stylized map of the Black Sea served as a setting for the pack of *Kapriz* papirosy. The colors indicated neither clouds nor smoke. If smoke, the clouds should have been grey on a field of blue, not blue on a field of grey. If sky, the clouds should have been white on a field of blue. Instead, this image appeared to be a map of the Balkans, with the three-pointed body of land to the left an echo of Greece, and the Aegean and Black seas to left and right respectively. The overlay of the tobacco pack onto the six-pointed star, a symbol of the Ottoman Empire, in the foreground of the abstracted map indicated the source of the tobacco as well as a hint of tobacco's role in empire. The ongoing activities of Russian forces in the Black Sea and Balkan regions, as well as the predilection for Crimean tobacco by Russian smokers, connected *Kapriz* to the nineteenth-century Russian imperial project. The use of the star, tobacco, and Cossack together implied an aggressive, even proprietary, attitude toward the area that made visual the Pan-Slavic rhetoric of the period. The placement of the smiling Cossack in the center, as well as the connection of the Cossack to the struggles in the region, indicated Russia's power over the stylized Balkans behind him.[85] He served as a gatekeeper, securing the imperial frontier through his papirosy and presence. Through him, tobacco made its way to the other men, and soon to be men, who surrounded him.

To further intertwine imperial domination and tobacco, underneath the puffing pantheon sat a poem by "Uncle Mikey," the pseudonym of the hero of the Russo-Turkish War of 1877–78, Sergei Apollonovich Korotkii.[86] The doggerel at the bottom spoke to the quality of *Kapriz*, and the healthfulness of the companion brand, exotically named *Kal'ian* (hookah), with its special "batting," a reference to cotton or other fibers stuffed in the cardboard mouthpiece to function as a type of filter. While the poem emphasized light brands, the empire-taming power at top did not seem a group that would need anything to buffer their smoke. Their shared strapping good health—even the man suffering from a toothache had a ruddy complexion—spoke of a society united by consumption of common, affordable luxury items that bound users in shared enjoyment. Just as the Cossack, star, and map behind united them in a vision of a greater, stronger empire, a simple *Kapriz* subjugated the area, secured the supplies, and harnessed the market.

Working as Uncle Kornei for Laferm and Uncle Mikey for Shaposhnikov, Korotkii wrote a great deal of advertising copy and gave his own likeness to numerous pieces. He even collected his poetry into volumes with titles like "Uncle Mikey Abroad" or "Uncle Mikey in the Countryside," which were then sold as stand-alone pamphlets or handed out as premiums.[87] In 1905, he applied to the government for the right to publish a journal devoted to tobacco and its enjoyment, though it was seemingly never published, and under his influence, the Shaposhnikov factory began to advertise to their own workers in 1910.[88] Korotkii's image and exploits often featured in the advertisements. He lived the life of the European imperialist, enjoying hunting expeditions into wild territories, meeting with foreign dignitaries, and securing the materials for more Russian smokers.[89] The poems of Uncle Mikey were ubiquitous and yet derided. Lev Uspenskii would later criticize another poet as "more Uncle Mikey than anyone of the classics."[90]

The branding of tobacco carried over the connections to the Imperial army as conquerors of the past became heroes of papirosy. Aleksandr Vasil'evich Suvorov (1729–1800) distinguished himself in the earlier Russo-Turkish War of 1787–91, which led to Russia extending control to Crimea. He also served the imperial cause to the west when he brutally snuffed out the Polish insurrection of 1794 and brilliantly led an attack on

French revolutionary forces in Italy in 1799. For his service, he was elevated to the exalted rank of Generalissimo in 1800. The cultural resonance of his deeds emerged in a papirosy named after him in the late nineteenth century. The choice of Suvorov, a man who had made his fame through expanding or controlling empire in battle, invested the product with meaning, as did the taste of the smoke, flavors of perhaps Crimean-grown tobacco chosen in deference to the papirosa's namesake. While manufacturers may not have always tailored appeals to consumers with their marketing, they most likely used advertising to try to draw in users and thought the values and actions represented by Suvorov would be attractive. Building on a tradition of creating snuffboxes with portraits of military and government figures to give out as gifts, the portrait of Suvorov on the pack, with windswept hair and a chest full of medals, enticed the viewer and connected the smoker and the product to men of empire and the fame, courage, and boldness they supposedly possessed. The imagery may also have served as a subtle inducement to users to join the imperial venture themselves in pursuit of similar glory.[91]

Fighting men of Central Asia and the Far East also got their recognition with packs of papirosy. A brand commemorated General Mikhail Nikolaevich Annenkov (1835–99) for his role as both an officer and an engineer in the conquest of Turkestan and the construction of the Transcaspian Railway. Another general active in Central Asia, Mikhail Dmitriyevich Skobelev (1843–82), earned his place in the tobacco canon by conquering the Khanate of Kokand and capturing Andijian. Tobacco products named after him gained popularity during the late 1870s.[92] Skobelev had further been a hero of the 1877–78 Russo-Turkish War and the siege of Plevna, commemorated in many popular prints of the period. In prints and stories, he was depicted as a romantic, glamorous free spirit.[93] In both cases, the connection of tobacco to empire was made explicitly with assumptions that users would quickly identify these brand names with regions, ideas, and quests that they had been part of, approved of, or might wish to join. Skobelev actually earned a second brand in his image in the Kolobov and Bobrov factories, *Belyi general* (white general). Under his nickname, Skobelev, pictured in the 1890 poster with sword drawn, stared at the viewer, his white horse caught mid-movement with only one foot on the ground (figure 1.3). Like the romantic portrait of Suvorov, no smoking appeared. The only thing for sale was valor.[94] As a pack rather than a poster, the appeal of the image came home with the users and followed them wherever they carried their papirosy, a constant reminder of the spirit and strength they were to associate with tobacco.

In advertisements from *Zoria* (reveille) and the factory-produced car-tridges *Zvezda* (star), military men appeared again as enticements to smoke, hinting at connections to empire (figures 1.4 and 1.5). *Zoria* from 1900 in-cluded in the crowd a gentleman of the Horse Guards, as evidenced by his elaborate, eagle-crested helmet and the cuirass (armored breast plate) that he wore. For *Zvezda*, the red jacket with blue cuffs would have aligned with

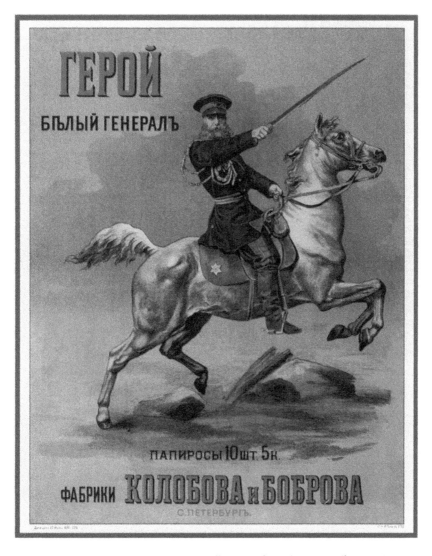

Figure 1.3   *Belyi general* poster. 1890. Collection of Russian State Library, Moscow.

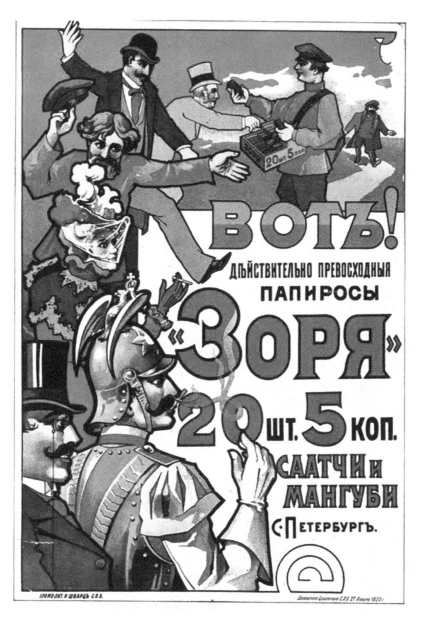

Figure 1.4 *Zoria* poster. 1900. Collection of Russian State Library, Moscow.

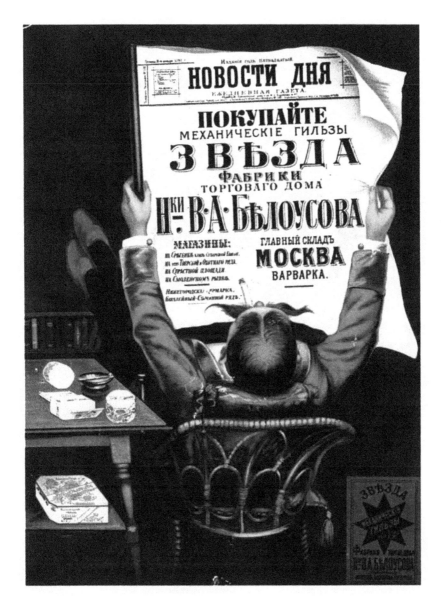

Figure 1.5 *Zvezda* poster. Prerevolutionary. Collection of Russian State Library, Moscow.

a uniform for a Russian Guard's Regiment, but the smoker sat in repose, with slippers on, papirosa accessories at the ready, and turned away from the viewer with his massive newspaper. In both cases, the soldier bridged the civilian and military world as a representative everyman who could still partake of a valorous smoke: with *Zoria* that smoke occurred in the company of worker, bourgeois, peasant, and even women; with *Zvezda* it happened during the intimacy of the evening and with refined and modern accessories. The poster for Kolobov and Bobrov's *Soldat* papirosy showed a similarly solitary smoker, but now updated into the newer uniforms of the early twentieth century (figure 1.6). Rather than relaxing in an interior or mingling with civilians, the hunched posture indicated he was grabbing a smoke while on the go. While nothing explicitly linked these military men to empire, the purpose of their existence in the nineteenth century and their patriotic value must have been readily apparent to contemporary viewers. Breaking the barrier between military service and society, the advertisements implied the suitability of smoking for all classes and genders, although the ethnic diversity of the group was limited. These images of the generic soldier seemed to be not Cossacks but European Russian males.

The *bogatyr*, an ancient counterpart to the heroic Cossack, appeared regularly in tobacco advertising, obliquely evoking nationalist myths and imperial visions. Revered for their loyalty and strength, the *bogatyr* defended ancient Rus' against the marauders of the early steppe. A poster for the papirosy *Vazhnyia* (great), with filters and a fancy case, depicted a *bogatyr* smiling with gentle joy over the mild, filtered papirosy of Bogdanov and Co. The advertisement still further domesticated him by juxtaposing the modern tobacco product and its tempering filters and fussy port cigar case with the rough axe and sturdy armor of a fabled hero (figure 1.7). Despite the tenderness of his smile and smoke, the vision of his massive hands as well as the battle-chipped bardiche propped against his shoulder suggested the same promise as the warriors of the *Zoria* and *Zvezda* advertisements. While in repose, not in battle, the *bogatyr* carried the same visions of a broad empire, which demanded battle readiness.[95]

Like the Cossack, the figure of the fighting *bogatyr* appeared regularly in advertising, in much the same way that it provided fodder for many artists of the late nineteenth century, like Viktor Vasnetsov (1848–1926) and Mikhail Vrubel (1856–1910). Brands such as Laferm's *Dobryi molodetz* (good lad) gained legitimacy with historical imagery or folkloric ideas.[96] The *bogatyr* fit well with the nineteenth-century imperial quest in Central Asia, where tobacco served as a way to claim and tame the new areas. After the conquest of Tashkent in 1865, the new region was harnessed to tobacco

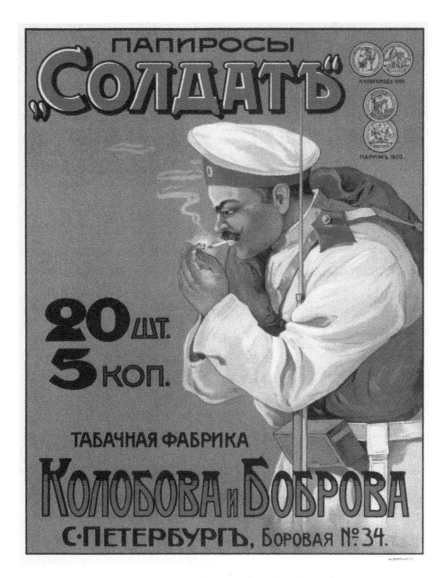

Figure 1.6 *Soldat* poster. 1900s. Collection of Russian State Library, Moscow.

just as Crimea had been a century before. Russia's foreign minister Aleksandr Gorchakov looked with interest at the ability of the region to produce not just cotton and silk but also tobacco. After the conquest, Russian officials introduced tobacco as a crop and taught the locals how to work with it. The new crop took root as a 1906 report to the prime minister Sergei Witte

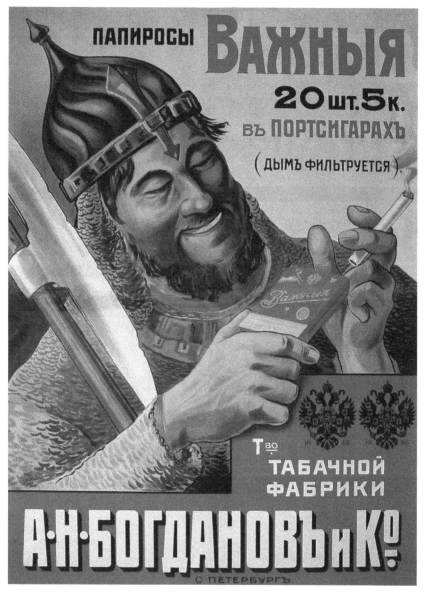

Figure 1.7   *Vazhnyia* poster. 1900s. Collection of Russian State Library, Moscow.

underscored the value of Turkestan's tobacco.[97] The invocation of mythic figures, even while using the styles of European art nouveau, allowed advertisers to elevate sales pitches for tobacco and other products and link them to a national cultural identity.[98] Images of strong, popular resonance could serve as rallying cries against foreign commodities.[99] The hint of humor brought on by the jarring juxtaposition of ancient figures enjoying modern products just added spice.[100]

In the 1900 advertisements for *Trezvon* (three bells) brand, again from the Bogdanov and Co. factory, the slogan at the top of the page made clear the relationship of tobacco, *bogatyr,* and empire (figure 1.8). With the addition of faith to the mix, the poster cried out, "The battle of the miraculous Bogatyr against the infidels." The composition echoed the famous painting of Viktor Vasnetsov, "After the Battle of Igor Sviatoslavich with the Polovtsians," yet inverted the hero from slain to slayer. Instead of all dead on the field, in this iteration, one stood triumphant as tobacco became a weapon in the fight against the infidel (*basurman*), as well as a shield to the larger-than life Russian hero.[101] In addition to his commanding pose, the *Trezvon bogatyr* towered over the competition in his bulk. His head alone appeared twice the size of any of the other papirosy men. Now rather than just a casual replacement for the weapon in hand, the papirosa became as large and lethal as a lance, as evidenced by the speared and slain competitors

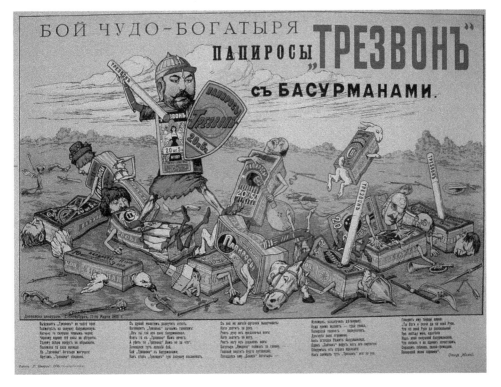

Figure 1.8   *Trezvon* poster. 1900. Collection of Russian State Library, Moscow.

scattered on the field. In addition to the stabbed and bludgeoned bodies, hacked off arms and legs littered the scene. Under the foot of the *bogatyr*, a hapless pack, ripped in two, languished with its innards now on display. The rival brands appeared as enemies of true faith in good tobacco. The image performed double duty playing on popular misgivings about Muslims in both the Ottoman Empire and Central Asia. The implication was that the consumption of this product would help tame the borders and strengthen Russian power.

The advertisement also displayed the work of the jocular "Uncle Mikey." Not only did Korotkii write the poem, but the face on the triumphant pack of *Trezvon* was that of Uncle Mikey himself.[102] Korotkii, a hero of tobacco, became the real-life, smoking Cossack and *bogatyr*—a valiant warrior of empire who smoked with verve, traveled the world looking for fine tobacco, and wrote poetry celebrating his passion for the habit.[103] Korotkii lent his personality to *Trezvon*, elevating it from a product to an autonomous entity—the Pinocchio of papirosy, a pack that became a man.[104] Uncle Mikey wrote his poem, at the bottom, in the style of a folk song, perhaps another nod to the ancient inspiration, and played on the theme, personifying the pack as a hero named *Trezvon* saying: "You run and gallop all over Russia" and "overcome the infidel . . . my fine papirosy."[105]

The empire of tobacco was not visible exclusively through military men of past and present. Advertisers connected Russian tobacco use to other symbols of the nation. A Dukat advertisement for 1912 noted the "the three sights of Moscow" as the tsar bell, the tsar cannon, and *Diushess* (duchess) papirosy. Another traded on the Bronze Horseman, the momentous statue of Peter the Great on horseback, which sat in St. Petersburg's Senate Square. There were limits, however, to how far such commercialization of the past could proceed. When Dukat tried to trademark a portrait of Peter the Great for their brand, the government balked. The Department of Trade and Manufacturing argued that while there was not a problem with putting Peter I on a label for a tobacco product, the trademarking of a historical figure was problematic because the image could not belong to just one company.[106]

Images of imperial dominance in the form of landscape pictures or idyllic vistas beckoned to users. Tobacco advertisements employed Egyptians, Bedouins, or camels, where a leisurely, pleasure-saturated East was contrasted with a civilized and modern West.[107] The 1912 advertisement for *Albanskii* (Albanian) tobacco featured camels, palm trees, minarets, and kaftan-draped traders in its vision (figure 1.9). In the copy, Uncle Mikey assured that the tobacco was loved "everywhere" and, the visual implied, with its shining pack levitating above the waters, a divine and inspiring tobacco experience. The choice of an Asiatic landscape with camels seemed rather incongruous for a tobacco named "Albanian," which was in fact most likely a Turkish blend like the other offerings of the Shaposhnikov factory.[108]

Tobacco advertisers also sculpted dreams of empire from women's flesh, the possession of females and their bodies standing for the conquests of lands and peoples. In tobacco art in the United States, exotic women, distant and unobtainable in real life, became the vicariously accessible female on a pack or poster.[109] Orientalist imagery was deployed in the Russian empire in multiple venues, including literature, and against many ethnicities, including the people of the Caucasus.[110] An entire genre of Russian tobacco advertising offered visions of the accessible, consumable, knowable "Oriental" female as enticement for their brands. For example, the Serebriakov

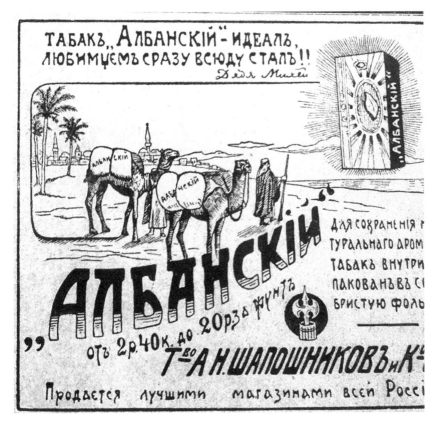

Figure 1.9 *Albanskii* advertisement. *Restorannoe Delo*, 1912. Collection of Russian State Library, Moscow.

factory of Omsk offered a beautiful smoking supine woman in Turkic dress as an inducement to its users (figure 1.10). Relaxed and smiling, she looked directly at the spectator while lounging on plush pillows and an exotic brocade chaise. Her tobacco use implied a slight intoxication, perhaps even a hashish-induced stupefaction, since hashish and opium were believed to be more prevalent in hot climates.[111] Whatever its source, her look beguiled the viewing male with its implications of relaxed resistance.

Sensory appeals saturated the poster. The odalisque motioned gently to the skyline while roses, fruit, and incense perfumed the scene. The seduction of flesh included a bare shoulder and turned ankle and arch thrust toward the viewer. This woman was an object of consumption as attainable as the tobacco she herself enjoyed, and one that provided a banquet of sensual pleasures. The visual invited the entirety of the senses to luxuriate in the smell of the flowers, incense, and tobacco; the feel of the supple fabrics and touch of her warm skin; the taste of the exotic fruits and their juices bursting and surging in the mouth; and the arousing sight of her soft eyes

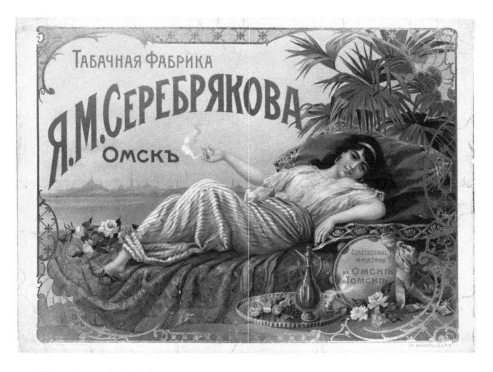

Figure 1.10	*Serebriakov* poster. Prerevolutionary. Collection of Russian State Library, Moscow.

and supple flesh. The excitation of the five senses was echoed in tobacco art in the United States as well.[112] The use of the sexualized female, alongside consumable items, linked lust to other bodily hungers, making the woman herself merchandise.[113]

More than a consumer product, she symbolized colonial areas open for possession, penetration, taming, and domination. The sexually available "Orientalist" female countered the image of the strictly controlled sexuality of idealized western-European females, and functioned as a mildly pornographic recruitment poster for imperial service.[114] As in the harem and tobacco paintings of nineteenth-century European artists, the waiting female in these advertisements anticipated the arrival of a male and placed the viewer in this role, thus entangling him in an elaborate colonial narrative. The image lacked a male figure, suggesting that the odalisque apparently awaited the European male who, it could be surmised, had either alluded or destroyed the Muslim man who had once controlled her. Thus the harem genre implied not just the domination of the female "other" but also the decimation of her male counterpart and thus successful imperial conquest.[115] The skyline in the back indicated exactly where this beauty awaited her Russian conqueror—Constantinople—bringing together the Pan-Slavic quest with smoking, sex, and sensuality.

The woman of the advertisement from Moscow's Gabai factory appeared similar in many ways to the woman of Serebriakov but stared more audaciously at the viewer with even a hint of challenge (figure 1.11). Next to her bed stood a hookah, which indicated not just that she smoked, but that she smoked with others, presumably other women of the harem. Perhaps soon, the image hinted, others might join the fabled orgiastic pleasures of the Orient. The image mixed sensual and rational appeals as it foregrounded not the woman and her enticements, but medals, awards, and samples of the product line. By bringing brands and accolades to the front of the advertisement, the artist catered to the viewers' connoisseurship rather than just base sensual appetites. Indeed, these items floated above and out toward the observer to command the eye.

The seals reflected another type of conquest, important in the atmosphere of industrial competition of the late nineteenth century—recognition as a quality product. In Russia and in international venues, tobacco merchants competed with zeal for industrial prizes issued by the government as incentives for technical innovation and development. In 1828, the tsarist government sponsored the first national industrial competition to issue such awards. At the fair, manufacturers could battle for the right to call their firm "purveyor to the Court of His Imperial Majesty" or to deploy

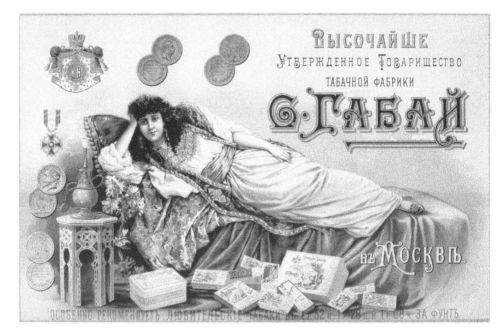

Figure 1.11   *Gabai* poster. 1890s. Collection of Russian State Library, Moscow.

the double-headed eagle of the state in their advertisements. The prizes became all the more important after the last All-Russian exhibition in Nizhni Novgorod in 1896.[116] In the Gabai poster, the seals of government approval and the packs of papirosy and tobacco appeared larger than life and dwarfed the promised pleasures of the odalisque. The sensuality of the Serebriakov advertisement did not disappear entirely, but intellectual arguments made by prizes of industry overshadowed the temptations of the harem and hookah.

The most brazen of Russian tobacco's consumable females came from Kolobov and Bobrov, a tobacco factory out of St. Petersburg (figure 1.12). While the advertisement was undated, the umber tones evoked a warm climate and the draped fabrics and coined necklaces of the woman called to mind the stereotypical accouterment of the Turkic people, implying the use of fragrant oriental leaf and an exotic sauce to highlight a Turkish-style papirosa. On its most basic level, the promise of pleasure was given to the viewer in the unspoken invitation of the half-naked, barefoot, and brazenly staring female; the warmth, languor, and carnal indulgence of tobacco all communicated in her gaze. The nude torso and gleaming skin invited the viewer's eye to drift over the limbs of the smoking woman and stroke her

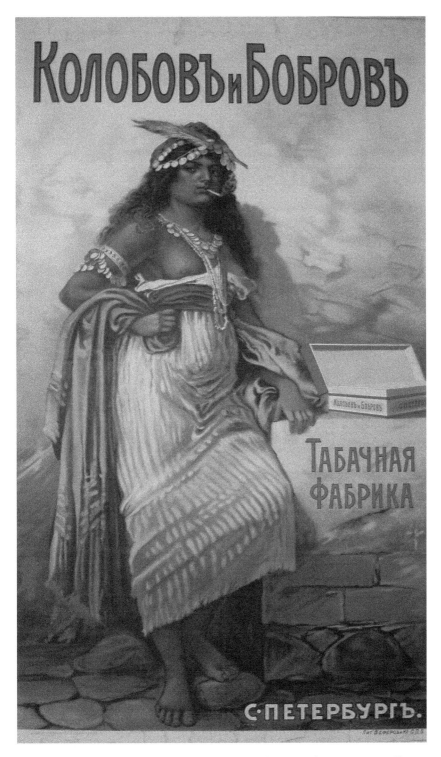

Figure 1.12 *Kolobov and Bobrov* poster. 1903. Collection of Russian State Library, Moscow.

with a gaze.[117] Her lack of clothing was typical of depictions of colonial women in European art, where nudity not only indicated that the woman was sexually available but also implied the Oriental female's assumed lack of sensitivity, modesty, and civilized behavior.[118] The setting suggested that her unbridled sexuality and unquenchable appetites had led her to the streets, beyond even the patriarchal oversight of the harem and its dissolute bacchanals, further inviting the viewer/consumer to contemplate the pleasures so presumably plentiful and available in the untamed Orient.

Perhaps the most striking elements of the woman in the Kolobov and Bobrov advertisement, aside from her large pelvic presentation, were her mannish jaw, shoulders, and biceps. The woman's physique and smoking connected her to masculinizing images of "primitive" women, such as the portrayals of African women in European art and advertising of the period. European artists struggled to contain the two visions of the primitive female—one where she was licentious, fertile, and abundantly female and another where she was robust, untamed, and able to work like a man. Artists vacillated between portrayals of colonial women as able to withstand grueling physical labor and as voluptuaries bent on hedonistic delights. Such portrayals of the "other" and her easy virtue served as an inducement to the men called to serve in these colonial areas. She enticed them to travel to the edges of empire to enjoy the easy romantic conquest of women outside the oversight of male authority and civilization, yet also assuaged any feelings of conscience over exploitation of colonial women by her seeming vitality compared to European women.[119] For the Russian male viewer, the implication was that the society of the Orient was so unhinged that woman's sexuality had no checks or boundaries of nature or state. The stabilizing influence of real men would help the area to progress. Kolobov and Bobrov presented a sexual recruitment poster for Russia's imperial campaigns.[120]

The raw sensuality of this advertisement was somewhat surprising given the censorship strictures in Russia in the late imperial period. Statutes in the nineteenth century set up strict guidelines for publishers to avoid offense to state, church, or individuals, and advertisements had to be pre-reviewed before publication. The implementation of the law was, however, arbitrary at times and poorly or incompetently enforced at others. It could be that this poster came out after the breakdown of the system in 1905, or perhaps the poster was pulled, never to be seen outside the archive. Usually, however, artists veiled the risqué implications of advertisements in order to pass the censors or so as to not risk offending, rather than enticing, customers.[121]

While the vision of the odalisque urged the male consumer to imagine himself the invader of the harem, Uncle Mikey, never shy to display his power or his visage, became the keeper of the harem himself (figure 1.13).

A two-page advertisement from 1912 showed Uncle Mikey in full costume. In this, and other campaign advertisements where he dressed in Orientalist clothing, he metamorphosed into a Russian soldier now elevated to the status of a ruler, the man who would be a tobacco king. For this piece, he took on the "costume of a Syrian Sheik," yet the drawing showed him looking

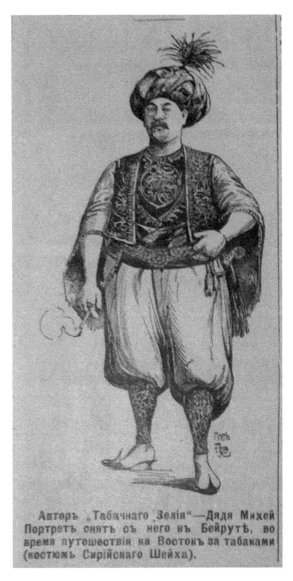

Figure 1.13   Uncle Mikey. *Restorannoe Delo,* 1912. Collection of Russian State Library, Moscow.

every inch the sturdy, Russian male. According to the caption, the picture caught Uncle Mikey on a trip to Beirut to purchase tobacco. In this and other such advertisements, he emerged the equal of royal heads of state, sitting among princes, and princesses, his unsmiling Russian mug balanced by turbans and kaftans.[122]

By the beginning of the twentieth century, the Russian imperial quest had pushed further still, and advertisers followed. Poster artists worked through the developing Russo-Japanese War in 1904 producing advertisements from the St. Petersburg factories of A. N. Shaposhnikov and Bogdanov and Co. (figures 1.14 and 1.15). The war began in January of 1904 when the Japanese launched an attack and siege on the Russians at Port Arthur, inflicting heavy damage. The tsarist government dismissed the incident and continued bombastically to declare their superiority, but words could not hide the inadequacy of the Russian military at its far eastern outpost. Popular support for the war soured quickly over the course of 1904 as battles in late spring and then summer proved Russian forces unable to stand up to the Japanese first in terms of numbers and then in training and material support. Both posters came before the humiliating surrender of Port Arthur in January 1905 and the subsequent disastrous Battle of Tsushima in that same year. They showed the still optimistic hopes of the state and the population for victory in the east coming from the work of soldiers on land—in both posters, the ever-prominent symbols of Russian tobacco, the Cossacks.

Vostochnyia (Eastern), the "new papirosy" from Shaposhnikov, presented war as pastorale (figure 1.14). A Cossack soldier sat relaxed and confident atop a horse that, if possible, looked even more assured than the soldier above him. Although an act of war had brought him, and presumably his tobacco, east, the soldier betrayed no panic. The image itself, in lush greens and blues, with fluffy clouds and placid waters, brought to mind not turmoil but tranquility. The fleet in the distance appeared strong and untouched while the port community sat verdant, well ordered, and peaceful. No hint of despair or possibility of trouble echoed in the figure or his environment.

In contrast, the poster for Bogdanov and Co., full of frothing seas and explosions, presented a much more traumatic visual for a casual consumer product (figure 1.15). At top, the devastating Japanese attack on the Russian Fleet at Port Arthur inspired patriotic fervor, harkening back to popular prints of military battles that became popular during the nineteenth century.[123] At the bottom, the stirring vision of a brigade of Cossacks charging to regain power on land countered the image of the tragic losses at sea. Symbols still embraced the packs of papirosy. This time instead of a star, a life preserver framed the boxes of *Kapriz*. The bridging of tragedy and hope

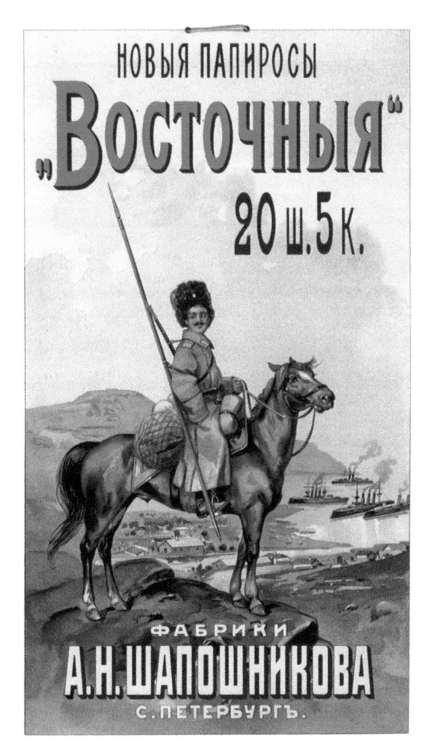

Figure 1.14 *Vostochnyia* poster. 1904. Collection of Russian State Library, Moscow.

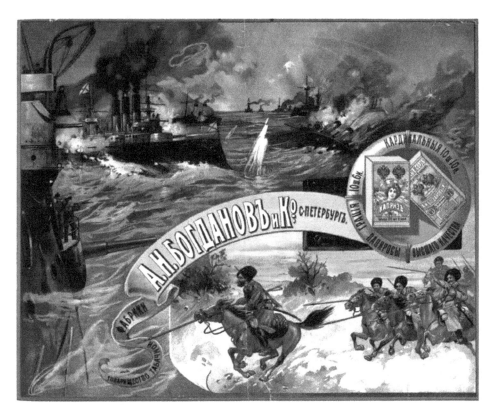

Figure 1.15   *Kapriz* poster. 1904. Collection of Russian State Library, Moscow.

with the papirosa, in the position of savior, appealed to the public in different ways. Perhaps the mounted Cossacks, so long associated with smoking, were now coming to the rescue enlivened by tobacco's energy. Perhaps the viewer, through their use of *Kapriz,* felt involved in the heroic deeds on both land and sea. In either case, a Bogdanov advertisement yet again connected tobacco, militarism, and empire in a vision where Cossacks guided consumer choices to valorous, patriotic, and imperial goals.

Smoking entailed a personal habit but also a social construct, a bodily enticement, a patriotic pursuit, and an imperial tool. The taste of tobacco, a construction of leaf from around the empire and sauce ingredients from around the world, merged in a brew that tasted, smelled, and smoked in a distinctly Russian fashion. The idiosyncratic sensory experience of Russian-made smokes at times repelled visitors and at others earned their praise. For Russians, the impression their tobacco made on others could not have passed unnoticed, and thus the smells, tastes, and peculiarities of the papirosa became also a way for Russians to display a national identity, distinguish themselves from others, and find their fellows by the telltale aroma, packs, and look of a Russian smoke.

Because of the political and economic implications of tobacco production for the tsarist empire, tobacco became enmeshed in the image of the soldier and especially the Cossack.[124] Advertisers built on these links, exploiting native warrior traditions and celebrating tsarist victories in their posters, copy, and branding. The Russo-Turkish conflicts especially spurred tobacco use and animated tobacco advertising, but so did engagements in Uzbekistan and the Far East. Tobacco merchants and marketers did not force these connections on the public. These ideas aligned with users' own understandings of market fluctuations, sympathies for Russia's imperial exploits, and the lived experience of many men who had served in the military.

Even if no setting was evident, the imperial context assured that when advertisers deployed an image of a Russian soldier, users associated him with manliness and vigor but also with nationalist pride, historic Russian greatness, and imperial dreams. The Cossack soldier, like the Russian peasant, was a stand-in for Russianness from the War of 1812 and beyond.[125] Russia's militarist vision of tobacco emerged in a mix of Cossacks, Crimea, the Ottomans, and Central Asia that was uniquely Russian.[126] In the process, advertisers and manufacturers commodified imperialism and projected a unified image of manliness and tobacco that included engagement with the tsarist vision for Russian expansion and empire.[127] In the United States, Native Americans served as a similar reminder of imperial visions, but without the strong connection of tobacco cultivation to the regions then held by Native Americans, just their origination of the practice. Native American women did not serve in similar fashion in advertisements in the United States. Instead, they became fierce hunters and warriors, but not sexualized consumables. African-American women did not feature in American tobacco art except as caricatures.[128] The harem women of Russian advertising, like those employed in European art, became not just a vision of tobacco's pleasures available at home, but an enticement to men to search for pleasure on the frontiers as a soldier for the tsarist army.

Papirosy scented Russian national identity, making it stand out from the rest of the world and connect intimately to imperial pretensions. Not only did smoking become a practice of empire, it held the promise of community in an increasingly fragmented society. For men recently returned from the Crimean War, the Russo-Turkish War, or the Russo-Japanese War, adrift in a world that changed without them and seemingly did not need them to move forward, a promised return of the feeling of being among friends, engaged in activities of a higher purpose, and working toward broader goals was just a few kopecks a way. The marketing of tobacco with soldiers undoubtedly would have appealed to soldiers and former soldiers, just as it served as an incentive to future soldiers.

2 : PRODUCED

Tobacco Queens and Working Girls

In 1881, Aleksandr Nikolaevich Shaposhnikov, owner of one of St. Petersburg's premier tobacco factories, died unexpectedly of typhoid fever, leaving his wife to take over the family business.[1] Not just a placeholder for her lost husband, Ekaterina Nikolaevna Shaposhnikova guided the factory to controlling membership in a massive tobacco trust with warehousing and diverse holdings by the eve of the 1917 revolution. Through the trust, she oversaw the production of paper, printing, and match factories; she gained a strong foothold in the Baltic, Polish, and frontier trade; and she had a grasp on 75 percent of the capital's tobacco market and nearly 30 percent of all of Russia's tobacco workers. Along the way Shaposhnikova fostered industrial innovation, establishing a factory technician with his own tobacco-machinery business that made him a millionaire. She ameliorated workers' conditions with an on-site cafeteria, clinic, free pharmacy, and a full-time doctor and medical assistant, while sponsoring a temperance society and social events for workers. Little wonder that at her death in January 1917 she was mourned as a Russian "tobacco queen."[2]

Shaposhnikova's story, and that of the factory she led, exposed many of the unique aspects of late-tsarist tobacco manufacture at both the national and international level. Peculiar to Russia was the low-grade makhorka tobacco, the cardboard-tubed papirosy cigarettes, the slow transition to mechanization in preference for cheap sweated labor, and the ownership of several large tobacco manufactures by women.[3] Typical was the largely female and underage labor force. Pitiable were the wages, working conditions, and living situations of these women and children. Shaposhnikova's factory pharmacy and cafeteria were trifles in the face of the industry-wide reliance on poorly paid handwork by women and children who toiled in difficult conditions at cramped factories or in tenements. Even as many manufacturers implemented progressive policies, child and women's labor focused unrest both within and outside the industry. The condition of the industry and its workers became integral to the outlooks of smokers and cessationists as the production of papirosy contributed to the social meaning of smoking.[4] Developing connoisseurship required that smokers know the composition and production methods of their smokes, including whether or not a factory used foreign or domestic tobacco, modern production techniques, and exotic flavorings.

Despite the comparatively small size of the tobacco industry, the women of tobacco had an outsize presence in the revolutionary movement. The vociferous working class assured that those who used tobacco had to be aware of the labor of women and children as well as the conditions in factories. Not just workers voiced concern. Many contemporary authors waxed poetic about the horrors of tobacco's child and female labor.[5] Workers were already well aware of the conditions of the factories, but perhaps the information on the abuse of women, and poor children's health, provided new insights for males and progressive intellectuals. Owners publicized their charitable actions, factory improvements, and worker programs in advertisements, press releases, and pamphlets, hoping to sway perceptions.

The story of the widow Shaposhnikova and the history of her business began this chapter, but the experiences of labor in the factory and the history of tobacco women in the era of revolutionary ferment conclude it. Starting in the 1890s and increasing through the post-1905 era, Russian tobacco workers agitated for greater rights. Despite being a largely female, supposedly quiescent labor force, tobacco workers engaged in fierce agitation, which the government brutally suppressed. The production of papirosy, and the subsequent experience of smoking, reeked of revolution.

TOBACCO, a product of the new world, appeared in Russia in the 1600s, but only in 1696 did Peter the Great (r. 1682–1725) legalize sales. With an eye toward import duties he made a trade deal with the English. Soon after, the tsar allowed the foundation of a factory for rolling and cutting in "the English style" under the purview of imported specialists. It closed within a year.[6] Another attempt in the early 1700s in Ukraine with Dutch support for tobacco "made in the German way" also languished.[7] Later efforts met with greater success. From the 1760s, Catherine the Great fostered Russian tobacco cultivation and production by allowing free sale of tobacco within the country with no tax. Over the next several decades, imports of Dutch tobacco provided for creeping growth in the number of users as Russian farming developed and the imperial hand grew stronger in Crimea.[8] By the nineteenth century, Russian agronomist K. Dmitriev contended that tobacco could be grown in almost every area of the empire.[9] Others argued it was as well suited to Russian cultivation as wine or even barley, and one insisted that since many regions had a climate similar to Virginia, Russian tobacco was already up to American standards.[10]

In the late eighteenth century, Russia briefly became a net exporter of tobacco by volume, but it was an uneven exchange of mostly raw, low grade Ukrainian leaf for expensive, high-grade, heavily-produced British, Dutch, and even Hungarian snuff. Snuff was the primary form of tobacco consumption in eighteenth-century Russia according to contemporaries, but this perception may have been created by the visibility of the product among the upper classes. Observers noted that the tobacco grown in the country appealed not to the cultivated tastes of the high-end enthusiast but to the needs of "simple folk." Use in the countryside by the common people, perhaps in snuff, or as crumbled tobacco for pipes, would have left their methods of consumption less visible.[11] In the early nineteenth century, imported cigars grew in importance, and, as one contemporary noted, a few million rubles a year went up in "foreign smelling smoke."[12]

The price of foreign tobacco incentivized the introduction of new seed to Ukraine, imported from Holland, Turkey, Persia, and America, and Russian leaf began to catch up in quality.[13] After 1812, the Russian minister of finance started a concerted campaign to import and distribute the best American seed. By 1845, an article in *Otechestvennyia zapiski: Ucheno-literaturnyi zhurnal'* (Notes domestic: A scientific-literary journal) claimed that Crimea had imported its tobacco from Turkey in 1820, but now the area supported its own supply and even exported it.[14] By 1899, the agricultural manual from V. G. Kotel'nikov augured a very different situation for Russian tobacco. Russians now grew profitable, desirable tobacco. Kotel'nikov urged peasants to include tobacco in a diversified list of crops. He argued, "Tobacco is one of not many goods which gives a peasant profitability for their labor. With just a little plot, he can receive a marketable good of a nameable sum." He cautioned peasants not to sow tobacco short-sightedly only when prices were high but to consistently work and improve their crops to be profitable.[15] Kotel'nikov did not advocate that peasants aspire to tobacco plantations of the American style. He advised small-scale, piecemeal cultivation.

Russia's internal tobacco-processing industry grew alongside the cultivation of native tobacco though in a similarly spasmodic way.[16] While there

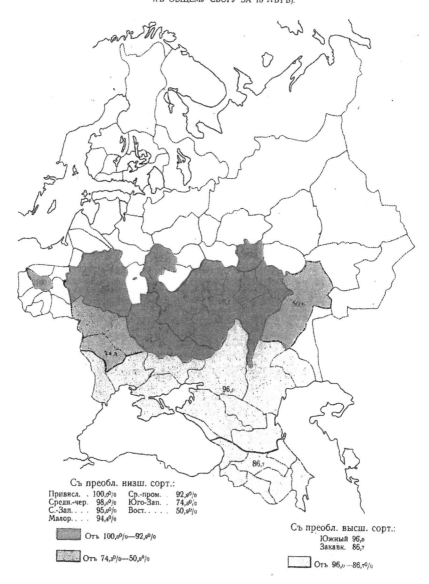

РАЙОНЫ СЪ ПРЕОБЛАДАНІЕМЪ СБОРА ВЫСШИХЪ ИЛИ НИЗШИХЪ СОРТОВЪ
ТАБАКА (%/ ОТНОШЕНІЕ СБОРА ТАБАКА ВЫСШ. И НИЗШ. СОРТОВЪ
КЪ ОБЩЕМУ СБОРУ ЗА 15 ЛѢТЪ).

Съ преобл. низш. сорт.:

Привисл. . 100,0%/o	Ср.-пром. . 92,8%/o
Средн.-чер. 98,0%/o	Юго-Зап. . 74,8%/o
С.-Зап. . . . 95,6%/o	Вост. 50,6%/o
Малор. . . . 94,8%/o	

Отъ 100,0%/o—92,0%/o

Отъ 74,3%/o—50,0%/o

Съ преобл. высш. сорт.:
Южный 96,0
Закавк. 86,7

Отъ 96,0—86,7%/o

Map 2.1 Higher and lower sort tobacco harvest by district, 1890–1904. Higher sorts are in the darker hues. N. I. Umnova, "Tabachnaia promyshlennost za 15 let' (s 1890–1904)," in *Sbornik statei i materialov po tabachnomu delu*, ed. S. S. Egiz (Petersburg: V. O. Kirshbaum, 1913). Collection of Russian State Library, Moscow.

were but six tobacco enterprises in the empire in 1812, by 1861 that number had reached 530. Enterprises remained small; the average 1861 factory employed thirteen workers.[17] The mushrooming of the number of tobacco businesses reflected both the ease with which a concern could be established, with only a few thousand or even a few hundred rubles, and the attraction of the growing market.[18] In the roughly fifteen-year period up to 1886, Russian tobacco use rose 76 percent even as French intake went up only 34 percent.[19] Admittedly, Russian tobacco consumption started from a lower point than French use, but the rise was still striking to Russian farmers and businessmen looking for opportunity.

Tobacco served as a model for the type of small-scale capitalist development that propelled post-reforms Russia. The Asmolov factory of Rostov-na-Don, for example, started small, but the factory became the largest makhorka enterprise in Russia in the 1880s. Asmolov began his venture with just three thousand rubles in 1857.[20] By 1913, the factory produced twenty-six billion papirosy.[21] V. I. Lenin used Asmolov as an archetype of Russia's entrepreneurial class in his *Development of Capitalism in Russia*, where he detailed how "Asmolov used to be a peddler's horse-driver, after a petty trader, director of a small tobacco workshop, and after owner of a factory with a turnover of many millions."[22] In an anniversary history of the factory, Asmolov himself marveled at the strength of the market for his products.[23]

While an Austrian would found Laferm, prerevolutionary Russia's largest tobacco factory, Russian Karaites (a Jewish sect) or ethnic Russians established many of the rest.[24] The Shaposhnikov family started small with trade and then diversified into production. Ekaterina Nikolaevna's mother-in-law Pelageia Stepanovna Shaposhnikova came to St. Petersburg from a merchant family in Kolomna, and when her husband died, leaving her with five children, she quickly established a store on Karavannaia Street for the trade of tobacco and other goods. From these 1853 beginnings, she expanded until in 1873 her son Aleksandr Nikolaevich took the next step and opened the tobacco factory, which he had just expanded into a new custom-designed factory building when he died in 1881.[25] The Dunaev factory of Iaroslavl, later to take the name of Balkan Star, followed a similar pattern of growth. After starting in grain trade and then diversifying into "tobacco and cigars, pipe stems, men's canes, pomade, perfume, pens, pencils, and various fancy goods," Nikolai Feodorovich Dunaev, a forty-nine-year-old peasant, moved into tobacco in 1849.[26] An 1860 law allowing tobacco sales in food stores enabled steady expansion.[27] Dunaev's factory worked in makhorka, brought from Chernigov and Poltava, which offered a number of

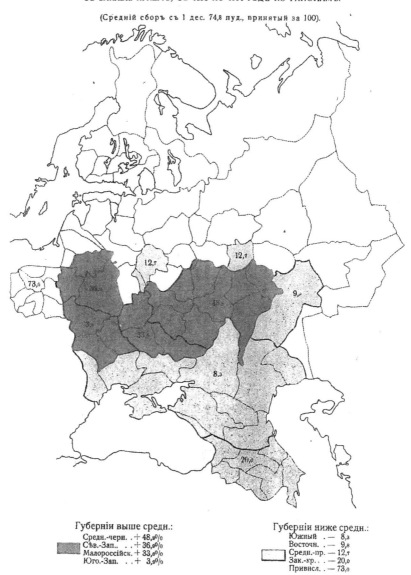

СРЕДНІЙ ЕЖЕГОДНЫЙ СБОРЪ ТАБАКА СЪ 1 ДЕС. ЗА 15 ЛѢТЪ (ПО ЕВРОП. РОССІИ СЪ ЗАКАВК. КРАЕМЪ) СЪ 1890 ПО 1904 ГОДЪ ПО РАЙОНАМЪ.

(Средній сборъ съ 1 дес. 74,8 пуд., принятый за 100).

Губерніи выше средн.:
Средн.-черн. . . + 48,в⁰/о
Сѣв.-Зап.. . . + 36,в⁰/о
Малороссійск. + 33,в⁰/о
Юго.-Зап. . . + 3,в⁰/о

Губерніи ниже средн.:
Южный . — 8,а
Восточн. . — 9,в
Средн.-пр. — 12,т
Зак.-кр.. . — 20,0
Привисл. . — 73,0

Map 2.2 Average harvest by district, 1890–1904. Higher and middling sorts are in darker hues. N. I. Umnova, "Tabachnaia promyshlennost za 15 let' (s 1890–1904)," in *Sbornik statei i materialov po tabachnomu delu*, ed. S. S. Egiz (Petersburg: V. O. Kirshbaum, 1913). Collection of Russian State Library, Moscow.

advantages including low material costs, stable markets outside the vagaries of war and tariffs, simpler production, and cheaper delivery.[28]

The focus on domestic tobacco like makhorka allowed Dunaev and other mid-century tobacco producers to weather the fluctuations brought on by war in the 1850s and 1870s, agricultural problems in the 1860s, and the excise tax system introduced in 1838 and refined in the 1860s.[29] Before 1838, the tobacco business in Russia, with a total of 120 factories, had no tax. In that year, manufacturers began to pay for the right to prepare and sell tobacco.[30] Tobacco was taxed at the point of manufacture, leaving un-refined or personal tobacco untaxed and uncounted in official statistics. Consequently, developed factories with established oversight experienced the greater tax burden as government analyses revealed that large amounts of the tobacco harvest went to local use to avoid reporting to the excise offi-cials.[31] The state did not seem to practice tax farming, but the tax system did nothing to stabilize the industry.[32] According to one historian, "The high excise rate, in combination with the weakness of the inspectorate for its receipts, opened the vast field to corruption and made the tobacco industry a source for wild speculation."[33] Despite occasional drops in revenue due to compliance issues, continued refinement of the system meant increasing revenue. The tobacco excise began in 1839.[34] From 1839 to 1899 the taxed amount rose fiftyfold.[35] By 1889 excise taxes generated 20,000,000 rubles with an additional 2.25 million rubles for imported tobacco.[36]

Complaints regarding the excise system continued to mount through the turn of the century, but one advocate argued that the taxing of tobacco was a net good because of its "convenience" and the "stable means of income." Unlike salt, tobacco was not considered a necessity, and, in contrast to alco-hol, there was no agreement that it was detrimental to the health of individ-uals or society. Taxing tobacco, a luxury good for the adult male population, allowed for a more targeted tax that could be further refined according to the quality of leaf so as to "consider the fiscal capacity of the taxpayers." The author concluded, "In technical terms, tobacco taxation has a serious ad-vantage especially in our decade of industrial development." Lax oversight constituted the only problem.[37]

In the 1860s, the fluctuation in the supply of tobacco and refinements in the tax system led to the fall of many smaller enterprises and consolidation by others.[38] The number of tobacco factories decreased by 25 percent and makhorka factories fell by 40 percent. By the 1870s, though many small manufacturers had disappeared, output increased and the character of Rus-sian tobacco production changed. Older, smaller light factories left the scene

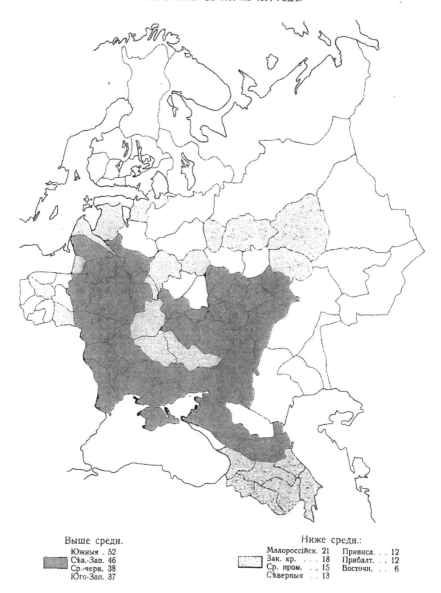

Картограмма № 3.

ЧИСЛО ФАБРИКЪ (ВЫШЕ И НИЖЕ СРЕДНЯГО ДЛЯ КАЖД. РАЙОНА)
ЗА 15 ЛѢТЪ: СЪ 1890 ПО 1904 ГОДЪ.

Выше средн.
Южныя . 52
Сѣв.-Зап. 46
Ср.-черн. 38
Юго-Зап. 37

Ниже средн.:
Малороссійск. 21
Зак. кр. . . . 18
Ср. пром. . . 15
Сѣверныя . . 13
Привисл. . . 12
Прибалт. . . 12
Восточн. . . . 6

Map 2.3   District factory numbers, 1890–1904. Higher sorts are in the darker hues. N. I. Umnova, "Tabachnaia promyshlennost za 15 let' (s 1890–1904)," in *Sbornik statei i materialov po tabachnomu delu*, ed. S. S. Egiz (Petersburg: V. O. Kirshbaum, 1913). Collection of Russian State Library, Moscow.

in preference for newer firms with larger capital investment. Production per factory increased 56 percent for tobacco and 104 percent for makhorka.[39] In addition to consolidation, the tax system encouraged expansion in lower, cheaper sorts of tobacco.[40] Even with lower taxes on inferior-quality wares, tobacco still made money for the state.[41] The Russian state's profit from tobacco followed international examples and finally fulfilled the promises for tobacco made in the seventeenth-century establishment of the trade.[42] Growth continued in the prewar years as seen in table 2.1. The precipitous increase in 1910 came as a result of changes in the system and rising taxes on higher sorts of tobacco.[43] Vodka revenues from the recently-established state monopoly dwarfed tobacco profits. In 1895, vodka produced 230 million rubles for the state, and in 1904, 576 million.[44] Comparatively, Russia stood in seventh place worldwide in the tax on tobacco, behind France, England, Spain, Austro-Hungary, Italy, and Norway.[45]

As Russian industry reorganized in the late nineteenth century, it also reoriented toward the production of ready-made papirosy. In the period from 1861 to 1900, the production of papirosy increased by thirtyfold, from .3 billion to 8.6 billion items, and the proportion of tobacco made into papirosy went from 5.9 to 12.7 percent.[46] In just the period from 1890 to 1900 the production of papirosy rose 167 percent. Urbanites and factory workers constituted the primary users and thus the rise in production came with the growth of the urban market.[47] As early as 1880, tobacco had taken over St. Petersburg, where every year inhabitants plopped down nineteen million rubles on the purchase of eight and a half million cigars and papirosy. The

Table 2.1   Excise tax receipts, 1904–13

Year	General sum of excise in 1000 rubles	As a percentage of total	
		Higher sorts	Lower sorts
1904	43,443	98.8	31.2
1905	44,523	68.4	31.6
1906	49,822	71.6	28.4
1907	45,319	69.9	30.1
1908	47,636	67.4	32.6
1909	53,042	69.9	30.1
1910	63,338	74.2	25.8
1911	67,862	76.0	24.0
1912	74,456	74.8	25.2
1913	81,465	76.3	23.7

V. N. Liubimenko, *Tabachnaia promyshlennost' v Rossii* (Petrograd: Komis. Po izuch. Estest. Proizvoditel'nykh sil Rossii, 1916), 65.

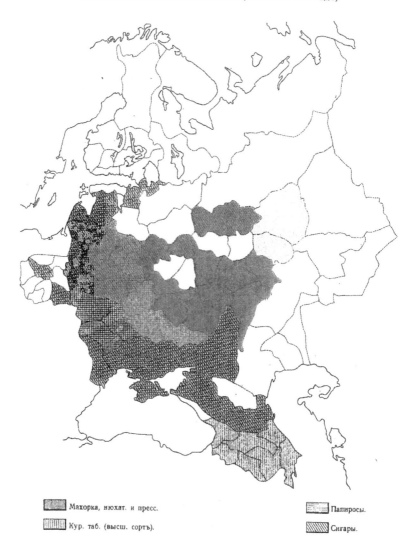

Картограмма № 4.

ВЫДѢЛКА РАЗНЫХЪ СОРТОВЪ ТАБАКА (СЪ 1899 ПО 1904 ГОДЪ).

Махорка, нюхат. и пресс.

Кур. таб. (высш. сортъ).

Папиросы.

Сигары.

Map 2.4 Tobacco processing by district, 1899–1904. Makhorka, snuff, and pressed tobacco (dark); Papirosy (horizontal lines), higher sorts of smoking tobacco (vertical lines), and cigars (diagonal lines). N. I. Umnova, "Tabachnaia promyshlennost za 15 let' (s 1890–1904)," in *Sbornik statei i materialov po tabachnomu delu* ed. S. S. Egiz (Petersburg: V. O. Kirshbaum, 1913). Collection of Russian State Library, Moscow.

figures translate into roughly nineteen rubles per person or, in low-grade tobacco, 380 packs every year. The source of this figure reported by a foreign observer was not attributed.[48]

No detailed consumption charts or figures appeared in any of the literature, and because of the tax system's centralization in more established factories and notoriously lax enforcement, production figures did not easily transfer into consumption statistics. A 1911 report pegged Belgian consumption at 2.5 kg per capita per year; Austrian at 1.5 kg, French at .81, and Russian at .83 kg.[49] Given that contemporaries recognized that large amounts of Russian tobacco were consumed where farmed or corrupt systems assured that much was transferred to small workshops to avoid taxation, this estimate based on taxed tobacco production likely missed a great deal.[50] In 1912 antitobacco author Dr. Tregubov appraised average per capita male consumption to be twenty papirosy a day (the modern equivalent of a pack a day). This figure also appeared in a 1909 pamphlet and lined up with other contemporary estimates.[51] If true, this would have put Russian consumption at 7,300 papirosy a year, or roughly 3.12 kg per year. According to another figure, the nineteenth-century smoker had thirty to forty papirosy a day, spending five to ten ruble a month on the habit.[52] This would double the estimate of Tregubov to 14,600 papirosy per year and thus 6.24 kg of tobacco. Each papirosa used approximately half a gram of tobacco (400 grams of tobacco produce 1000 papirosy), thus estimates for Russian consumption ranged from 1,619 papirosy per year to 14,600 per year.

Official records showed consumption at nowhere near the above estimates. In 1913 output in papirosy from tobacco was 47,634,000 and 21,800,000 from makhorka. These production numbers likely did not reflect large amounts of tobacco used in the region of production, which even on the eve of the war still evaded official counts.[53] If taken against the total population of the empire, official counts would allow for less than one papirosa a year per capita and not more than two for adult males. By comparison, per capita consumption in the United States in 1930 was 1,500 cigarettes a year and, by 1960, 4,000 a year.[54]

Anecdotal evidence from outside observers upheld larger contemporary, eye-witness estimates over official tax figures and painted a vision of a mass of smoking males in Russia. A western representative from the paper trade remarked in 1907, "The quantity of cigarettes smoked in Russia is almost incredible, as they are practically the only form of smoking indulged in by all classes, and it is not too much to say that the average number smoked would not fall short of 150 a week for every male over 15 years of age."[55] The

American's estimate would put average consumption at a little over a pack a day for all mature males. The foreign trade representative reflected the opinion of many Russian observers that it seemed everyone, of every class, smoked papirosy everywhere.

Russian contemporaries depicted increased tobacco use not as a problem but as a sign of progress that indicated Russia's growing inclusion in Western development. An 1896 essay detailed Russia's place within a smoking world by citing the rapidly rising consumption, noting that while smoking was more prevalent in the West, Russia had its own zones, particularly in the south and in areas of Ukraine, where tobacco use was common.[56] Small-scale statistical surveys backed a vision of a Russia cloaked in smoke. An 1891 article in *Vrach* found 68.1 percent of military men smoked, and among officers, smoking reached 78.7 percent. The average consumption per month was about two packs a day.[57] The large numbers of smokers in the military likely meant greater pressure on nonsmokers in the ranks to start and underscored the connections of militarism, manliness, and tobacco outlined previously.

By the turn of the century, smoking had taken off. As N. O. Osipov reported in 1901, "The greatest rise in production of tobacco products occurred in the greatest way in the production of papirosy, the number of which between 1890 and 1899 more than doubled. Obviously in the last twenty years the form of tobacco use has undergone a complete change, not to mention that with every day the pipe is disappearing, the people are more and more accustomed to the use of ready-made, factory-produced papirosy."[58]

Production figures backed a vision of increasing use of factory papirosy. In 1908 papirosy constituted 28.5 percent of all tobacco worked; by 1913 this doubled to 46.3 percent.[59] As tobacco production grew, increasing amounts went to papirosy, as seen in table 2.2.

The growth in tobacco production, especially in the low-grade makhorka tobacco, was striking in the late imperial period. Authorities, in turn, attempted to move the market through tax changes into higher-end tobaccos, as shown in table 2.3.

The taxes resulted in an increased emphasis on loose tobacco over papirosy and decreasing the amount of "pure" tobacco per papirosa.[60] By 1904 pure tobacco content decreased to 81 percent of 1890 levels for first sort papirosy and to 72 percent for third sort papirosy.[61] Producers chose to decrease quality rather than increase price, and their continued move in this direction indicated that they did not suffer any major repercussions on the market.

Table 2.2   Tobacco production, 1890–1914

	Smoking and snuff tobacco produced in thousand pounds		*Items produced in millions*		*Total weight of products in thousand pounds*
	Higher sort	*Makhorka*	*Cigar/ Cigarette*	*Papirosy*	
1890	26,064	92,016	203	3,739	126,540
1895	28,260	102,096	181	5,687	140,364
1900	67,716	73,188	179	8,616	149,976
1904	33,876	142,668	157	11,818	185,040
1910	24,804	152,676	143	133	208,944
1914	26,316	206,784	133	29,772	265,500

V. N. Liubimenko, *Tabak* (Petrograd: M. S. Sabashnikovy, 1922), 25.

Table 2.3   Tobacco produced by type, 1910 and 1911

	Amount worked in factories in pounds for entire Russian empire	
	1910	*1911*
Tobacco—Smoking	24,799,032	24,479,280
—Papirosy	19,796,004	21,346,596
—Snuff	6,372	6,480
—Cigars	1,348,092	1,363,104
—Cigarettes	45,144	43,992
Makhorka papirosy	88,488	45,684
—smoking	153,197,208	152,801,424
—snuff	8,793,684	8,759,016
—pressed	876,960	987,624
TOTAL	208,950,984	209,840,400

V. N. Liubimenko, *Tabachnaia promyshlennost' v Rossii* (Petrograd: Komis. Po izuch. Estest. Proizvoditel'nykh sil Rossii, 1916), 59.

Russians of the nineteenth century clearly distinguished cigarettes from papirosy. To construct a papirosa, handworkers, usually women, used a round form to twist the paper of a cartridge, gluing the last millimeter to form a tube that was filled with tobacco, to which they attached a mouthpiece of twisted, trapezoidal-cut cardboard. For the Russian of 1901, "A cigarette is a papirosa without paper; the tobacco leaf forms its cartridge. Usually a cigarette is formed of beaten, crumpled American tobacco. This material is wetted, pressed into a dense mass and divided into chunks."[62] In factories in the city and in small workshops in their villages, groups of women produced the tobacco cartridges for papirosy. In the 1880s, costs made it more economical to send materials to the village and set up a small shop for several peasant women and girls to roll tubes with minimal training and oversight. Supplied with the paper, cardboard, and rudimentary tools, village women spent up to thirteen hours a day, thirty-five weeks a year producing tobacco cartridges for a largely urban market. Observers reported that all except the very old participated.[63]

Starting in the 1880s, mechanical innovations allowed for the reduction of handwork in tobacco processing elsewhere around the globe. James Bonsack of Virginia patented the first cigarette-packing machine in 1881.[64] The first in Mexico came to *el modelo* in 1884.[65] James Duke brought his to production in the United States in 1885.[66] Russians innovated production, but later, more gradually, and with the focus on their particular style of smoke. Crumbling tobacco with steam machinery allowed for preparation of smoking tobacco as well as papirosy, but only a little over half of factories had steam machinery as late as 1904.[67] Cartridge machines enabled production without glue, but caught on slowly after their appearance in the 1890s.[68] The majority of factories employed a mix of machine and handwork, with higher-quality tobacco factories mechanizing more quickly than those working in cheaper makhorka.[69]

Before 1900 most Russian factory owners increased output not by experimenting with new and costly machinery, but simply by employing more women and children and replacing expensive male employees, as shown in table 2.4. Factory owners saw no profit in investing in pricey machinery that required oversight by trained technicians. In Bulgaria, a similar process occurred as women went from 10 percent of the workforce in 1900 to 70 percent by 1908.[70] The cigar industry in the United States also feminized in this period.[71] Mechanization did not fuel the boom in Russian tobacco consumption. Russia had enough cheap female and child

Table 2.4   Number of factory workers by gender and age, 1800 and 1900

	Number of factory workers		
	1800	*1900*	*Number of increase*
Grown men	10,866	10,967	121
Grown women	18,922	23,121	4,199
Underage m/f	2,818	4,818	2,000
All	32,606	38,926	6,320

M. V. Dzhervis, *Russkaia tabachnaia fabrika v XVIII i XIX vekakh* (Leningrad: Akademii nauk SSSR, 1933), 100.

labor to enable manufactures to exploit rather than mechanize and create modern products with old techniques.[72] As one 1933 industry history
noted, "Simple arithmetic showed factory owners the advantage of using
cheap hand labor in comparison to increasing production with expensive
machinery."[73]

The overall number of tobacco workers in 1900—just under forty
thousand—was smaller than that of many industries. Textiles employed
475,537 workers in 1900, and from just 1887 to 1900, one million workers
joined the Russian labor force overall.[74] Despite the low numbers, the tobacco workforce held distinctive features, making it more visible. Indeed,
the fact that so many stories and events featured tobacco workers despite
their low numbers indicated a larger impact from this group than their size
would have suggested.[75]

By the turn of the century, women made up 85 percent of St. Petersburg
tobacco workers and 60 percent of Moscow's tobacco industry.[76] Despite
the available machinery, 93.2 percent of factories still relied on hand work
in the 1890s and only 13.2 percent of tobacco or makhorka factories employed gas or steam machines.[77] Over the course of the decade, however, the
number of steam-powered tobacco crumbling machines increased. Only
292 factories had them in 1890, but by 1899 445 did. Makhorka factories,
already at the low end in supply costs, did not mechanize at the same rate,
and in some cases enterprises even fell back into greater use of handwork.[78]
This led to regional variations so that areas of higher-end production tran-
sitioned more quickly than the rest of the country toward mechanization.
For instance, Nizhnyi Novgorod moved from 108 handwork stations in
1880 to only forty-nine by 1894.[79]

Ol'ga Petrovna Ogarenko, who began work at the Asmolov makhorka
factory in 1898 at the age of eleven, noted that at that time, "all work was
done by hand. Tobacco was cut with a knife. Cartridges glued by hand. *Papirosy* packed by hand. The instruments for preparing papirosy were iron
(or copper) 'machines' resembling a pipe and stick."[80] In 1898 the factory
installed its first tobacco-packing machine. In those factories where machines did appear, a reduction in handwork did not necessarily follow.
Adding mouthpieces and tobacco to the cartridge still required hand labor.
Instead, overcrowding of the factory occasioned by the machines led to
the handwork being put out into apartments. Overall, the industry saw no
major increase in per worker productivity. As one Soviet historian put it,
"If tobacco production all the same triumphed, then it triumphed at the
cost of cruel exploitation of worker strength and indeed the same conditions of labor."[81] The addition of packing machines to the shop floor did

not improve conditions for workers, but instead led to overcrowding, the devaluation of handwork, and unemployment.[82]

The Shaposhnikov factory stood at the forefront of technical innovation in the tobacco industry at the turn of the century because of the foresight of its owner and her attention to the work of one of her employees—I. A. Semonov. With the support of Shaposhnikova, Semenov became the Russian Bonsack, creating a number of machines, including one for cartridge production that won grand prize at the 1900 World's Fair in Paris, as well as a machine that produced both the cartridge and mouthpiece together, which appeared in the same year.[83] Semenov, with the sponsorship of Shaposhnikova, opened a shop for the production of tobacco machinery and quickly became a major supplier. Cheaper, less reliable competitors appeared, finding buyers in the lower tobacco market, but Semenov became quite wealthy.[84] With these innovations, many Russian manufacturers, like their comrades in Canada and Britain, began to claim the distinction of products made through modern means without glue.[85] *Katyk* cartridge advertisements crowed that they were made "without hands"— calling up the miraculous Russian Orthodox image of Christ and making instead an icon for the machine age. Kolobov and Bobrov of St. Petersburg trumpeted their "mechanical" papirosy.[86] A 1901 poster for Laferm celebrated the new six-story factory for not just the latest electric machines but also for the three million "white" papirosy and cartridges it produced a day—each "without human touch."

After the turn of the century, papirosy production mechanized slowly and the number of factories continued to decline, but output did not fall. Increasing employment of women and children maintained production and pricing. The Asmolov factory stood at the forefront of this process, installing machinery from the firms of Semenov as well as those of Vlodarkevich and Sekliudskii yet still relying on a large number of female and child laborers. The combination allowed for a massive increase in production, which was visible not just in the empire but also around Western Europe, where Asmolov brands appeared with increasing frequency. As a history of the company published a year later stated, "According to the amount of tobacco produced, Asmolov [was] the premier private tobacco factory in the world."[87]

The slow-rising mechanization of the industry took place against the background of economic strategizing by the larger firms for increasing concentration. As small firms fell off, others were purchased and consolidated. A number of tobacco firms had already founded joint-stock companies, such as Laferm in 1870 and both Dukat and Brothers Shapshal in the early 1900s.[88] The greatest impact came from the creation in 1913 of the Russian

Tobacco Company, a freestanding corporation established in Britain but composed of Russian manufactures and financing.[89] The Russian Tobacco Company brought together leading tobacco firms from all over the empire, including the St. Petersburg manufacturers Laferm, Ottoman, Brothers Shapshal, Bogdanov and Company, Shapohsnikov and Company, and Kolobov and Bobrov; the Moscow factories of Dukat and Gabai; and the Rostov-na-Don companies of Kushnarev and Company, Brothers Aslandi, and Asmolov and Company. The company also made a stab at vertical integration by adding in the companion industries of Iogansen, Kosheleff, Russian, and Tchernoff paper factories; the Russian Printing and Publishing Joint Stock Company, and the Dunaeff Tobacco and Matches Company, adding a sugar company in 1915.[90]

The group, for whom Ekaterina Nikolaevna Shaposhnikova served as managing director (*director-rasporiaditel'*), announced its intention to use its combined power to allow the joint purchase of raw materials at lower prices so as to decrease the prices for tobacco and papirosy.[91] Perhaps a more realistic reading would be that the concentration of industry allowed the factories to stop lowering prices to compete for market share, squeeze farmers for lower raw material costs, and gain greater profits for their companies. Competition with foreign trusts, especially the Americans, provided a major incentive for Russian organization according to reports from leaders of the trust.[92] The outcomes for industry were greater concentration and more emphasis on papirosy. By 1912, the trust accounted for 49 percent of all yellow-leaf tobacco worked in Russia.[93] By 1917, almost 70 percent of Russian papirosy production came through the trust.[94]

By 1914, the production of papirosy increased by over seven and a half times its 1890 value as the average production per factory rose by 350 percent and the number of workers per factory rose by almost 40 percent.[95] Not all of this production was for the Russian market, and exports were made to the southern border (Persia), the east (Mongolia and China), and the west (Germany and Finland especially).[96] From 1890 to 1904, exports of papirosy alone increased by 1100 percent, according to a 1913 study.[97] Overall, the export of papirosy increased dramatically, as shown in table 2.5.

While the mass export might have been novel, Russian papirosy were nothing new to Europe. In his 1861 history, Henry Sutherland Edwards noted, "The introduction of the Russian *cigarette* into England is one of the unexpected results of the Crimean war. . . . It may be said that the *papirosses* have already gained a large amount of public favour."[98] By 1915, an American tobacco connoisseur declared that Russia was Europe's largest

Table 2.5   Export of papirosy in millions, 1890–1909

1890	27
1895	40
1900	152
1904	820
1909	1006

V. N. Liubimenko, *Tabak* (Petrograd: M. S. Sabashnikovy, 1922), 33.

producer of tobacco, and while the common Russian leaf was "coarse, dark and heavy" like French tobacco, the leaf grown in the South from Turkish seed was "fit for cigarettes."[99] Russian firms also set up abroad and made a name for themselves. In New York, over one hundred small Russian factories on the east side made cigarettes with tobacco blends that were valued for their aroma.[100] The Russian firm A. Lopato and Sons set up in Harbin in 1898 as the railway moved to the east.[101] The Russian brand *Zarina* advertised in American papers in 1900 that "clean healthy girls" rolled their products.[102]

The growth of the tobacco business became evident in the grueling conditions for laborers. A tobacco worker's shift could stretch to as long as eighteen hours, although after 1897 legislation limited the workday to eleven and a half hours, with a commute, usually on foot, on either end.[103] For most, the workday began at six or seven in the morning with a prayer and continued through a lunch break of an hour and a half at midday until a quitting time of seven or eight in the evening, with a prayer and either a hymn or song for the emperor.[104] Because of the oversight by a government official necessary for the excise tax system, tobacco factories could not operate legally over holidays or overnight.[105] Still, there was fluctuation according to the seasons and for market days. Elizaveta Viktorovna Torsueva, a worker in the Asmolov factory, remembered, "In winter, we worked fourteen and in summer eighteen hours and during the time of the Makareevskii market we worked without lunch break."[106]

The factory building transformed, too. More successful owners invested in new premises, like Shaposhnikov's stone or Laferm's six-story showplace. Most manufacturers, however, just converted houses, with production broken into a few different rooms. The lack of preplanning made for inefficiency, poor ventilation, and overcrowding. The factory of Konstantin and Pavel Petrov, founded in 1864, followed this pattern. The three-story stone home held different operations on its various floors—drying ovens, cartridge machines, accountants, rollers, and even a cafeteria for workers.[107]

The transport of tobacco between floors, or from the warehouse to the shop floor by the rollers themselves, was done by hauling tobacco in bundles on the head, adding labor and time.[108] The days were long and the circumstances less than desirable. In an interview collected years later and perhaps colored by a desire to trumpet Soviet power, worker Solomon Egorovich Maier of the Shtaf factory in Saratov recounted, "To work there was completely impossible. It was stuffy and dark with tobacco dust and soot. That is what we put up with then, though it is incomprehensible now. The work was difficult . . . we breathed almost only dust."[109] According to Torsueva of the Asmolov factory, "The working conditions were indeed hard. Ventilation was nonexistent in the shops. . . . The supervisors were rude and cynical." She continued, "The hard conditions awoke deep resentments in workers and gave us a theme for conversations."[110] A lightly fictionalized story from a former worker began with the ventilation being so poor as to necessitate intervention from the city government.[111]

Workers considered certain spaces in the factory especially hazardous. Ivan Alekseevich Galaktionov of Saratov remembered,

> The most dangerous place for work was drying. It was a square room of five to six meters with no windows, and two security doors. The brick floor was laid with tiles, and fires burned under the floor. On the walls surrounding were . . . lattice iron shelves. There the crumbled tobacco laid for drying. The tobacco spilled in layers on the floor and the lattice shelves. After that, the doors were secured and the drying began.[112]

Inside the room, temperatures began at an unbearable 50°C (122°F), at times climbing higher over the next twelve hours. This was a particularly hazardous job. Galaktionov continued,

> Workers had to check periodically. . . . At the time there were no respirators. . . . The majority could not take it. Every time they went into the room, they would vomit from tobacco fume poisoning. The fumes from the dryer distributed throughout the whole factory and, on top of the tobacco dust, even more strongly poisoned the air.[113]

A coworker corroborated the especial dangers of the drying room in his testimony.[114]

Workers remembered the omnipresence of dust, the unendurable heat, the insufferable fumes, and the lack of proper ventilation. In winter, windows were closed to obstruct the cold. In the summer, they were closed to keep the tobacco from becoming too dry.[115] The result was dust that one worker described as "so heavy it was like a cloud and I could not see."[116] A journalist visiting a tobacco factory in 1887 reported,

> You enter the factory, and look at the dark basements without any hint of ventilation, where pillars of fine tobacco dust stand. . . . You see a swarming crowd of people with plugged noses, ears, and mouths. They work for fourteen hours a day and breathe what? It is completely inconceivable. I cannot be in that basement for five minutes. The owner says, "You adapt." Perhaps so, but who can make it to that point?[117]

Elena Stepanovna Shtengel, who worked in prerevolutionary Saratov, remembered that workers suffered splitting headaches because from "light to light [they] breathed in tobacco dust, smelled the soot of the lamp wax."[118] Even sales workers, often housed in a factory shop on the premises, complained of the "suffocating tobacco fumes" that filled the air.[119] Another worker blamed the unhealthful atmosphere for the prevalence of tuberculosis, noting that "up to the revolution that terrible scourge took to the grave many tobacco workers."[120] Different types of dust increased the danger. Galaktionov of Saratov continued his description of the most hazardous areas of the tobacco factory with the snuff department, where powdered nettles employed to strengthen the mix "clouded above and left the room in darkness."[121]

Health researchers like Dr. M. K. Valitskaia worried over the dust at workstations and over food as many workers ate directly at their station when a factory did not provide a cafeteria.[122] Others argued that even a designated cafeteria did not stop the tobacco dust from covering all the food, which they implied was unhealthy.[123] Dust presented problems not just within the factory. A commission of doctors and factory inspectors in the town of Iarloslav put the owner of the Balkan Star factory on notice that his factory befouled the air of the city.[124]

Overcrowding exacerbated air problems as cramped and dangerous conditions in shops revealed the ways manufacturers shoehorned new machines into preexisting buildings. The ever-moving belts that turned the machinery caught up workers' fingers, arms, legs, or clothing, pulling them into gears and mechanisms and resulting in maiming or death.[125] Maier of the Shtaf factory recalled the horrific death of a coworker who became entangled in machine belts. Flesh and chunks of brain flew through the shop as he was ground into the device: "By the time the machine stopped he was already dead." As a boy from the factory recalled, "You had to work quickly; the machines did not wait."[126]

Increasingly women and child workers endured these conditions. In 1900, one in four factory workers were female, with 31 percent female by 1914.[127] The concentration of women in tobacco was much higher, never falling below 50 percent and in the last years of the nineteenth century reaching even higher numbers.[128] Tobacco work, especially the rolling and stuffing of papirosy, perfectly matched the perceived skills and deficits of women.[129] Because they were in labor that was designated neither physically nor mentally demanding and that took advantage of their "agile and dexterous hands but weak bodies," women were paid far less.[130] The low skill level of the employment also meant a more easily recruited labor force and consequent disinterest from employers in stability or care for workers. Employment was erratic.[131]

While employers might consider the work unskilled, to be able to roll papirosy at a sufficient rate to make a living wage actually required a good deal of talent. According to Mariia Ivanovna Kuznetsova, a worker at the Saratov Shtaf factory, despite the stereotypes, the labor was indeed difficult: "To glue a cartridge was not so easy. You must twirl the mouthpiece, then twist the paper onto it and glue it. And the rice paper is thin and so delicate that it almost rips."[132] Russian and East European hand rollers were recognized as some of the best in the world. When Duke started his cigarette business in the United States, he imported over one hundred East European Jewish rollers because of their recognized speed and accuracy. His first was a Ukrainian Jewish man named Gladstein, but he brought on others from Poland as well as a manager from St. Petersburg. Soon thereafter, Duke liquidated his Jewish hand-rolling group because of twin pressures of mechanization and the perceived greater radical volatility of the East European workforce.[133]

Although in Russia employers considered rollers "unskilled," Duke's efforts indicated this was not the case, and Russian tobacco factory owners took extra measures to attract workers. An 1881 contract between the Asmolov factory and a Sofiia Nikiforovna Baranova of Tsarskoe selo elaborated the incentives and expectations for a potential worker. Asmolov promised paid transport as well as a return ticket after a year, both to be taken from future earnings. The company asked of Sofiia Nikiforovna obedience, attendance, "clean and accurate" work, no fighting, and no "contradictory behavior."[134] Women who entered into the factory from the countryside might come from families that were comfortable enough to have females go earn extra income or that did not have land to work.[135] Either way, the women who entered into these positions found an entirely new way of life in the city, away from home and in the predominantly female workspace.

Contemporary authors depicted the lives of tobacco women as degrading and difficult. Tolstoy wrote with fervor of the mortifications of tobacco work for women in his 1886 essay "Tak shto zhe nam delat'?" (What Shall We Do Then?), an extended discussion of the evils of capitalism and the connection between consumption and consumer. He accused smokers of complicity in the plight of tobacco workers. He derided those who argued that, if not they, then others would surely buy these items, retorting that this was the same logic of the mob. In a florid bit of prose, Tolstoy compared those who would argue they could do nothing against systemic oppression to a person who indulged in cannibalism even after knowing his cutlets were made of human flesh.[136]

To support his argument, Tolstoy described the two *papirosnitsy* (women who rolled papirosy) working for an acquaintance's private order, saying that both, the woman and child, appeared "thin, yellow, and old." He described their work:

> Quickly, quickly, she worked with her hands and fingers on the table, nervously twitching in some type of fit. Diagonally sat a girl who similarly worked along with the same fits. Both women seemed to be under the power of St. Vitus's disease. I walked closer and looked at what they were doing. They glanced at me with their eyes and all the same intently continued their work. Before them was scattered tobacco and cartridges. They were making papirosy. The woman rubbed the tobacco in her palm, packed it in the machine, filled the cartridge and passed it to the girl. The girl twirled a paper, thrust it on the cartridge, threw it down, and reached for another. All of this was done with such speed, with such intensity, that it is difficult to convey it.[137]

Tolstoy complimented their speed, and the woman replied, "Fourteen years I have done only this." Concerned for the two, he asked how they made on with the work, to which the woman answered, "'Yes. It hurts in the chest, and the smell is oppressive.'" Tolstoy said he could see the degenerative effects in the woman—"a strong organism which has already begun to collapse."[138]

Tolstoy's friend employed women not even afforded the comparative stability of a factory job. Itinerant papirosy workers lived on the edge of society, often sleeping in doorways, grabbing tobacco and paper to roll outside and then selling them loose on the street.[139] Street selling was associated with marginalized groups—women, orphans, and Jews—and became a ready marker of the ways in which tobacco use fed into exploitation. The street seller became a constant reminder on the boulevard for smokers of the ease of indulging their habit and the socioeconomic costs of its production and distribution.

A photo from the 1912 S. An-sky ethnographic expedition put on display the look of the provincial street seller (figure 2.1). The photographer for the expedition, Solomon Iudovin, captured images that combined the impulse to document a time, place, and people with artistic training that framed his figures in light and compositions similar to those of old masters. In the photograph "Tobacco Peddler," taken in the western Ukrainian town of Starokonstantinov, the tobacco seller posed outside in a muddy spot along a wooden gated wall in a complete outfit of tie, vest, collar, and jacket. His groomed aspect matched his aspirational ensemble, though a hole in the left toe of his worn galoshes indicated that he was attempting to project a status more affluent than he lived. His well-worn case held the standard display of his trade—packs of tobacco and accessories arranged in ashtrays shaped like shells. The mobile display allowed the opportunistic sellers to move to the smokers, yet also made them easy prey to theft or graft. The lock on the case likely discouraged but did not stop property loss. It was a life on the margins of order, safety, and stability.

Despite the plentiful number of street sellers and low-cost laborers ready to roll custom papirosy or sell loose tobacco on the streets, most users purchased factory-made papirosy. "Factory-made" often disguised, however, a tenement-style system where dozens of women would roll tobacco with the same single-minded ferocity, but in a room with oversight. Piecework rates, not hourly wages, determined their take-home pay. Another photo from the An-sky expedition captured the look and feel of one of these workshops (figure 2.2). In the composition, four women and one young man sit inside a workshop and behind a long table on which papers, tobacco, and finished papirosy were all lined up in piles. As with Iudovin's other images, composition, lighting, and setting were all carefully considered not just to document the Jewish experience but also to convey a feel for the life of these laborers. Here, the close, communal aspect of tobacco work, and especially rolling papirosy, came through clearly, as did the typical gender and age composition of the workforce.

In An-sky's earlier commentary on the tobacco workshop experience, he noted the ways in which the workers shared labor and poverty: "The women toiled in small workshops that had two, three, or five workers. The owners of the workshops, for the most part, toiled alongside the workers. Their wages were incredibly low. The best women workers . . . received five and a half rubles a month. The assistants received a ruble and a half

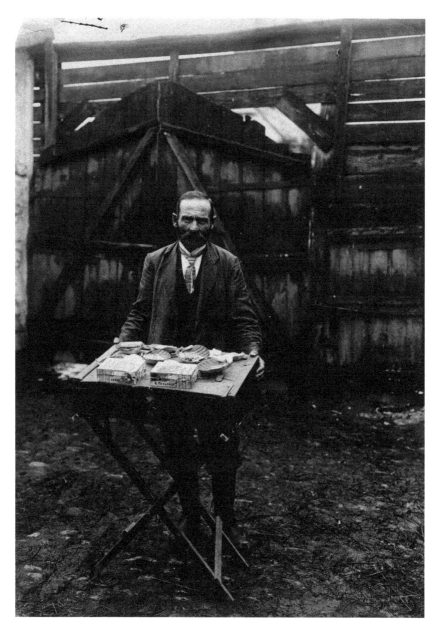

Figure 2.1   Tobacco Peddler. Photo by Solomon Iudovin, 1912. Collection "Photo-Archive of An-sky's Expeditions." Courtesy of the Center "Petersburg Judaica."

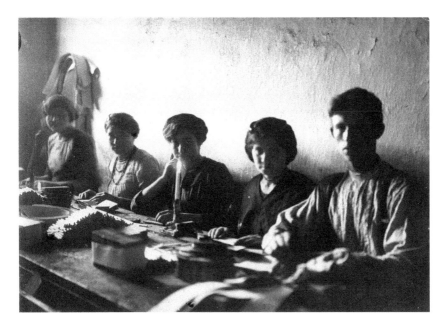

Figure 2.2   At a cigarette factory, Starokonstantinov. Photo by Solomon Yudovin, 1912. Collection "Photo-Archive of An-sky's Expeditions." Courtesy of the Center "Petersburg Judaica."

a month."[140] The closeness of the shop floor may have bred solidarity. The American labor leader Samuel L. Gompers recalled in his autobiography his own experience as a cigar roller in the United States among the tenements of New York: "A good cigarmaker learned to do [the work] more or less mechanically, which left us free to think, talk, listen, or sing. . . . Often we chose someone to read to us who was a particularly good reader, and in payment the rest of us gave him sufficient of our cigars so he was not the loser. The reading was always followed by discussion, so we learned to know each other pretty thoroughly." While no memoirs recorded a similar shared reading system among *papirosnitsy*, undoubtedly in such close quarters the women would have been able to talk as they worked, exchanging ideas and building solidarity. Although Gompers lamented the feminization of his own shop making worker organization impossible, the later history of Russia's tobacco industry indicated that worker volatility was not a problem.[141]

Low wages followed from the doubly denigrated nature of handwork and women's labor. Wages for women averaged about one-half to two-thirds that of their male counterparts across all industries.[142] In tobacco, males earned about fifteen to twenty rubles a month, women eight to ten, and children two to four and a half.[143] Most *papirosnitsy* earned too little to allow independent lives. Usually a woman worked alongside her father, husband, or siblings. Maier of the Shtaf factory remembered that as a child he worked alongside his father, brother, and three sisters, and despite the poor pay, it was worth it for the family, for "it's one thing to live on twelve to fourteen rubles a month, another to live on twenty-four to forty-eight."[144] This allowed employers another means to exert pressure on workers as supervisors considered families less of a flight risk than individuals and could threaten expulsion of all for the infractions of one or to pressure another.[145] To earn the higher wages, women had to provide around two thousand papirosy in a fourteen-hour day.[146] Few adult women could meet that quota, and some would negotiate with the paper cutters to take home materials to prepare cartridges for stuffing and twisting on the mouthpieces the next day.[147] One worker remembered helping her mother, who worked days at Laferm, to glue cartridges together at night—sometimes well past midnight—before her mother would return for her shift the next day.[148] Factories also employed children on an ad-hoc basis to roll papirosy outside the shop walls.[149]

Within the factories, younger women and children worked in a system of apprenticeship, which assured that they would earn even less, if at all. At the Kushnarev factory in Rostov-na-Don, girls as young as nine glued cartridges; during their first month of training they earned nothing. After becoming apprentices, they earned fifty kopeck a month, which rose to one ruble fifty kopeck once they could add the mouthpieces. The move from student to master usually took about three years, and during that time, apprentices crouched under the worktable gluing and twisting cartridges and mouthpieces for their masters above.[150] While called an apprenticeship, the apprentice often learned very little, simply completing the preparatory work that allowed masters to produce enough to make a living. Apprentices endured harsh discipline, frequent beatings, and attempts to prolong their period of training. One worker testified to five years as an apprentice at poor wages, even though she was doing the same work as her higher-earning master.[151] Another said that "older female workers hid the methods of working from newcomers out of fear of competition."[152]

The tobacco industry dodge of using the apprentice system as a way to exploit youth for cheaper labor appeared in other industries.[153] The instruction of the apprenticeship diminished more and more, and the opportunities for advancement and higher wages faded.[154] In many cases, apprenticed children found they owed their masters for room and board. While the law supposedly protected children, workers remembered that this was easily circumvented. Girls under fifteen were restricted to an eight-hour workday, but they would often toil for ten to twelve hours without the promised longer breaks for lunch.[155] Another worker recalled that inspectors came to the factory, but "if they even see a child, they never ask how old they are."[156] Children did not silently endure the abuses of the system. In 1902, St. Petersburg tobacco apprentices demanded an increase in pay for assisting their masters. When denied, they went on strike.[157]

Child factory labor increased dramatically over the course of the nineteenth century. Whereas at mid-century, about 15 percent of industrial workers were aged sixteen or under, by 1879–85 around 33 percent of Moscow Province workers had entered the industry before the age of twelve.[158] Attitudes changed over the course of the nineteenth century to an understanding of factory labor as different and exploitative. A law in 1882 limited child workers and by 1900 the number of children in the work force was stabilizing. Owners employed women at an increased rate, however, to keep labor costs down.[159]

Both women and children were subjected to physical abuse and intimidation on the shop floor. A 1912 *Pravda* article described the harassment of women at the Ottoman tobacco factory by male higher-ups that left "the women in tears, and the men in hopeless drunkenness."[160] In 1914, an article in *Rabotnitsa* recounted the "Old Don Juan" of the Bogdanov tobacco factory, who regularly threatened women who resisted his advances and of whom everyone had a "salty story" to tell.[161] According to another story, an owner attempted to press her female workers to roll papirosy for her with hardly any pay. They eventually defied her, burning down the building, and forcing her to flee in just her nightshirt.[162] A worker recalled his supervisor beating him.[163] Another child worker described the owner slapping him.[164] One young girl remembered the shop supervisor propositioning her with the promise of lighter work at higher pay if she came to his house.[165]

Bruises were visible, but the health effects of tobacco production remained elusive. Although an 1871 pamphlet detailed the dangers to both human and horse in the factory, not all were convinced that tobacco manufacture harmed man and beast.[166] An anonymous author in 1905 claimed that "thousands of people poison[ed] themselves preparing poison for others," but health experts in Russia and elsewhere disputed such claims.[167] Another author claimed that "workers at tobacco factories often [forgot] the name of the street where they [lived]," citing this as proof of the dangers of tobacco work for the nervous system.[168]

As Dr. V. V. Sviatlovskii noted in his 1889 investigation of tobacco worker health, over one hundred years of research had yielded wildly different conclusions, ranging from those who saw tobacco work as dangerous to those who said it strengthened workers or even protected them from "cholera, neuralgia, rheumatism, and many other diseases."[169] Sviatlovskii cited research from German, French, and Russian doctors before ultimately concluding that for most, "healthy lungs splendidly combat the effects of the dusty production. . . [but] the weak and the ill of course quickly go subject to the effects of tobacco dust" and experience many problems related to the "nervous system."[170] Sviatlovskii did concede that the lack of infectious diseases among tobacco workers might have been because they stopped work, not because of therapeutic effects. Still, he concluded that consumption and chronic lung lesions were "almost unobserved" among tobacco workers, and he observed that, based on anecdotal reports from records at the Asmolov factory, not only did any irritation from tobacco dust clear up rapidly, laborers who appeared at work with catarrh found themselves quickly healed. Citing a Dr. Chugin, Sviatlovskii conceded that worker headaches could come partly from "inhalation of drifting bits of aromatic tobacco" but noted this was also met by the workers' own faults as it resulted "in part from poor sanitary levels of home life."[171]

An 1886 history from a Dr. Rokau recommended a French prophylactic against dust—drinking "water with vinegar and sugar."[172] In an 1887 article for the journal *Vrach*, the author noted that "the inhalation of dust and smoking are, of course, far from the same thing." The article listed the many conflicting conclusions—from the finding that chest complaints were prominent in tobacco factories to a study demonstrating that children nursed at the breast by tobacco workers died at higher rates than those raised on the maligned chew-teat (*soska*—a suckle of chewed bread wrapped in cloth) and another that saw no difference in tobacco working women from other factory women.[173]

Other argued for tobacco work's healthful effects. The author of the 1852 *O razvedenii i fabrikatsii tabaka* (On the cultivation and fabrication of tobacco) reported that French doctors found that "tobacco only in the rarest circumstances causes a noticeable effect on a worker—only in snuff powdering and tobacco drying." The author wrote that Russian experience bore out these conclusions. For most workers, the first week or two might mean a headache or loss of appetite, but after that, problems occurred only for the exceptional worker in certain factory areas: "Tobacco work might act as a balm for the health of workers, just as is true of the majority of medicinal items whose effectiveness comes from poisonous qualities. Workers find that tobacco fumes are a preventative to rheumatism and when suffering from aches from a cold consider a good sleep in a tobacco leaf pile the best remedy."[174] He concluded, "Tobacco factories must be considered a protective, even salvific, force against many well-known diseases."[175]

The most often cited work from medical authorities was the thorough research of Dr. M. K. Valitskaia, a "woman doctor," whose posting as a practitioner in tobacco factories became the basis for a one-year health study of almost one thousand workers at twelve factories, including those in Rostov-na-Don, Taganrog, and Kharkhov. Valitskaia argued that the literature from France and Russia had heretofore neglected questions of nerves, but that this was "amazing" since smoking and inhalation of tobacco dust were "almost identical." Valitskaia discounted many illnesses other doctors attributed to tobacco, observing that she had seen no change in skin color, inflammation of lungs, or gastrointestinal issues. She documented a persistent cough among almost all workers and reported that she rarely encountered older tobacco workers. Only in newer workers did she see any of the expected symptoms of nicotine poisoning—nosebleeds, headache, nausea, vomiting, diarrhea, sleeplessness, dizziness—and these were especially evident among women. She concluded that after a time, the body "visibly becomes accustomed."[176]

Valitskaia found one symptom at odds with all existing literature—the pupils of tobacco workers were wider than those of non–tobacco workers. She posited a type of contagion in this condition, spreading from workers to coworkers as well as acquaintance and family members: "I observed this phenomenon of this worker in the members of his family not even at the same factory but living in the same yard and in the excise clerk working strictly in the general room at the factory on the manager, in supervisors, in a word all tobacco personnel involved."[177] A higher percentage of makhorka workers suffered, though it was also evident in less dangerous zones of the factory. Onward from dilated pupils, other nervous disorders followed in her observations, including tremors, tongue spasms, leg cramps, and heart palpitations, but she said she had found only two cases of angina.[178] Valitskaia concluded that children should only be in packing and taxation departments and pregnant and nursing women should have their time in the factory limited. She underscored that the weakness of women and children caused problems, not the dangers of working with tobacco.[179]

Intriguingly, Valitskaia argued that those who saw miscarriage and infant death as linked to tobacco were generally mistaken. While high, she claimed, the number of miscarriages and infant deaths could not be attributed solely to tobacco use but also to the squalid conditions of labor and home life.[180] This divergence of opinion suggested a view of workers as less civilized, a distrust of women workers' behavior, or a belief that the miscarriages were actually abortions or infanticide. Perhaps this prejudice came from the perceived dissolute behavior of *papirosnitsy*. In 1886, tobacco factory women gave birth to about half of all illegitimate children born to factory women in the city.[181] Beyond illegitimacy, *papirosnitsy* were often seen as only steps away from prostitution. Workers testified to this in their memoirs. One worker, recounting the poor wages, lamented, "And some women workers, in order to support their families, had to 'go on the street.'"[182] More infamously, when the women of the Laferm tobacco factory of St. Petersburg went on strike over wages, the hardhearted mayor, Victor von Wahl, suggested the women "augment their earnings by walking the streets" if they were unhappy with their pay.[183]

Valitskaia intimated that the ethnicity of owners and workers, rather than work conditions, led to health problems. She further judged, "The majority of tobacco factories in Russia are extremely primitive and unworkable. Especially bad are the small, principally Jewish factories.[184] She was not the only doctor to attribute worker health problems to the ethnicity of owners and workers. Jewish bodies were seen as more susceptible to factory pressures but also more capable of spreading contagion onto the produced goods. Another health writer noted, in an aside, that the "density" of workers, especially of Jewish workers, could be complicit in the ventilation problems of factories.[185]

Some went from blaming Jewish workers for their ill health to calling tobacco a Jewish industry that endangered all, just as many accused Jews of orchestrating the drunkenness of the population by producing alcohol and luring Russians into taverns.[186] One antitobacco tract took a break from its diatribe to add an anti-Semitic note, claiming that nine-tenths of tobacco factories "are in the hands of the Jews."[187] While the author meant this as an attack on the industry, the ownership of tobacco concerns by Jewish entrepreneurs in Russia would have followed European trends. In Mannheim, where Jewish people constituted only 4 percent of the population, they owned 40 percent of tobacco companies.[188] In Russia, Jewish laborers did constitute a large portion of the tobacco work force.[189] One business observer argued that the trade in cartridges flourished in Brest because of the large percentage of Jews who worked in the industry very cheaply.[190] The leap from Jewish workers being susceptible to illness to their being a danger to society emerged in perceptions of these workers as prone to radicalism. An 1871 report from the governor of Vilnius testified that a Jewish worker encouraged a recent strike in imitation of events in Odessa. He proposed transferring the worker to Archangel.[191]

Worker testimony avoided discussing the health dangers of tobacco production, Jewish or otherwise, but instead focused on conditions evident across industries, such as overcrowding, the lack of maternity leave, and the dangers of bringing children to work or leaving them at home. A prewar article on the Sheremetevskii tobacco factory in Grodno argued the epidemic typhus grew from the overcrowding of the workers into filthy living situations.[192] Agrippina Filipovna Pavlova of the Shtaf factory in Saratov told of how she worked "right up to the moment of birth," nearly having her child on the shop floor and only barely managing to make it to the factory yard. Returning to work, she remembered that she "took him to the shop, laid him in a basket of some sort, and . . . worked. And [she] was not the only one like that. At Shtaf factory almost all the women worked with nursing babies in baskets."[193] According to a 1912 survey, three-quarters of women worked right up to birth. For most a break of two or three days was all they got. Laws regarding pregnant workers did not appear until the 1890s, and then at the local, not national, level. In St. Petersburg, a factory of more than a hundred women was required to employ a full-time midwife, but generally there was little interest and lax enforcement.[194] Most bemoaned lack of childcare rather than natal care. One *papirosnitsa* argued that the return to the shop floor with a nursing child sitting in a basket below while the mother completed a twelve-to-fourteen hour shift led to the high infant death rate.[195]

No laws required that factories provide childcare, and without options many women brought infants to work or left children at home with little supervision.[196] Fedor Fedorovich Tsveitsikh, also of Saratov, noted that bringing children to the factory was permitted but dangerous. With the machines packed together, without any safety guards, the floor could be very hazardous. Leaving the children at home with a nanny was no great choice either. In some cases, the nanny was an older sibling not yet allowed to work, perhaps seven or eight years old. As Tsveitsikh reported, "The nanny was such that she herself needed her own nanny."[197] Another worker mourned, "Many children left with such 'nannies' died."[198] Elizaveta Filippova Tsittel' remembered being lent out by her father as a nanny before she was old enough to work. A child herself, she brought little care to her charges. She recalled that she would have much rather gone to school, but as the child of a widowed father there was no choice. Even after her father remarried, she continued to work. She recollected, "The five of us earned thirty rubles a month. In our courtyard we were considered rich because once a week we could buy meat and each of us had shoes. Other worker families lived worse than we did."[199]

Tobacco laborers left the dangers of the factory only to meet the hazards of crowded, overpriced lodgings with poor ventilation, inadequate sanitation, and insufficient lighting.[200] With no running water or sewage provision, the verdict that workers grew sick from their domestic situations may have held some truth.[201] Evdokiia Vasil'evna Nosanova remembered working from age ten at the factory, but spoke with particular disquiet about the worry of losing that job. Her mother had been unable to provide for the two of them even with her additional wages. At one point they got thrown out of their lodgings and had to make do in an earthen dug out. When her mother married again, their lives did not improve. The second husband was a drunkard and with now four children in a small apartment, conditions were hard. One of the children died of hunger, yet even with these troubles, Nosanova regarded herself as lucky; "Others lived still worse."[202]

Workers spent by far the largest part of their budgets on food—30 to 50 percent. In some tobacco factories, cafeterias provided meals for workers, but in most they made their own arrangements at local taverns or brought food.[203] Activists pointed to the lack of cafeterias as a factor in worker health, but workers themselves argued that factory provision of food was less desirable because it came with additional pressures born out of debt and supervision.[204] The same could be said of factory housing provided by some enterprises.[205] By the 1880s, the majority of workers at the Dunaev factory lived in a wood building on the factory lot.[206] The attractions of housing and cafeterias were outweighed for some by the added coercive power for owners.[207]

Conspicuously lacking in worker testimony were charges of tobacco work leading to tuberculosis. Only one mentioned this, noting simply, "The majority of them fell ill with consumption."[208] This could be a reflection of genuine disinterest, but given that many of these testimonies were collected in the 1930s, when improvements on the shop floor still lagged, it could be that this was a conscious editorial choice. A more consistent health complaint of workers was the effects of "dry food," by which was meant "bread, onions, herring, eggs, etc.," or other foods not served hot and considered "especially bad for children's bodies."[209] Another worker told of how, for a few kopeks, one could have the glue workers tend a bowl for hot food on their work stove among the pots of adhesive.[210] This worry over the health effects of cold meals and eating at workstations was echoed in the statistical study of Dr. Valitskaia, who connected "dry food" and poor worker health.[211] The lack of not just cafeterias but also available hot water entered into many discussions of health and factory amenities.[212]

Factory medical experts and workers might have disagreed on the health danger in tobacco work, but authors of antitobacco literature showed none of their reticence. They claimed that a tobacco factory worker suffered more the ill effects of tobacco than even a user because of the long hours in the dust.[213] As Dr. A. I. Il'inskii argued in his 1888 *Polezno, ili vredno kurit', ni-ukhat' i zhevat' tabak* (Is it healthy or dangerous to smoke, snuff, and chew tobacco?), "All the workers of a tobacco factory are pale, anemic, sluggish, gaunt, very susceptible to a number of illnesses and often suffering from those that are caused by the slow poisoning by tobacco . . . loss of appetite, cough, catarrh of lungs and stomach, and nerve disease."[214] V. Mikhailovskii's 1894 pamphlet, which enjoyed at least five printings, reported that tobacco degraded workers' hearing, lungs, and even blood. N. M. Druzhinin's dissertation, a pointed investigation of women's and children's labor referenced in many other works, argued of tobacco work that, "in sanitary terms, it is one of the most hazardous. Poisonous dust settles in the lungs, and asthma, chronic bronchitis, angina, and tuberculosis rage among the female workers."[215] Druzhinin said that this could be traced to the fact that "women are physically weaker than men."[216] Druzhinin thus wed the view that tobacco production endangered workers more than other labors with the idea that the laborers were constitutionally unable to stand the danger.

The suffering of children animated many antitobacco tracts with arguments about miscarriages, infant death, and child labor, supported with a mixture of anecdotal evidence, moral handwringing, and selective use of contemporary science. Archpriest Evgenii Popov gave as evidence the testimony of an unnamed scientist, coupled with the cases of three women whose collective history consisted of one miscarriage and nine live births that all ended in the death of the infant, to prove that the main factor leading to the death of children was "the nicotine that hung in the air of the tobacco factories."[217] In the 1904 pamphlet *Perestanem kurit! Shto takoe tabak i kakoi vred ot nego byvaet* (Stop smoking! What is tobacco and what type of danger does it hold?), A. Appolov held that the working of tobacco was more dangerous than smoking it and that the production of tobacco caused miscarriages, still births, and ill children.[218] Another pamphlet cited a study of 126 newborns to tobacco factory workers, of which seventy-two died. Some authors went on to further note that the nicotine poisoned amniotic fluid and breast milk.[219] One author alleged that the infant death rate among tobacco factory women who nursed their children was a full 10 percent higher than the death rate among those children who were wet-nursed.[220] Not all experts agreed, however, and some cited studies that found instead of increased miscarriage among tobacco factory women no differences between their constitutions, menstruation, or infant survival and those of other factory women.[221]

Authors of antismoking literature implicated tobacco users in the harm done to women and children in an industry of death. Dr. Il'inskii bemoaned the work of children and youth at the factories and asked rhetorically of his audience, "How many children and young people have paid with their lives working at a tobacco factory!"[222] The moral effects on society as a whole also featured in pamphlet critiques. Druzhinin claimed that the detrimental consequences of labor on women and children became evident in the economic and moral destruction of the family and visited themselves on the next generation as well, thereby becoming a problem for the nation as a whole.[223] S. A. Beliakov in his 1904 pamphlet *Tabak i vliianie kureniia ego na zdorov'e cheloveka* (Tobacco and the effects of smoking on men's health) leveled a singular recognition of the dangers to male tobacco factory workers, arguing that working in the industry made them sexually weak.[224]

Antitobacco tracts often added a companion villain to their attacks on tobacco and the labor of women and children—the match factory. Appolov commented that smokers used many matches, and they needed to consider that match factories were also dangerous.[225] The development of the match industry contributed to the spread of cigarettes in the west, allowing an easy light for the modern smoke, but the difficulties for workers were infamous.[226] The self-lighting match came first from Warsaw in the years of Tsar Nikolas I, but required a bank of poisonous phosphorous to light.[227] Protections in production were lax, leading to worker exposure, and phosphorous poisoning led to wasting, yellow skin, stomach problems, breathing issues, trembling, and general debility.[228] Despite the dangerous nature of the work, in Russia children under twelve composed about half the workforce in match making. Sometimes children as young as four or five labored in the poorly ventilated shops starting at five or six in the morning and working until eleven at night.[229] St. Petersburg was a pioneer in the field, with already nine factories by 1842.[230] Most Russians continued to use a flint for lighting until a safety match without phosphorous appeared.[231] The government issued a tax on matches in 1887 to improve conditions in factories, and further laws forced smaller, nonhygienic shops to close.[232] The crossover between the igniter and the act of smoking came out in business partnerships.[233] The Russian Tobacco Trust owned match factories, and Nastas'ia Fedorovna Bogdanova, the wife of tobacco owner Aleksandr Nikolaevich Bogdanov, was herself the owner of a Petersburg match factory.[234] By 1914, lighters began to appear on the market, allowing for easier smoking, but these did not quickly displace matches.[235]

Protective legislation rolled out for all types of industrial labor starting in 1835, but making laws met with resistance from industrialists and enforcing legislation remained a difficulty. A factory inspectorate designed to oversee implementation of regulations did not appear until the 1880s, and it was imperfectly deployed in factories and missed entirely small shops.[236] From the 1860s, increasing disquiet about labor conditions spurred by reformers, worker activists, and economic theorists filtered out into public opinion, regarding not just child labor, but all industrial conditions. Popular literature from authors like Tolstoy, Anton Chekhov (1860–1904), Fedor Dostoevsky (1821–81), and Maxim Gorky (1868–1936) spurred public interest in factory reform. The agitation yielded fruit in an 1882 law with restrictions on child labor and requirements for factory children's education. The law was revisited in 1884, 1885, and 1897, and according to inspectors' reports the number of children working in all industry rapidly decreased.[237] Reformers pushed for legislation in the late nineteenth century to remove youth from industries like matches and tobacco that they considered especially hazardous.[238] The vision of the horrific plight of children in the match industry—making and selling—came out in European labor critiques too, such as the maudlin story by Hans Christian Anderson, "The Poor Little Match Girl" (1845).[239]

Perhaps the reform movement led to the public face presented by many factory owners. The booklet celebrating the twenty-five-year anniversary of the Shaposhnikov factory praised the founder not just for his business acumen but also for his conviction that it "was his duty to improve the lives of, and care for, his workers."[240] The author goes on to extoll Shaposhnikov's "expansive Russian nature" that pushed him to found a kitchen and cafeteria for his workers and remunerate them generously, as "their established pay was always higher than the workers of all other Petersburg factories . . . from this it is understandable why many workers related to their owner with respect and love . . . and why a significant number of men and women workers, there at the foundation of the factory, stayed there for twenty-five years on duty."[241] His wife continued these efforts, creating a public image as a philanthropist as well as a caring owner. She served on the society for the care of poor and sick children and worked as a temperance advocate. Like her husband, she claimed to pay her workers better than those of other ventures and tried to dispel the worst dust in the factory through the installation of closed drums for tobacco crumbling. Beyond the shop floor, cafeteria, and kitchen, she added a new dormitory to the factory grounds in 1897 constructed "to all sanitary and hygienic norms of the time."[242]

Other factory owners also made efforts to improve factory conditions out of altruism, guilt, or calculation. Dunaev pursued a number of charitable endeavors, establishing a hospital, a school, and an orphanage at his factory, and giving money to the poor. In addition to a dormitory, he added a bathhouse and paid his workers a bit more than average.[243] Asmolov and Co. installed new ventilations systems, onsite medical care with a doctor and a physician's assistant, and a pharmacy. According to an 1889 report from the factory, the workers only called on the medical assistance forty three times, indicating either their lack of trust for the care, disinterest in it, or distaste for it.[244] The Kushnarev factory, out of Rostov, funded construction of a large iconostasis, and on the fiftieth anniversary of the factory's founding in 1853, the owner pledged 65,000 rubles to charitable works and 35,000 to a worker's aid fund.[245] A 1938 history of the Asmolov factory charged that the medical service of the prerevolutionary period at the plant was provided by "one, always drunken, 'general' feldsher," implying that the care given was substandard in training (a doctor's assistant, not a doctor) and quality.[246] In the twenty-year anniversary history of the Asmolov tobacco factory, the author lauded the extensive work being done by the owner to help worker health and wellbeing with a hospital and school under construction for workers and their families.[247]

Shaposhnikova publicized her piety and charitable endeavors in her 1890 pamphlet, which began with details of the elaborate prayer ceremony she commissioned for the anniversary, underscoring her strong connections to religious and national traditions.[248] Her efforts were like those of many business owners of the time who employed charitable works and prayer ceremonies or sponsored art and theater as a means of building their public image.[249] A 1912 advertisement penned by Uncle Mikey further spread the good word of the Shaposhnikov factory. The piece told the story of a Syrian loader, who credited Uncle Mikey with being such a good boss that, in return, the Syrians gave him the finest tobacco "that Allah provided" for Shaposhnikov's *Osman* and *Melanzh* brands.[250] Shaposhnikova, in the guise of Uncle Mikey, presented herself as a friend of workers internationally and a fair employer at home. Workers seemed less than convinced by their employers' philanthropic gestures. As one later said, "It seems that Asmolov had two faces: One—for advertisements—fine-looking, sweet, which one could place among icons; and a second which was greedy, rapacious, and thieving."[251]

Attempts to improve worker conditions did not hold back worker discontent. One early-twentieth-century investigator of women's and children's labor argued that owners hired them not just for monetary considerations but because they considered women "generally more attentive, industrious, and abstemious than men. They constitute a more calm and conservative element."[252] Employers attempted to keep workers quiescent in innovative ways. The ministry of finance singled out the Zhukov factory of St. Petersburg in 1840 for their unique approach to trying to quell worker discontent. Zhukov saw as dangerous the urban environment and its pressures for overindulgence in food, drink, goods, and services. To keep his workers more rooted in the village and the values he thought preferable, he made them regularly return to their homes in the countryside.[253]

Despite this, women and children did not remain quiet. Tobacco workers in particular took a notable role in strike activity beginning in the 1890s and moving through the revolutionary year of 1905 and into 1917. Their anger roiled over in spots across the empire from St. Petersburg to Odessa and from Kiev to Baku.[254] As one historian judged, women tobacco workers presented a "remarkably volatile, militant, and tenacious" group in comparison to women in other industries. This might have been a result of the peculiar composition of the tobacco work force, because while the industry was overwhelmingly female and low-wage, the proportion of urban-born women was higher in tobacco than in textile mills, and tobacco workers tended to be more literate and older than women in other industries.[255]

Georgii Plekhanov (1856–1918) reported the first mass tobacco strike in 1878, though an earlier strike of just five workers took place in Vilnius in 1871.[256] The 1878 action occurred when the women of two St. Petersburg tobacco factories walked out over lowered wages. Discontented with the response of management, the strikers then threw machinery and furniture out the window. The strike concluded successfully for the women when management broke and acceded to their demands. Plekhanov, revealing the condescension from radicals toward female workers, noted that the activity "was all the more interesting because it occurred in an exclusively female setting."[257] A Moscow strike in 1884 of over five hundred workers over low wages, shortened hours, and material slowdowns forced the city to call in mounted police and reserve forces. They arrested over fifty workers.[258]

The first strike at the Asmolov factory came in 1884. Militancy there continued through the work of Elizaveta Viktorovna Torsueva (aka Bystritskaia) a founding member of the first Social Democratic (SD) circle in Rostov in the 1890s. Part of a family of revolutionaries, Elizaveta had a brother active in the railway industry, a far from unique situation. The women of the Rostov tobacco industry shared strong ties with the railway workers of their city, oftentimes, like with Elizaveta, familial. While women labored in the tobacco factories, their husbands, brothers, sons, or fathers would find work in the better-paying, greater-skilled, and highly radicalizing main railway workshop. These women stood at the forefront of the first large socialist-aided mass workers' movement of the 1890s, centered in the industries of Rostov.[259]

The rapid industrialization, urbanization, and social dislocation of the late nineteenth century led to discontent throughout the empire. Famine hit in 1891–92, and harvest failures continued in the succeeding years. While tobacco production continued to grow, so too did discontent, and the 1890s saw widespread worker resistance.[260] In Odessa, all 150 workers of the S. I. Asvadurov factory walked out in protest over their wages and stayed out for two weeks. Workers voiced their discontent, and then they organized and prepared for more intense attacks. In December Odessa tobacco workers walked out again, helped in their protest this time by a newly established strike fund.[261] In other regions the anger was similarly intense. A Moscow propagandist journeying to Taganrog found a ready group of women in the tobacco factory interested in learning how to read and then moving into active agitation.[262] The strike of tobacco workers at the G. and L. Edel'stein factory of Vilnius was the largest strike in the city in the 1890s.[263]

The women of Laferm, a factory located in the heart of St. Petersburg on Vasilevskii Island with an easy walk across the Palace Bridge to Palace Square and Nevsky Prospekt, proved central to many worker actions.[264] In late 1895 St. Petersburg, 1,300 of the 1,435 workers at the Laferm tobacco factory walked out. When negotiations began to go poorly in early 1896, the strikers broke the windows of the factory, defenestrating raw materials and furniture and necessitating the intervention of police, the mayor, the militia, and two fire department units. As one witness noted, "They threw thousands and tens of thousands of cigarettes into the street. Afterwards I never heard, in Petersburg at any rate, of workers trying to destroy machinery (probably this would have been difficult for women), but the sight of huge boxes of cigarettes being thrown into the street—it was frightful."[265] The police held six to eight hundred women in connection with the disquiet and arrested twenty-seven of the group, dismissing another thirty. While the strikers did not have their demands met, the administration did budge on the allocation of moneys collected from fines.[266] The victory did not long placate the women. Three years later a strike at another St. Petersburg factory resulted in more property damage, defenestration, and four hundred angry female workers. Two hundred tobacco workers took to the streets again in 1898 in St. Petersburg over wage rates brought down by mechanization. Owners promised new techniques and machinery would allow women to make up the costs of wage decreases, but women did not believe the promises of factory leadership and at times destroyed machinery.[267]

Workers remembered the Laferm strike as a triumph, as a 1907 letter to *Zhizn' Tabachnika* (Tobacco worker life) attested, and members of the radical intelligentsia used the Laferm strike to encourage workers of other factories.[268] The Petersburg "Union for the Struggle for the Freedom of the

Working Class" distributed a leaflet asking, "What do the women workers of Laferm factory want?" The leaflet listed complaints over equipment
problems, fines, low pay, and the "rude address" of factory administration.
An 1896 May Day leaflet from the union, this one with Lenin's imprint,
trumpeted the actions of the Laferm workers in a general heralding of
workers' actions that showed the growing consciousness of Russian laborers.[269] The union put out the pamphlets, but they were not active organizers
of the strike, as the union had made no moves to recruit women. Since the
arrest of the Brusnev circle in 1892, women had not been targeted for organizing, and efforts from the group to get either metalworkers or printers to
ally with the striking *papirosnitsy* foundered. Despite the visible and violent
actions of tobacco women, so embedded was the belief that women were
backward that one female revolutionary concluded, ironically, "It was easy
to understand that cigarette-makers and weavers cannot readily be made
into activists whereas metal workers and typographers were ready-made
revolutionaries."[270] Despite the disinterest of the revolutionary groups in
females for radical agitation, the women of Laferm seem to have come to
their own conclusions regarding the relationship of labor to owners.[271]

Radical groups might have seen women as less promising strikers, but the
authorities did not treat them as any less dangerous. Government forces vi-
olently stopped the 1897 strike at Moscow's Gabai factory. The overwhelming majority of the workforce had taken to the streets in protest of lowered
wages, and the city called Cossacks on horseback to disperse the strike,
incarcerating the "trouble makers" in the Butyrskaia prison for a week.[272]
Such strong-arm tactics did not halt worker agitation. In Rostov, the SDs
distributed leaflets to the Asmolov factory workers in 1901 complaining
of the dust and child labor of the factories and asking for better wages and
"polite treatment."[273] Grigorii Vasil'evich Cherepakhin remembered helping his father distribute literature around the Asmolov factory even though
he was underage. In 1902, when the railway workers of Rostov-na-Don took
to the streets, tobacco workers were one of the first groups to join them.[274]
Female tobacco workers displayed solidarity in other actions as well. In a
Kiev province strike of 1903, the women created a strike fund to sustain
their comrades through weeks of unemployment.[275] A testimony from a *papirosnitsa* in a Grodno factory, however, noted the difficulties of getting information across large factories such as the 1,500-employee establishment
where she was employed. There, a strike was broken because information
did not make it across departments.[276]

Owners responded with increasing violence and intimidation tactics. When thirty thousand workers went on strike in November of 1902

in Rostov, the military was called in to break the strike, killing eight and wounding twenty-three. Fearing there would be violence at the funeral, the authorities responded by bringing in Cossacks to quell the crowd. The owners of Asmolov attempted to forestall further unrest by forcing their workers to sign a pledge that they would not strike further.[277] SD activists distributed a leaflet to the Asmolov factory workers on July 18, 1903, declaring, "For 30–40k/day the factory takes your strength, health and youth . . . female workers you must know this. You must understand that you are people and that you have honor and conscience." The leaflet went on to detail a charge against a supervisor: that he had tried to pressure a female worker into sex and then fired her when she would not consent. It ended with an attempt to embarrass the female workers into activism: "Is it possible that you do not understand that you shame and dishonor yourself by allowing yourselves to be so treated?"[278]

In the early twentieth century, government sponsors attempted to unite workers so as to channel their energies into approved activities and perhaps also smooth controversies. Sergei Zubatov, head of the Moscow city security services tried to create labor groups across the city's industries that would encourage peaceful worker activity and provide legal means to improve their material circumstances. Women of tobacco participated in small numbers, yet radical operatives still used the Zubatov organization to infiltrate some tobacco factories. An SD group began at the Dukat factory under the cover of the Zubatov groups. These early experiences in the Zubatov movement became formative for later organizers of tobacco workers.[279]

Not all government-sponsored activity retained a pacific demeanor. Activist Vera Karelina featured the humiliating tactics of management along with the endemic sexual harassment of the industry in her work with Father Gapon's Assembly of Russian Factory Workers. The assembly formed as an outgrowth of the 1901 tsarist initiative to lure laborers away from revolutionary groups, but their work quickly became a complicated mix of paternalist intent, worker discontent, and organizer activism. Karelina utilized a short story called "In the Courtyard" to rally women to action in special circles set up for them after the larger assembly proved hostile. She would read the story, set in a tobacco factory, and recount the actions of a cruel factory administrator, who resorted to a forced, degrading public search of a female worker when she would not acquiesce to his advances. Two guards groped the woman and exposed her breasts as they rifled through her blouse and turned out her pockets looking for stolen goods. The story served as a gateway to discussions of the further degradations of women in industry and a rallying point for Karelina's women's groups.[280]

Karelina began the women's groups because she argued that male resistance, women's illiteracy, feminine timidity, women's membership in worker groups near their homes rather than near their factories, and the double burden of work and home kept women from fully participating in other groups. Karelina pointed out that in addition to the actions of sexist employers, male workers harassed women. She recalled, "When I myself worked at the factory (Laferm), it would happen that I would leave after a fourteen-hour day on the machines . . . and then still have vulgar mockery hurled at me as I left."[281] Sexism featured in the tobacco industry of other countries. In the Ottoman tobacco industry, a similarly volatile group of workers with large portions of women and children rebelled against lowering wages and harsh conditions. There, male workers pushed at times not just for economic concessions from owners, but also for them to stop employing women and children.[282]

Father Gapon's organization proved central to the events that ignited the revolution of 1905. On January 9, 1905, the government met a peaceful march of Gapon's workers, who were carrying icons and singing hymns, with violence. In the days after the attack, known as Bloody Sunday, tobacco workers rose up. For some, this would be their first strike. Aleksei Petrovich Sadovnikov recalled that at the Shtaf factory in Saratov, the conditions had been so awful that "the thought never occurred that they might somehow organize."[283] But in 1905 they walked out.

Success met several of the tobacco workers' strikes. In September 1905, the Moscow tobacco factories of Dukat and Gabai both went on strike. Led by the combined forces of SD and Socialist Revolutionary (SR) groups, the workers demanded an eight-hour day, sick pay, the abolition of night shifts, and the regulation of child labor. Despite an initial arrest of two strike leaders, the workers held on for three weeks until the management agreed to their demands. The strike at the Dukat factory continued for forty-two days as the administration refused negotiation. Workers from other firms contributed to the strike, and this solidarity forced an agreement from management for a ten-hour day and rehiring those previously dismissed.[284]

The ties forged in September led to the creation in November of the Union of Tobacco Workers. Menshevik sponsored, though officially non-affiliated, the group counted 1,000 members and was closely allied to the Gabai and Dukat factories. I. Ia Tikhomirov, a former Zubatov group member, served as the first president of the organization. Although dwarfed by groups like the printers with eight thousand members, or the metalworkers with almost five thousand, the tobacco union claimed 30 percent of the city's tobacco industry and came in on par with construction workers and plumbers in terms of numbers. Skilled workers unionized more readily, and tobacco work was considered semi- or unskilled, with a consequently low percentage of unionized laborers.[285]

Organizers lamented the lack of participation by women in some areas, but the percentage of women in tobacco unions was higher than in any other group. In 1907, women made up 44 percent of the Moscow tobacco union. While this did not reach the gender distribution of the labor force, which had 60 percent women, the magnification of women's voices, simply by virtue of their number, made for a singular platform for women workers' issues.[286] This stood in stark contrast to other unions. For instance, tailors had 66 percent female labor but only 13 percent female membership in the union; and in the candy industry they were 53 percent of labor but only 3 percent of the union.[287]

In October of 1905, a general strike took hold of the entire city of St. Petersburg. Karelina said that it began the same way at most factories, with soldiers lined up around factories, and she put the women of Laferm front and center in the activities:

> It would go like this. The women would walk as a mass out of the factory and one of the girls would carry and drop a pack of proclamations in the middle of the line of soldiers, and she would herself hide in the crowd. This happened at the tobacco factory Laferm on Vasilevskii island. . . . Never were there places where women did not appear in the strikes. . . . When the general strike began in October, the women of Laferm tobacco factory . . . were first on the street . . . I remember on the morning of October 18 the manifesto of the constitution from Nicholas II came out and almost all factories and mills, as if they knew, began to strike again. . . . All were excited, joyous, as if they wished that the tsar had truly given a constitution. . . . They made way to the Laferm where work was still ongoing. Just as the crowd came to the factory and workers came to the window and saw the red flags they left work and came to the street. . . . Not one woman stayed at the factory.[288]

The turmoil of the strikes of October resulted in the organization of the St. Petersburg Soviet of Workers' Deputies, where Vera Karelina again emerged as a leading spokesperson for working women. The workers of Laferm tried to nominate her as their delegate to the Soviet, but when she refused, since she did not actually work there, they chose another woman, Anna Afanas'eva, to be their delegate. Of the over five hundred deputies, seven women first served, and by December when the police made arrests, eighteen women were members, though most were intelligentsia.[289]

The workers of Rezhi tobacco factory in Petersburg selected A. M. Barkova as their delegate to the first St. Petersburg Soviet, and she moved into a slot on the executive committee. When she was arrested, the workers sent another tobacco worker, Anna Sigova of Laferm, to take her place. Evading prison time in 1905, Barkova set up an apartment on Kartashikhina Street where female tobacco workers being aided by the Bolsheviks could meet. Eventually she was imprisoned, exiled, escaped, and went on to agitate for the Bolsheviks in Finland and elsewhere.[290] These radical beginnings held long influence. A 1908 secret police survey found that St. Petersburg tobacco workers still gravitated toward SD groups.[291]

Not all workers found success in strikes. The workers of Asmolov returned to find a sign on their factory gates: "All workers are fired. The factory is closed."[292] In June of 1905 tobacco workers in Tashkent went on strike, but with little coordination with other industry groups.[293] Barkova remembered that while the tobacco workers of her factory picked deputies for the Soviet, when they returned to the work, they found their factory closed and their delegates, including a woman of fifty, were arrested.[294]

The workers of the Asmolov factory, always one of the more active groups, met in 1905 with vigor. The factory administration and authorities responded with violence. When, in November of 1905, the striking workers marched to the mayor, the peaceful group, mostly women, was attacked by police and mounted Cossacks with whips. They had asked for shorter hours and greater pay. The owners agreed to the money but not the hours, and the city came to a standstill. As the couplet went, "The Asmolov girls asked for a bigger pay pack/ Asmolov angrily sent them a Cossack."[295] In Rostov, the attack on striking workers led to the election of many women into the city's Soviet, especially representatives from the female tobacco worker strike committees. According to one local organizer, in Rostov there were more female deputies to the Soviet than in many of the textile districts where women made up a larger portion of the work force. Across the empire, women's agitation from the tobacco industry was noticeable.[296]

Worker Tsittel' remembered the poor conclusion of the 1905 strikes in Saratov, where the crowd of strikers, mostly women, fled the scourges of the Cossacks: "We walked to the second gate and saw that along the street Cossacks galloped. Half the workers behind the gate left. The Cossacks caught them with whips. . . . The gate closed and the Cossacks flogged our comrades on the street. There were screams, cries, and moans. We lost our heads and did not even try to open the gate. The workers that were on the street ran to the gate but the gate was closed and the Cossacks overtook them and whipped them."[297] Not just beatings met the strikers of Saratov. Evdokiia Iakovlevna Stepanova recalled shootings.[298]

In addition to the police, owners, and authorities, workers also encountered the repressive forces of the Black Hundreds, a group of ultranationalist vigilantes who took up arms to support the tsarist government in the aftermath of the October Manifesto. The perception of tobacco as a Jewish industry may have made it a particular target of the virulently racist, antiworker, antirevolutionary thugs.[299] Agitation from the Black Hundreds overtook the Dunaev tobacco and match factories.[300] Tsittel' of Saratov recalled her father's advising her to stay off the streets in the aftermath of 1905, as "it would be better for [her] to not go out anywhere as [she] would be beaten on the street as a Jewess."[301] She further remembered a pogrom where the Black Hundreds damaged property, drank, and beat people, and she discouraged a coworker from burning down the factory on an attacker's suggestion.[302] Another Saratov worker spoke of rioters closing in on a meeting of strikers: "Suddenly we saw coming from the city a procession with music. It was the Black Hundreds. . . . They walked with an orchestra, icons, portraits of the tsar and sang hymns. . . . The drunken among them were many and all with sticks. The sticks were decorated with three strips of color—blue, red and white—to echo the Russian flag."[303] The Black Hundreds and the crackdown on activists chilled revolutionary fervor and seemed to dissuade women especially. The union paper *Golos tabachnika* (Voice of the Tobacco Worker) recounted difficulties as late as 1907 in attracting women to their ranks.[304] This disinterest may have also been due, however, to the already well-documented sexism women of tobacco had encountered among activists and from other male workers.

Some tobacco workers continued in active resistance. In 1906, fifty engineers at Laferm walked out over the hiring of a mechanic whom they considered not their choice. Workers joined the action, pushing for their own agenda regarding piece rates and general authority over work conditions and hiring and firing of others. The 1906 Laferm strike displayed the solidarity across skill and gender divisions present in some tobacco works and indicated the desire for worker control in even highly feminized industries and shops.[305]

By the eve of World War I, more workers started agitating for better pay and benefits. A *Pravda* article of June 1912 urged the women of the Shaposhnikov factory to rise up and unite against injustices like a factory supervisor who "fined women left and right" even as they earned only forty-five kopek a day.[306] An article a month later revisited the theme.[307] A June 1912 piece complained of the horrible wages and conditions for women of the Laferm factory and noted that many of the workers were coming to a consensus. Their demands included a nine-hour day (or eight hours of night work), a twenty-kopek raise for all (thirty for skilled workers), "cheerful interactions" with managers, improved medical care, and sick pay.[308]

The celebrations of International Women's Day provided a rallying point for women from feminist and socialist groups. The first Russian celebration of the holiday took place in 1913. Anticipating police interference, it was staged on February 17.[309] Women's journals and Menshevik and Bolshevik papers all worked to agitate among women's groups. Increasing strike activity was evident in tobacco factories around the empire. In 1913, *Pravda* reported a small strike in April, and in March a strike of six hundred workers at the Shapshal factory, the majority of them women, over the ill treatment and firing of a technician, included calls for a boycott.[310] The dismissal of a worker at the Asmolov factory for being a correspondent to a worker paper caught ire from the publication *Severnaia pravda*.[311] In St. Petersburg, the anger of the workers was especially evident in the firms of the Russian Tobacco Company, including Laferm and Shaphosnikov. In June and July 1913, the workers of Laferm walked out, the majority of them women.[312] Male laborers were sent in as scabs and not only did the women bar their entry, they published their names and called for a citywide boycott of the factory products. Later that year, Laferm workers organized money for comrades striking at the Gavanera factory, and in September, they went on strike over the arrest of political activists.[313] In January 1914, they again took to the streets. This time, 2,000 of the 2,400 workers walked out in commemoration of Bloody Sunday. In March of 1914, workers from both Laferm and Shaposhnikov joined a citywide group of 27,000 workers protesting health issues for their comrades at the "Treugol'nik" rubber factory. Another factory illness brought them to the streets again.[314]

Over the course of the period, female tobacco workers became, according to one historian, "exceptionally assertive."[315] After 1905, an observer of the Moscow tobacco workers' union commented that most members saw the organization as a means to provide protection rather than as a place for struggling against the regime. But that was not universally true, and the lean of tobacco workers toward socialist and Marxist parties became marked. According to a secret police report of 1908, the Petersburg tobacco union was under the influence of the SDs.[316]

Despite the volatility of female tobacco workers, and the high percentage of them in actions, the raw numbers of those involved in politics remained below those of other industries. For example, the number of unionized metal workers in Petersburg in 1917 was 140,000, while that of tobacco workers was only 14,000.[317] The number of tobacco activists connected to Bolshevism was low. Only 1.6 percent of female Bolsheviks were tobacco workers.[318]

Tobacco workers did try to send Bolshevik party members to the Soviet, but as with the case of Laferm's choice of A. M. Barsakova, this did not always succeed.[319] The lack of a strong Bolshevik contingent did not mean that tobacco workers were apolitical, backwards, or complacent. Partially this reflected an issue of affiliation and the silencing of Menshevik and bourgeois feminist voices in later histories.[320] This may have led to their actions having less impact on the construction of the narrative of the revolution.

TOBACCO production came to Russia in the 1600s, but exploded in the late nineteenth century. Russian industry grew in a piecemeal way, under government oversight from a tax system that encouraged consolidation. As production burgeoned and use skyrocketed, tobacco laborers came into increasing focus because the Russian industry's reliance on low-cost hand labor from women and children brought more intense scrutiny. Factory conditions reflected this push for cheaper, more, and faster, but the abusive, unhealthy, and dangerous conditions of the tobacco and companion match industries did not go without comment. Essays by popular authors on the production, labor, and consumption relationships established in the late nineteenth century had profound effects on how smokers and antismoking forces conceptualized the habit.

The labor relationships of Russian tobacco workers—their feminization and agitation—were not without parallels. While the United States and other western manufacturers mechanized and diffused the worst exploitation in tobacco, in countries like Russia where labor was cheap and production not mechanized, the factory conditions and low pay yielded worker agitation. The feminization of Russia's tobacco workers made this agitation different. Russian activists did not consider women a revolutionary force, and yet women of the tobacco industry in Russia participated in political activism in larger and larger percentages and with increasing organization, solidarity, and violence, contributing measurably to the general turmoil that succeeded in the eventual overturn of the tsarist system.

Female laborers and children, considered unskilled and unenlightened workers, showed remarkable solidarity and attention to labor issues. They went on strike early and often, and by 1905 female activists were organizing female workers into discussion circles and mutual aid groups and even encouraging them into labor unions. Many systemic and cultural restrictions kept women's activism low in most industries, but female tobacco workers participated at a higher percentage than others did. Like male workers, they were subject to the same crackdowns that led to a scale back of revolutionary activity in the post-1905 period, but by the eve of World War I, they returned to the streets.

From Tolstoy's denunciation of smokers as near cannibals to the paternalistic cries of pamphlet authors and on to the tales of exploitation in the radical press, smokers had to be aware of the social, economic, and cultural costs of their habit. Despite these horrific tales and the disquieting sight of women's violent agitation on the streets, production and consumption estimates back a vision of a population steeped in nicotine and constant smoking. Users at all levels confronted details of the manufacture of their smokes in popular culture from literary figures, manufacturers, strike reports, and worker activists. Certainly some did not care about the plight of workers. The clouding of the issue by medical authorities who blamed worker lifestyles over work styles perhaps gave them comfort, or the publicized charitable activities from owners may have provided cover for users to indulge in their habit as a net good. Given the high nicotine content of Russian tobaccos and the new potent delivery style of the papirosa, it might also be that the addictive qualities of tobacco trumped appeals to the conscience. Whatever the case, the ghosts of production's evils hovered over the smoker like a cloud.

3 : TASTED

Distinctive Smoking and Social Inclusion

The playful cockerel of *Peri* brand papirosy certainly commanded the viewer's attention when he appeared in the 1910s (figure 3.1). Named for a Persian winged fairy, this half-man, half-rooster looked comfortably situated in the bourgeois society of late imperial Russia. A decidedly masculine figure for a brand named after a sprite, he straddled boundaries between male and female, human and animal, and urban and rural, just as his namesake Persian pixies trembled between the poles of good and evil and the worlds of God and man. Beyond the mythical sphere, the rooster built on the already masculine image of tobacco as the soldier's friend and played on connections of virility from farm life, where the cock—*petykh*—ruled the barnyard. He was so vigorous as to satisfy not one but a bevy of hens. This manliest of animals, symbolic of virility, strength, and potency, stared straight out, papirosa firmly gripped in beak, fully erect and preening while sucking on a phallic substitute. A manlier poster for smoking may not exist. While the Marlboro man symbolized masculinity, he did not enjoy a similar dual meaning as the cockerel of St. Petersburg's A. N. Shaposhnikov poster.

The well-dressed rooster displayed prosperity as well as machismo. Sporting a jaunty outfit of vest, jacket, boutonnière, cufflinks, gloves, spats, cane, and monocle, he destroyed his rivals with his fashionable dress, and completed his ensemble with smoking. The rooster's celebrated actions as the herald of the day connected him to the pace of the modern as well as its style. He told the time and did so with a power that brought the humans around him to heel, signaling the breakneck rhythm of a new, industrial, modern day—*ot petukhov do petukhov*—from rooster crow to rooster crow.

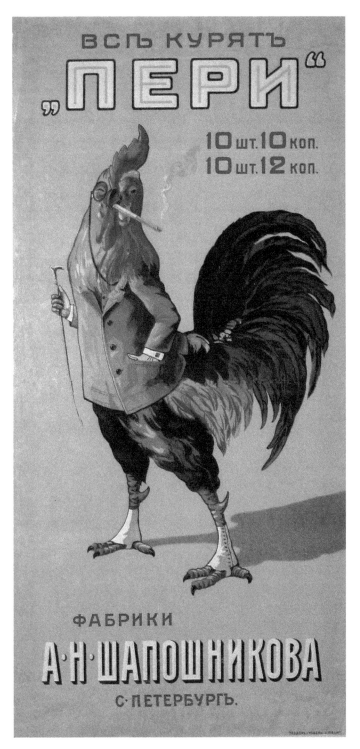

Figure 3.1 *Peri* poster. 1910s. Collection of Russian State Library, Moscow.

Despite the bravado, *Peri*'s rooster revealed anxiety as well as excitement for the denizen of the late-imperial city and its rapid industrialization and urbanization producing massive social mobility, dislocation, and disquiet. Like many an urbanite and despite the glories of his haberdashery and habits, *Peri*'s cockerel remained at base a creature only recently removed from the farm, and even a bit of a joke. He might have acquired the outward look of a dandy, but underneath he was a rube from the countryside afraid of being exposed, shunned, and expelled. In a piece of sly, back-handed humor, the poster poked a bit of fun at the smoker, teasing that clothes could never fully hide their rude origins. The brand name hummed along to the same theme. In operas, literature, and other entertainments, artists, in Europe and in Russia, employed *Peries* as stand-ins for romantic, tragicomic, fairy figures fluttering about at dissonance with modern life.[1] Like these other liminal characters, Shaposhnikov's rooster struggled to fit in. Isolated in the frame, he was not integrated fully into the urban milieu.

Shaposhnikov's poster, however, promised to alleviate the isolation of the lonely transplant. The slogan above him provided hope. "Everyone smokes *Peri*." Like many advertisements of the period, the poster producers incorporated appeals that their product was fashionable, ubiquitous, and necessary, assuring consumers that with purchase and use they could belong. Like other brands, *Peri* could serve as a silent signal of social status, aspirations, and desires. Packaging and paper quality visibly marked brands for consumers and onlookers. Smell carried information to bystanders, implying the quality of papirosa, leaf, blend, and smoker and serving as a sensory signal only intelligible to others in the know. For truly universal brands, simply saying the name could be an invitation to smoke or a denigration of another, a code incomprehensible to nonsmokers. Nothing could signal more to an outsider that one had made it than the ability to exclude others with secret languages, jokes, and symbols.

Smoking showed strangers that one fit in while providing confidence and means of assimilation for the newly arrived—all at one kopek per papirosa. Tobacco could range from affordable to luxurious, serving, as one historian put it, "either as an exotic indulgence to the very rich or as an everyday luxury to the hardworking poor."[2] The outfit of our protagonist and the relatively high pricing of *Peri* indicated this was either an aspirational brand for the less affluent smoker or an advertisement aimed at the higher-end market. Either way, a simple papirosa quieted fears of being bereft and alone on the shores of modernity. If consumers visualized themselves as the well-appointed rooster, then *Peri* held the assurance of material success in a period of chaotic economic change. In the poster, the stylish air of *Peri*'s dandy caught the eye of a passerby, demonstrating how consumption could be about standing out as well as fitting in.

Posters, literature, memoirs, and art depicted educated consumption as a way to develop distinction in the rapidly expanding urban environment of late-nineteenth-century Russia—a setting of danger and opportunity that brought worries over anonymity as well as fears of exposure.[3] The city allowed an "ocular freedom" for new inhabitants where they could vicariously live the "other," invade their space, judge and be judged.[4] It also allowed consumers of lower status to occasionally or vicariously enjoy high-culture entertainments. A once-a-year excursion to the theater or purchase of a gramophone to listen to recordings of an opera blurred distinctions of clientele so that a lower-class consumer could develop the taste, or even exceed the knowledge, of someone of higher status.[5] By consuming particular brands, smokers could develop both a gustatory experience and a cultivated taste and do so as an act of confident connoisseurship. Undoubtedly brands tasted differently according to leaf quality and the many technological and production changes of the period, but the smell of tobacco, the accessories for its use, and the language and knowledge deployed in discussing the merits of one's preferred papirosy exhibited the taste of a user to those around him or her. Taste became a communal experience, learned by example, shared with those around, and judged by their reaction. The display of taste was socially orchestrated. Smoking, with its multiple actions—choosing, lighting, inhaling—was not intuitive and had to be learned from imitation or through tutelage, guaranteeing a communal origin for the individual habit.[6]

Brand, smell, language, accessories, and spaces signaled the type of smoker and their social standing. Cultural figures implied in their memoirs, poems, and novels that tobacco freed the intellect and exposed progressive sensibilities. By developing taste, the newly arrived and the tenuously situated could prove they deserved the station they had achieved by demonstrating their refined sensibilities. Smoking promised entry into exclusive social spaces, a vibrant consumer society, and a liberating political ideology, and, not surprisingly, others wanted in. Russian workers, peasant migrants, women, and children shouldered their way into the cultural representations of tobacco to indicate that they were mature, public, active, and political citizens of a modern state. This quest for inclusion did not, however, come without some chafing from the establishment. Just as some historians argue that alcohol was not a problem until middle-class concern over lower-class disorder brought it to the attention of social reformers, so too did lower-class smoking garner the attention, disapproval, and disquiet of the upper classes when it intruded into the privileged spaces or offended their sensibilities.[7]

Social pressures may have made smoking seem a way to belong and cultural figures might have trumpeted tobacco as liberation, but more than imagery fed into the creation of the habit. Advertisers served up social anxiety as a way to manipulate consumers in the late tsarist period, but unlike cosmetics or clothes, tobacco included chemical dependency, enthralling its users in addictive cycles that in turn propped up the perception that tobacco made one belong. Nicotine withdrawal brought on feelings of disquiet, even as advertisers promised smoking would eliminate other worries. Tobacco's addictive properties, the psychological dependencies of the habit, and the social benefits of inclusion meant that advertising often followed rather than led smokers' desires. Papirosy production burgeoned before advertising in Russia really got off the ground, showing that increased smoking did not arrive simply through advertising and better manipulation by marketers of popular fears. The apprehension and restlessness that nicotine withdrawal brought on, and that smoking alleviated, existed before *Peri*'s cockerel even donned his spats. Papirosy were both the cause of anxiety and its promised cure.

DESPITE efforts from late tsarist authorities to maintain tranquility while modernizing, the social impact of emancipation and industrialization reverberated throughout the late nineteenth century in the form of rapid urbanization and colossal social and cultural upheaval.[8] The transition provided further fodder to the discussions of Russia's liberal educated elite classes regarding the direction of the country that found expression in calls for national retrenchment, massive change, or even withdrawal from the path of Western-style development.[9] Russian intellectuals did not confront these changes alone. Recently developed industries brought more people to the city, provided them with lower-cost goods, afforded them novel entertainments, and introduced them to a new urban lifestyle. By World War I, about 15 percent of the population lived in urban areas, and Russian mass consumption developed in a hothouse atmosphere as recently urbanized, newly literate, barely proletarianized, and freshly radicalized citizens became first-time consumers at the same time. In the simmering cultural hubbub, what one chose to do, how they did it, with whom, and while using what marked identity or aspirations.[10]

Many of these new consumers bought tobacco. Options barraged the smokers throughout their day, be they advertisements on the street, displays in stores, offerings from coworkers and flatmates, or smokes shared with friends and family. Advertisers played up the perceived fashionable omnipresence of smoking and urged urbanites to see themselves as part of a community that almost required smoking, although not just any pack would do, and usually, they added, the crowd clamored for more. In the 1914 advertisement for *Zolotyia* (golden) brand of Bogdanov and Co., a crowd of men gathered around a street seller on a downtown street within sight of the Kremlin wall (figure 3.2).[11] All levels of society were present according to the semiotics of haberdashery: the seller himself in peaked cap, along with two others similarly attired; two bourgeois males in bowlers; a peasant in a woolen hat; a soldier in great coat and military cap; a gentleman in woolen suit with tweed topper; and a man in the back with moustache and an exotic, perhaps Cossack, fur cloche. At the top of the advertisement, a couplet underscored the democratic, public, and modern aspects of *Zolotyia*:

> Near the street-stand the people crowd
> Like at the bar and all around,
> All of them yell and shout excitedly
> Give me "Golden" papirosy!![12]

The street seller catered to the buyer on the way to work who needed a convenient source for his daily pack, but the mention of bar and pub in the

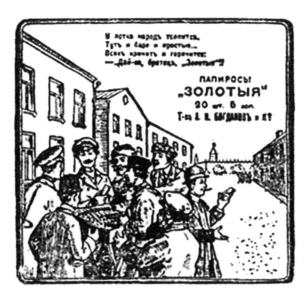

Figure 3.2   *Zolotyia* advertisement. *Put' pravdy*, 1914. Collection of Russian State Library, Moscow.

poem brought to mind the opportunities for leisure in the city. The couplet and visual together connected *Zolotyia* to urban life both day and night and showed the ease of buying tobacco in urban areas. Often homeless women or street children would wrap papirosy and then sell them in the market squares or along the streets making sure that day or night a smoke was always close at hand.[13]

The egalitarian appeal of smoking echoed through other advertisements. The 1900 poster for *Zoria* (reveille) brand gave a visual representation of the "everyone" who smoked (figure 1.4). Worker and soldier, young and old, male and female, bourgeois and peasant, all enjoyed the "truly excellent" papirosy from St. Petersburg's Saatchi and Mangubi firm. All looked fashionable and healthy in their stereotypical representations. The upper-class male and female both appeared ready to attend some evening entertainment. Again, an artist employed a monocle, this time along with top hat, to signal a man of means. The woman in plumed chapeau with veil and lace bolero jacket held her papirosa in an immaculately gloved hand while the man in ceremonial guard's uniform clenched his in his mouth. Even the bearded peasant looked prosperous. The far background of the advertisement implied a distant pastoral countryside, with a wide blue sky and green fields. Simultaneously, the red-shirted peasant's invitation to the viewer, given with doffed hat and outstretched arm, indicated the gateway from the peaceful background to the tumult of people, through the red-shirted street seller. Purchasing and consuming *Zoria* ushered the user from the countryside to the urban crowd. The man in bowler behind the peasant similarly beckoned the viewer to step forward into the modern with his smile and gesture. Color, style, and figures all summoned the smoker into an exciting urban milieu.

The 1896 advertisement for *Furor* brand dispensed with the detailed picture of the different types of consumers for the product, and instead, taking a cue from the brand name, depicted a mass of arms from a nameless crowd jostling, pushing, and eager for a taste of the "newly re-released" papirosy that one could purchase "everywhere" (figure 3.3).[14] The disembodied hands engaged in kinetic action, and grasping at the packs promoted a message of mass consumption enabled by new mass production. Such appeals appeared in other advertisements where manufacturers trumpeted their sales figures, implying, like *Furor,* that demand for their product indicated its quality.[15] *Safo* papirosy similarly claimed a mass following with a 1912 advertisement, which featured a globe with the brand and price superimposed (figure 3.4).[16] The slogan at top contended that "now everyone smokes Safo," giving voice to an international reach made visible in a globe under the sway of *Safo.*

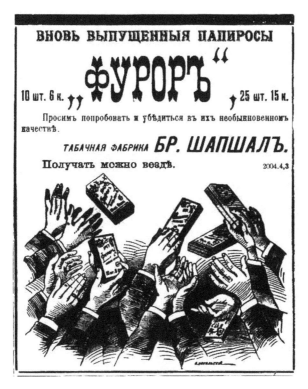

Figure 3.3   *Furor* advertisement. *Moskovskii listok*, 1896. Collection of Russian State Library, Moscow.

The common perception, and advertised promise, that everyone around the world of all classes smoked did not translate into marketers pushing revolutionary visions of an egalitarian society. In the advertisements that featured actual figures, not globes or disembodied hands, class markers appeared prominently. Smoking did not overturn the existing system as much as reinforce it by repeating visual markers of the divisions of class, gender, and geography even as all pictured consumed a common item and brand.

Some papirosy were double the cost of others. The difference in price points emerged in targeted messaging. *Zoria* and *Zolotyia*, which featured varied groups united by smoking, were cheaper brands.[17] More expensive tobacco brands tended to depict dandies or women of fashion without companion images of lower class figures enjoying the product (figures 3.1, 3.11, 3.12, 3.13, 3.14, 3.18, 3.19, 3.20, 3.21, 3.22).

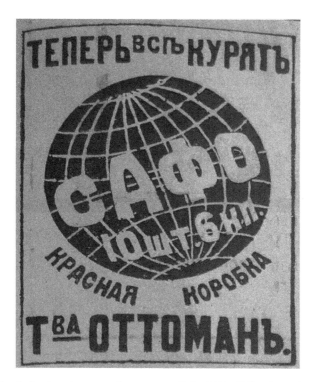

Figure 3.4 *Safo* advertisement. *Restorannoe Delo*, 1912. Collection of Russian State Library, Moscow.

Table 3.1 Papirosy by price range

.25 kopek per papirosa	.3 kopek per papirosa	.6 kopek per papirosa		1 kopek per papirosa
Gadalka	Kapriz	Desert	Golos	Peri
Sigarnaia	Kometa	Fru fru	Furor	Diushess
Sladkiia	Kair	Kabinetnyia	Safo	Brom
Vazhnyia	Bar	Al'dona	Iar	Smirna
Zoria	Desert	Bosonozhka	No. 6	Evropeiskiia
Trynkia	Dukat	Ada	Nora	Grafskiia
Tary Bary	Roskosh	Narzan	Bebe	No. 100
Taras Bulba	Diushess	Novyi Vek	Kado	Teremok
Urkainskii		Roskosh		Peri
Zolotyia			Vostok	Modnyia
Vostochnyia	Pushka (.4k)			Kliko
Soldat	Suvorov (.5k)			

Although smoking brought users together in a common action, the bonds this may have created were strained constantly from the difference that delivery type, leaf quality, brand choice, and production brought to the tobacco experience as well as the variations that smokers themselves cultivated through language, accessories, and etiquette. By emphasizing social distinction built on the taste of tobacco as a gustatory experience and articulated in a language that provided evidence of a user's distinction, users and marketers resisted the leveling effect the availability of cheap tobacco might have afforded. Types of taste depended heavily on context. Technological changes, cultural shifts, dietary modifications, and intellectual associations assured that experiences of taste diverged. Cultural and natural differences affected the appreciation of flavors—such as bitterness, so that black bread might be a staple of Russia, but foreigners considered it unpalatable and indigestible.[18] Biology, habit, heredity, ethnicity, and age individualized taste, and over the decades, the connection between scent and taste and the nuances that, it was implied, were available only to connoisseurs created further peculiarities.[19]

Nineteenth-century discussions of taste suffered from a general denigration of it on a hierarchy that favored sight and hearing as the most civilized, enlightened, and therefore most human (that is, not brutish) senses.[20] Disquiet with physical sensations of taste emerged from the connection of smell, taste, and touch to animal instincts, lust, and gluttony. Connoisseurship liberated the physical experience of taste from its animal origins by splitting low- and high-quality leaf, celebrating etiquette over boorish behavior, trumpeting the spiritual and intellectual benefits of use, and distinguishing upper- and lower-class brands. By bringing rationality to consumption, connoisseurship allowed Russian elites to indulge in a common habit without descending into being common, imbuing products that industrial capitalism had made affordable to the masses with symbolic value.[21] As mechanization and low-cost labor brought down the costs of papirosy, such distinctions became more important to solidifying status.

The Russian upper classes in the nineteenth century displayed status through consumption and ostentatious spectacles of material goods. When pressed, they sacrificed well-being in favor of appearance—for example, privileging serving ware for public use over bed linens for private comfort in the early nineteenth-century capital. Attention to estate-specific displays of status, including body language, public space, and servant entourages, continued even as the influence of the aristocracy declined.[22] In the village of the 1880s, manufactured goods like lamps or samovars indicated relative wealth and signaled status to others.[23]

Tobacco wove through the language of class and distinction. According to an 1845 essay on "Tobacco Production in Russia," Catherine the Great had noted that while tobacco could be grown in Russia, the quality and workmanship made it suitable only for "simple folk." The essay's author concluded that this was no longer the case and that while many people might swear they were unable to smoke Russian tobacco, once the government permitted the tobacco master in Petersburg to use a "German or Dutch signature and coat of arms," most of these smokers were placated, showing either that their skills of discernment were not so well-honed or that the Russian tobacco had reached an adequate level of quality.[24] The article detailed changes in tobacco over the period that went deeper than the seal on the package. The author observed that tastes had changed and now Russians "smoke a lot and the tobacco is light, almost without scent." The author depicted the scent of Catherinian tobacco as intoxicating and noted how older smokers, who came off as true specialists, could distinguish their own brands from thousands of others by the perfume of their tobacco and their "passion" for the product.[25]

A foreign observer argued that by the turn of the century in Russia, by taste either developing or devolving, "The best of society smoke[d]."[26] Turkish tobacco, and that grown in Russia from Turkish seed, enjoyed the most praise. The upper class mixed Turkish tobacco with native tobacco grown in Odessa, Kishenev, and Dubossarakh.[27] A 1916 manual carefully laid out the hierarchy of tobacco according to region and leaf choice, so that tobacco from Yalta and American were at the top, while German and Chernigov tobacco occupied a middle ground, and Russian and Kavkas makhorka indicated the lowest sort.[28]

According to V. E. Ignatiev's 1896 entry on smoking in the Brokgauz and Efron encyclopedia, "pleasant odors" came from leaf choice, but manufacturers worked over the blend in secret recipes "in order to give them the appropriate taste and prevent the rapid combustion of tobacco or rot." The sauce was typically a mixture of "two or three things, such as: saltpeter, table salt, potash, honey, sugar, spirits, raisins, chicory coffee, coffee grounds, incense, anise, dill, etc." This potpourri of ingredients enhanced the smell, taste, and the burn of tobacco so much that it exuded, "while burning, various odors, which are so valued by smoking lovers; but at the same time they need not spoil the natural flavor of tobacco." In all, Ignatiev provided a detailed picture of the sensory experience a connoisseur should aspire to: "Good tobacco must have a natural color, a sufficiently acrid (*ostryi*) smell of the smoke, moreover the taste need not be bitter, scratchy, or burning; the smoldering of tobacco must proceed slowly, without crackling, the color of the smoke must be bluish, and the remaining ash must have a whitish color. The cinders of higher sorts of tobacco are often markedly whiter than lower."[29] Even those bent on exposing tobacco's danger dwelt on its sensible intoxication. For example, Vitol'd Khmelevskii's doctoral dissertation, which focused on nicotine levels in the corpses of animals poisoned by tobacco fumes, contemplated tobacco's more pleasant odors, noting that it was "essential to not just impregnate it with aromatic items, but also to remove from it that which might occasion bad smells."

Connoisseurs knew good tobacco by its scent and could similarly identify bad tobacco by its stench. Makhorka, the tobacco of the people, was marked by its disagreeable odor, taste, and strength, according to its detractors. These qualities were reflected in its low cost, but also occasioned revulsion from those around the smoker. As one antismoking author commented, makhorka's odor was "disgusting." Interestingly, the author also noted the inelegance of its delivery, as makhorka was increasingly sold as "'bag' [*kartuznyi*] tobacco . . . smoked more in the village and countryside." The author concluded that in the city users gravitated to papirosy, presumably a sign of their sophistication.[30] Despite the distaste of some, the market share and production of makhorka still rose. By 1900, the growth in cheaper papirosy was about 10 percent a year, and that of loose-leaf makhorka, largely for the rural market, nearly 6 percent.[31]

The expansion of tobacco use in the late nineteenth century can be viewed through the increasing agitation against it, manifested in attempts to regulate its smoke and smell.[32] The worries over smoke carried more than simply fear of disease. At different times tobacco was seen to soil the soul, weaken the will, strengthen manliness, connote working-class origins, or signal military inclusion, and the smoke of others promised to visit these connotations on those around them in a way akin to older ideas about infection and dependent on newer concepts of smell. Nineteenth-century reformers, worried over disease drifting along in scent, sought to deodorize the city, especially the poor, to stop epidemics, and tobacco odor got caught up in these efforts.[33] Smoke-free carriages in trains, smoking parlors in homes, and smoking jackets for the well-heeled male all implied a concern for controlling the effects of tobacco that wafted in the air.

Smoke served as an odorant even as bourgeois ritual increasingly stressed deodorization. Though a studied, artful "lack" of odor became the norm for bourgeois etiquette, and sight grew to supersede scent as the sense of science and Enlightenment, still odor held cultural significance and retained power in literature.[34] When the urban milieu threatened to overwhelm the developing self with anonymity, tobacco brand choice, and the smells accompanying it, could push out to others and signal social status, aspiration, or character to even the most casual observer. For instance, works by Charles Dickens (1812–70), Émile Zola (1840–1902), and Dostoevsky used the semiotics of scent for quick character development. According to one scholar of the sensory, Russian literature overflowed with fragrance, even more so than contemporary German and English works. The scant 160 pages of Ivan Turgenev's (1818–83) *Fathers and Sons* contained over twenty references to aromas that expressed politics, generation, gender, and the West, and tobacco played its role as a pungent symbol of the conflict between young and old, new and conservative, and son and father. For example, Arkady's cigars caused his father to turn his face from the lad—their smoke as disturbing as his nihilism. In Dostoevsky's *Crime and Punishment*, the stench of St. Petersburg, and urban corruption generally, perfumed the novel, and corpses befouled the atmosphere.[35] When Raskolnikov went to kill the old woman, he distracted her with a papirosy case, and then later he complained of the aggressive effrontery of the prosecutor, who smoked during their meeting.

Scent occupied the Russian intellectual milieu, and smoke provided a new and easily observable intrusion. In passages from Russian literature, medical tracts, magazines, etiquette manuals, and advertising, the scent of smoking was commented on and found both praise and condemnation.[36] Tobacco's odors signaled social status, aspiration, or character. Consumer behavior served as a point for identity creation, and smoking allowed production of self through consumption and display of it with the smell that remained even after use.[37] Tobacco aficionados bragged of their ability to identify brands by their scent, and certain mixtures became popular rages. But while connoisseurs waxed lyrical over blends, and advertisements celebrated smoke with depictions of rings, tendrils, and billowing clouds, antitobacco advocates emphasized the foul, unpleasant nature of the exhalation. As the urban arena brought people shoulder to shoulder with habits, odors, diseases, and dirt, fear of contagion also rubbed off.[38] Tobacco smoke—wafting on the breeze—could settle on the clothes, hair, and bodies of others and linger in their identity. To smell of tobacco might enmesh the consumer in unwanted associations or indicate bad manners. Etiquette manuals for theatergoers specified that it was poor behavior to smell excessively of perfume or have breath smelling of beer or tobacco.[39] Smoke and its odor was the most evident indicator of the use of a commodity that people worried penetrated far deeper than skin and held changes more permanent than scent.[40]

The taint of smoking was visited unequally on the classes. Men of means could afford separate smoking areas and special protective clothing, but those of the lower orders often smoked in venues like the tavern, where the whiff of societal opprobrium mingled with the odor of tobacco.[41] Scent marked off spaces in the city as respectable or dangerous, and tobacco smoke participated in these sensory delineations of respectability.[42] The areas without tobacco contrasted markedly from the taverns and clubs that, according to all contemporaries, reeked of smoke.[43]

Scent did not stand alone in smoking's sensory aftermath. Technological innovations brought variations to the flavor of smoking in the nineteenth century. Users would notice the absence of glue, along with the introduction of newer and better papers, because these changes affected burn and scent, essential components of taste. Burn quality for both cigars and papirosy merited extended discussion in articles on tobacco production, where details on which chemicals aided burn, or hindered it, and how these affected not just the flavor of the inhalation but also the smell of smoke and the color of ash took up paragraphs.[44]

Users could taste, smell, see, and feel the modern in the product, and marketers told them how to explain that change. In their 1896 advertisement, the cartridge maker Katyk and Co. crowed that their product was made mechanically "without glue" and from the best French papers.[45] "The smoke is filtered," proclaimed the refrain under the smiling *bogatyr* in the poster for *Vazhnyia* (figure 1.7). While the technology was not explained, the slogan implied that the feel of the inhalation would be smoother, with perhaps a milder taste. Even for those who detected no difference, the language provided by manufacturers suggested ways for users to articulate how their consumption was better than that of others.

Attention to taste distinguished cultured smokers and protected them from one of the dangers of the modern market—falsification. While a rural inhabitant would grow and process their own tobacco, the urbanite was prey to the vagaries of a market where sourcing was at times unknown and quality often uneven. Anxieties revealed themselves in allegations of impurities in mass-produced tobacco and papirosy. According to an 1883 article in *Zdorov'e* (Health), the public recognized falsification as a problem in milk, bread, wine, and vodka, but few knew that tobacco and coffee could also be tampered with almost undetectably. The author argued that some of this might be due to leaf quality since the level of manipulation necessary to enhance European plantation tobacco, which was not as naturally aromatic and distinctive in its taste as Turkish and Asiatic tobacco, led to problems. While he noted that the tobacco used in Russian papirosy was healthier, he concluded that the "Papirosa paper of Russian fabrication [was] often, visibly, not safe."[46] Ignatiev focused on the dyes used to make papers to appear white or yellow and the leaf of cigars look dark. He cautioned that such alterations might fool the eye, but they did not alter the quality of leaf and might carry poison with them.[47] In Canada, such discussions led to large-scale investigations regarding the quality and safety of cigarettes in this same period.[48] In Russia, antismoking advocates frequently featured adulteration in their litany on the evils of tobacco.[49] One racist rant connected falsification to the Jewish ownership of factories, writing that "counterfeiting of tobacco happen[ed] at its point of production," which was "in the hands of Jews," and price was no guarantee of quality.[50]

At times, the difference between adulteration and processing was lost on antitobacco advocates. One author concluded, "It is well known that the more fragrant the tobacco, the more expensive, and the more poisonous items in it; in other sorts of tobacco, there may be less real poison (nicotine), but there are more mix ins which are no less poisonous."[51] He continued by arguing that adulteration, saucing, and marketing all colluded in tricking consumers, so that they would be "more likely to consider Russian makhorka less dangerous than other so called 'Turkish tobaccos' with enticing slogans and pictures on the boxes."[52] A 1916 tobacco manual argued that the most common form of deception was to make cheap tobaccos seem more expensive by adding perhaps cherry leaves or rose petals. The author noted, however, that for the "experienced smoker it was easily evident by taste" and therefore could not be widely practiced.[53]

True tobacco connoisseurs had to avoid the glitz and purchase products revealing the full provenance from cultivation to production to sale to assure the highest standards had been met and that a quality product was consumed. Falsification was presented as a problem for mass-market, uneducated consumers. A connoisseur understood, as Ignatiev pointed out, that the "quality of tobacco depend[ed] on place of growth, climatic levels, soil on which it grows, methods of culturing, and in the end, those methods of working, which determine the way of use and taste of tobacco."[54] An educated smoker understood the qualities of place and climate, *terroir,* which similarly fascinated the oenophile. Attention to *terroir* and concern for falsification and insufficient production oversight inevitably brought users to confront political and social questions of the day, such as the costs of imperial expansion, horrific working conditions, exploitation of women's and child's labor, lagging agricultural development, insufficient industrial oversight, burdensome taxation, and governmental inefficiencies. Thus Tolstoy's contemplation of the papirosy rollers played a part in the construction of connoisseurship, as did the imperialist pretensions of Balkan Star and Shaposhnikova's advertisement of her programs for workers.

Consumption of tobacco enjoyed other political associations resulting from the way it was introduced into Russia in the seventeenth century. Viewed by many as Western, against tradition, and sinful, smoking coincided with the impulse of the *intelligentsia* toward secularization and progress and against traditional society and its restrictions.[55] More than simply an idealized vision of smoking, tobacco access formed a crucial connection to freedoms lost or rights desired for prisoners, student, and workers. The socialist M. V. Butashevich-Petrashevskii (1821–66) recalled that during his stay in the Peter and Paul fortress the smell of tobacco smoke reminded him of liberty and led him to ask that the guard take a few rubles from his coat to buy him a pipe and some Zhukov tobacco.[56] Seminary students recalled stolen moments in the lavatory to enjoy a smoke, and the right to smoking breaks appeared in striking workers' demands.[57] Perhaps in a nod to the common belief that tobacco helped focus, student cooperative associations included tobacco in the list of necessities for serious study alongside food, lodging, and books.[58] Intellectuals wrote of not just the freedom to smoke, but the freedom that came from smoking. The Russian Romantic Alexander Bestuzhev-Marlinskii (1797–1837) gave smoking as the attribute of the enlightened man when he quipped, "'I think, therefore I am,' says Descartes. 'I smoke, therefore I think,' say I.'"[59]

The connection of tobacco to mental labor in various contexts added to the imagery of tobacco as a bourgeois pursuit. In his 1907 contemplation of tobacco use, *Zagadka kureniia* (The mystery of smoking), S. Tormazov regarded the smoker and their habits, connecting certain social groups and activities definitively to smoking: "If we follow a clerk, creating a report, or students, writing a dissertation, or a lawyer, preparing a petition or talk, or a book keeper tabulating accounts, then we can observe that the ashtray sitting before them during that work fills with a large number of papirosy butts and in a different time, when the work is harder or when it is more interesting, then during that work the smoking is less visible."[60] In addition to mental labors, discussions of "political, economic, and philosophical" characters also brought forward the greater tobacco use, as Tormazov recalled of just a few years passed: "If there were a few *intelligentsia* come together in a room, the smoke would get so thick that, according to the saying, you could cut it with an ax, and you could be sure that there was hot bickering of some general question." If mental labor led to smoking, physical labor, he argued, instead weakened the desire for tobacco. Thus tobacco use might spread to all classes, but the pull to smoking was visited only on the thinking man rather than the laboring one.[61]

Freedom of thought as well as freedom more generally became party to the imagery of tobacco in the "other."[62] The Bogdanov and Co. factory's poster for their papirosy *Sigarniia* (cigar) featured an African-American male holding bright yellow tobacco leaf (Virginia) out to the viewer (figure 3.5). American tobacco was often depicted with African-American or

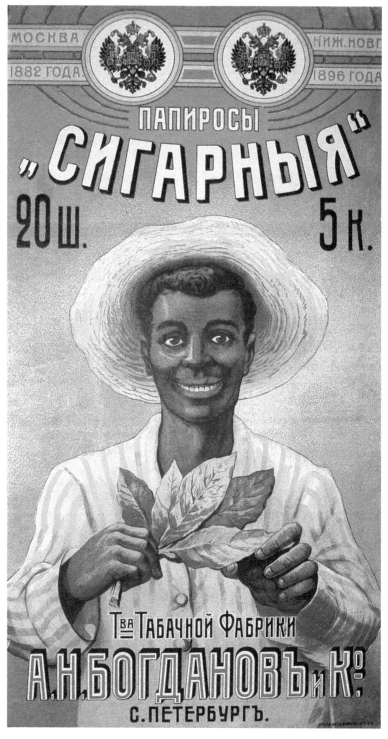

Figure 3.5 *Sigarnaia* poster. Prerevolutionary. Collection of Russian State Library, Moscow.

golliwog images in the global market, but the smiling tobacco worker would have had a strange resonance in Russia, where earlier political allegory had often employed the American slave as stand-in for the Russian serf. Images of black males, representing African-American, Caribbean, or African producers or users, stood outside tobacco shops from the early eighteenth century in Russia.[63] Certainly emancipation in both Russia and the United States had tempered that relationship but had not obliterated it.[64] In the post–Civil War world of which this poster was part, the African-American male, depicted here as both producer and dealer of bright leaf, brought to mind both economic and political freedom, aligning tobacco with liberation as well as Western production and American democracy.

The use of a racialized "other" for the sale of tobacco served as a variant of the orientalist vision of the odalisque and the Cossack, but here conquest was not on the table. The advertisement was not a wholesale adoption of American imagery, but rather, like the papirosa itself, a blend. The name itself transgressed the boundaries between different tobaccos and styles of smoking—a cigarette that was a cigar?—but there were other subtle changes as well. The borrowing of an American image was made Russian in three ways—the poster nodded to the St. Petersburg base of the Bogdanov concern by featuring the city name at the base of the poster; the name of the papirosy implied the use of Caribbean tobaccos or additives to impart a cigar-like flavor; and the top of the poster featured seals gained from Russian national manufacturing competitions (Moscow 1882 and Nizhnyi Novgorod 1896). *Sigarnaia* were thus a foreign and domestic product, emerging as a mixture of associations that the consumer could purchase.

Authors used tobacco to signal change and character attributes, indicating that readers readily understood the distinctive styles of use and assumptions that should come from these. Early on, snuff became the habit of the older and unfashionable generation; by 1904 one author observed, "Snuff is mostly the habit of wretched old men and women for whom the joys of life are few. They stuff their noses with tobacco and from that receive a little tickle in the nose which gives them some enjoyment."[65] Over the course of the century, the more fashionable cigar and then papirosa took over from the pipe as the symbols of independence and thought and, from their availability to all classes, held some indications of democratic pretension. For the generation of the 1860s, class associations became distinct as cigars came to symbolize upper-class indulgence and papirosy youthful vigor, social modernization, and the ethos of the Great Reforms. When Alexander II lifted the ban on smoking in the streets in the 1860s, the new freedom to walk and smoke became associated with the general atmosphere of reform. For instance, the Russian poet Nikolai Nekrasov (1821–78) equated his ability to smoke in the street with that of writing without censorship.[66]

Nekrasov and his public embrace of smoking lent tobacco use a reflected glory—a type of celebrity status. Others openly offered their devotion for public comment. Peter the Great's tobacco habit, picked up from his Western friends, was legendary. Catherine the Great was known to take snuff. Sergei Witte, the Russian minister of finance from 1892 to 1903, was an inveterate smoker who supposedly spent much of his time at the Russo-Japanese peace conference of 1905 with a papirosa in his debonair holder, despite his push for increased taxes on tobacco and matches.[67] The philosopher Nikolai Chernyshevsky (1828–89) quelled his nerves with papirosy, Anton Chekhov smoked, as did most of his characters, and Dostoevsky was known to chain smoke Saatchi and Mangubi or Laferm papirosy as he wrote.[68] The poet Zinaida Gippius (1869–1945) caused waves by bending gender expectations in her open relationships, unconventional fashion, and provocative smoking habits.[69] Even fictional characters' smoking preference gained prominence. Chernyshevsky's prototypical radical Rakhmetov from *What is to be Done?* (1863) denied himself all luxuries in pursuit of revolution except cigars. For the educated consumer, knowing the history of their product and the history of its greatest consumers—fictional or historical—became important to the display of their own status.

Manufacturers capitalized on the public's interest in celebrity by issuing brands named for well-known figures and with the inclusion of cards in packs with portraits of actors or artists. In 1905, Gabai tobacco put out a round of cheap papirosy called *Slava Rossii* (the glory of Russia) that featured a portrait of Tolstoy in a peasant shirt as part of the brand advertisement, an ironic choice given his denunciations of the habit.[70] For the Pushkin centennial in 1899, tobacconists released papirosy, loose-tobacco, rolling papers, and matches in his honor.[71] In addition to literary figures, tobacco card series featured portraits of famous composers or men and women of the stage.[72] The celebrity endorsement could become a game. A Shaposhnikov contest in 1912 allowed readers to guess which famous unnamed figure was pictured in their regular advertisement. The winners took papirosy as prizes along with the affirmation of their educated status.[73]

Ever the emissary of cultured consumption, Uncle Mikey, pointed out the royal users of Russia's tobacco firmament in his 1912 advertisement, "Tobacco in Russia: An Historical-Poetic Investigation." Not content to let his pseudonymous self get all the credit, he appended his real name, S. A. Korotkii, to the piece, lending a certain gravitas to this advertisement. In rough couplets he joked that feeble-minded Tsar Fedor (r. 1584–98) heard bells but nothing about tobacco and assured readers that even in the face of Tsar Mikhail's notoriously cruel seventeenth-century ban, Uncle Mikey would take the punishment rather than give up tobacco. In his historical riff, Korotkii gave smokers a basic knowledge of tobacco's rise in the world and in Russia in particular. He told of early tobacco terminology ("drinking" tobacco meant smoking) and how the "tsar-carpenter" Peter I took up smoking in Holland with his friends and returned to Petersburg to spread it to all of Russia.[74] Korotkii wove tobacco through Russia's history, to make smoking the national pastime.

Tobacco posters based on famous art works similarly tried to borrow the glory of Russia's history and great works in the service of tobacco promotion. Two paintings by Ilia Repin made appearances as tobacco posters, the already viewed Zaporozhian Cossacks (figure 1.1) and the *Volga Boat Haulers,* painted in 1870–73, where the third, harnessed peasant puffed on a pipe.[75] The veiled references to the poem "The Lay of the Host of Igor" as well as the painting of it by Vasnetsov play across the image of the Trezvon advertisement of brave *bogatyr* (figure 1.9). By appropriating works of art, historical treasures, and celebrated figures to their cause, manufacturers bonded their consumer products to milestones of Russian culture, just as Uncle Mikey tied tobacco to the tsars and military themes entwined smoking with empire. These works of art became part of the smoker's lexicon, and knowing them gave smokers claim to connoisseurship but also made their habit something more—a celebration of nation and spirit.

Artists, in turn, used papirosy within their works to illustrate characters and comment on current behavioral norms, many of these establishing types of smoker well before advertisers employed them. Pavel Andreevich Fedotov (1815–52) utilized tobacco to signal means and attitudes in his densely narrated paintings of the nineteenth century. In *The Aristocrat's Breakfast* (1849–50), the artist depicted a young man surrounded by fashionable trappings of the stylish gentry, including rolling papers strewn across the floor, a smoking jacket with oriental cap, and an ashtray at his elbow with smoldering papirosa (figure 3.6). The painting, a commentary on the superficiality of the young dandy who tried to hide from his entering visitor that, despite all the trappings of wealth, all he had for breakfast was a humble piece of black bread and a papirosa, showed the centrality of smoking to his personae and lifestyle. While critics made much of the meager breakfast, the evidence of his smoking was left unspoken but was evident everywhere— the tobacco that began the day, the smoking cap to cover the smell, the thick robe to shield clothing from smoking's aftermath, and the pack at the

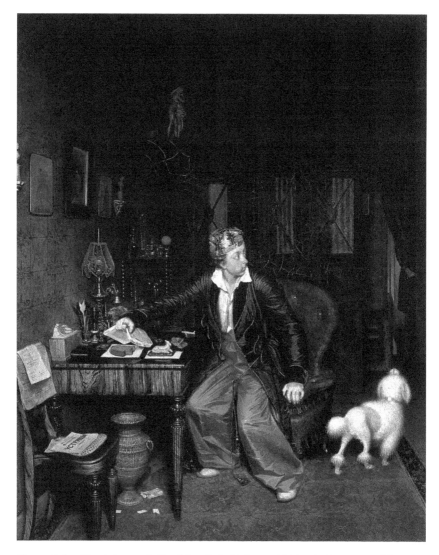

Figure 3.6   *The Aristocrat's Breakfast.* P. A. Fedotov, 1849–50. Courtesy of the State Tretyakov Gallery, Moscow.

ready yet also so disregarded as to let fall to the floor.[76] Like the connection of Cossack and smoking, the fashionable implications of tobacco and dandyism had been well established before marketers ever caught hold of it.

Vasili Gregorievich Perov (1834–82), another astute observer of Russian life in the nineteenth century, portrayed the social aspects of smoking—solidarity, masculinity, and leisure—to such effect as to create a vision of the smoking break that became iconic and often reproduced in later years for smoking paraphernalia (figure 3.7). His 1871 painting *Hunters Stop to Rest* showed three men sitting in animated conversation, surrounded by the evidence of their manly activity, which was demonstrated not just by the rugged landscape but also the confirmation of a successful hunt in the forms of the dead game and guns at rest in the foreground and the relaxed positions of the men. No alcohol aided the vision of male sociability. Instead, a single papirosa, consumed by one of the listeners, became the accompaniment to manly social activities. This painting, from a period when Perov moved away from social critique and instead toward a celebration of the mundane joys of daily life displayed across classes, showed the early centrality of tobacco to constructions of Russian male rituals and identity. Further, the rugged landscape, meant to invoke the wild Russian countryside, tied into national celebrations of the glories of the Russian land during this period.

The symbiotic relationship of literature, history, marketing, art, and tobacco displayed the ways that the simple papirosa became invested with cultural meaning. The placement of papirosy within not just Russian history

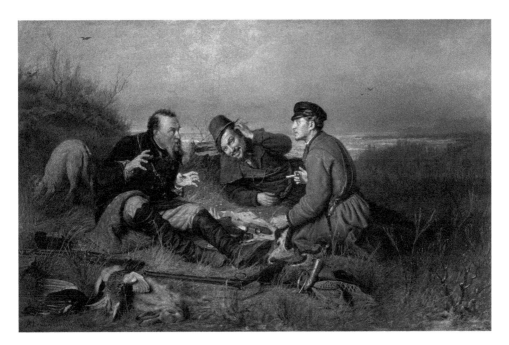

Figure 3.7   *Hunters Stop to Rest.* V. G. Perov, 1871. Courtesy of the State Tretyakov Gallery, Moscow.

but also the global history of use similarly laid claim to a grand legacy for the product while educating the viewer and providing them a means of cultured consumption. The 1903 poster for Ia. S. Kushnarev's factory jubilee created a vision of not just Russian tobacco, but especially Kushnarev tobacco in the saga of tobacco's global progress (figure 3.8). The artist N. N. Karazin signed the poster in the bottom left, an unusual move, and perhaps a testimony to the aspirations of the manufacturer. Rather than just borrowing from a work of art by a famous painter, the manufacturer commissioned a canvas specifically for their factory. The elaborate design was pregnant with meaning. At center, two visions of the factory guided the viewer through fifty years of industrial progress—from the factory's foundation in 1853 to the current day's iteration of 1903. The factory at bottom, one story and only two buildings, contrasted markedly with the classically square, symmetrically pleasing lines of the new factory, which maintained a bonded, strict order compared to the chaotic images of the margins. Trees in regular plantings with common height frame a building of multiple stories, metal roofs, elaborate entrance gate, and tree-filled courtyards. In place of the horse and cart, a smokestack belched progress and indicated modern power at top. Figures with pipes and water pipes, as well as the loose tobacco and papirosy arrayed in packs at the bottom, indicated the many ways to ingest tobacco.

The size, symmetry, and classical presentation of the 1903 factory intimated that the development of new, more modern production processes, adept management, and the strong market for Kushnarev tobacco allowed for such growth. The imperial seals at top and the large array of different goods at bottom both indicated their quality. In the background, images of tobacco plants called to mind the scientific and botanical works of the period, placing the advertisement in the realm of popular science and not just commercial endeavor.

The historical primer of tobacco provided by the images of men and women of all nations enjoying tobacco to right and left of the factory further elevated the marketing appeal by making it an ethnographic album as well as advertisement. Stereotypically depicted Native Americans, Chinese, Turks, and Central Asians all admired the vision of the developing factory, a trope of European imagery—primitive peoples awed by industrial might in a way that itself harkened back to religious paintings of pagans overwhelmed by the glory of Christ. Tobacco's imperialized meaning appeared in full detail. A Cossack stood, back to the viewer, in the right foreground, chatting up the odalisques sitting beside a water pipe attended by a eunuch, indicating his conquest of these women and, by extension, their country.

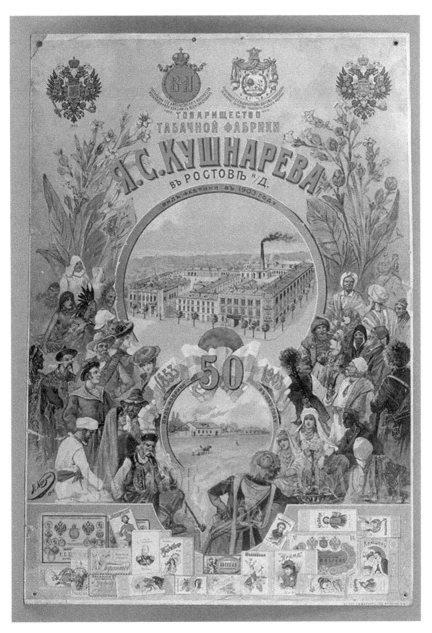

Figure 3.8 *Ia. S. Kushnarev* poster. N. N. Karazin, 1903. Collection of Russian State Library, Moscow.

Their sheik was placed behind, pipe in hand, admiring the new factory and seemingly content in his loss of power, if it meant the boon of tobacco. Behind this tableau, other peoples of the expanded Russian empire regarded the factory—a man and woman in the antiquated dress of boyars, a peasant woman in elaborate flowered headgear, another in a red scarf, a Muslim woman in hijab, and a Muslim male in fez. His back to the viewer, a military man of the Caucasus donned a typical fur hat as well as a gun strapped to his back. The Russian empire's history of tobacco contrasted with that of the world on the other side of the factory inset. On the left a group of Native Americans, a British tar, another soldier in a pith helmet, a moor, a Chinese man, a Turkish man and woman, two European women of fashion, and several others admired the Kushnarev factory. Russia's imperial history paraded by as the equal to the entire global history of tobacco on the other side. Russia was a world unto itself.

Like the history developed by Uncle Mikey and the appropriation of works of art by Ottoman and others, the elaborate presentation of tobacco as a commodity of deep impact and global span allowed users to see themselves as part of something bigger than the purchase of a pack of papirosy. The elevation of tobacco was also evidenced in the personification of tobacco as a beautiful woman, a love, or an item of worship. In Britain, this tendency led to odes to tobacco as a "divine weed" that could take the form of a lover or a god.[77] In Russia, mythic women served similar ends. A Shaposhnikov advertising couplet invoked the *houri,* the nymphs of Muslim paradise, to imply that the brand was a gift from the heavens: "'Golden straw'—tobacco flower / strong smelling and gentle, like rose flowers / *Houri* of paradise bring you greetings / such papirosy have never been seen in the world."[78] Russia, spanning the border between Europe and Asia, implied tobacco's divinity in depictions that borrowed from Christian, Muslim, and Hindu traditions, yet again emphasized the global pretentions of Russia's tobacco empire.

Utilizing the *style moderne* with its ready application to mythic themes, poster advertisements wove elaborate fantasies of female nymphs, sprites, and goddesses who personified tobacco's seductive qualities.[79] The genre elevated tobacco not only through its imagery but also through its quality. The artists of the *style moderne* were considered progressive because of their mission to transform life by bringing art to the everyday.[80] A dreamy advertisement for the papirosy and loose tobacco of Shaposhnikov featuring two alabaster-skinned goddesses typified this style (figure 3.9). The duo faced outward, at the viewer. One looked off to the left, but the other directly regarded the consumer. They embraced in an otherworldly romantic

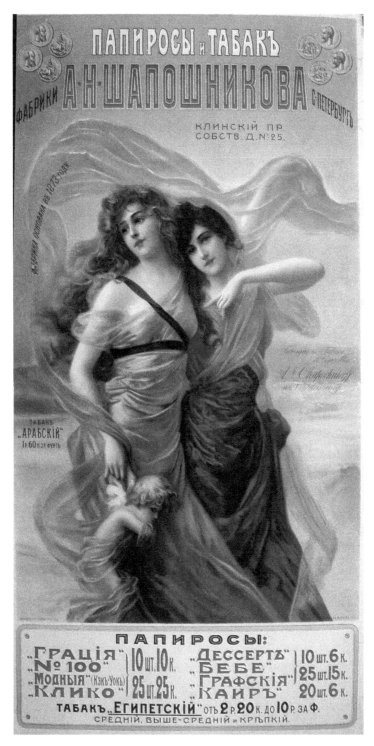

Figure 3.9 *Gratsiia* poster. Prerevolutionary. Collection of Russian State Library, Moscow.

setting, draped in rich colors and ensnared in tendrils of gauzy, smoky fabric. Below, a cupid cowers in the skirt of the golden-haired beauty. The gorgeous poster could have hung on the wall of a home or store, and many of these posters may have doubled as domestic art. More than just providing titillation, these women, enveloped in misty fabrics and sheltering a cherub, became tobacco personified—the golden leaf of the West and the dark leaf of the Turks. Wrapped together in a twisting film of otherworldliness, they enticed the viewer to partake in an experience sumptuous, exotic, and sexual.

The poster for Laferm's *Fru-Fru* (frou-frou) brand, with its gold leaf and heavy-stock paper, was elaborately and expensively produced (figure 3.10). At ten for six kopeck, *Fru-Fru* sold at a higher end of the market, but not at the most expensive point. *Fru-Fru* took its name from the French term coined to describe the sensuous, rustling sound made by women's silken skirts as they walked across a room. The visual of the swirling, roiling smoke on the poster echoed the name's evocation of the intimate swooshing of women's clothing twining about their legs and body. Thoughts of intimacy and sensuality drifted in the sinuous smoke alongside the writhing, golden-haired nymphs. Seven of the eleven seemed to be clothed only in smoke, and the transparent shifts on the others covered little. Three held packs of papirosy in their hands as they squirmed in the smoke, making the connection to the pack of *Fru-Fru* at right explicit. The love for smoke presented here moved beyond the seemingly chaste affair of the Shaposhnikov poster and on to barely shrouded carnal desire. Here, the fleshly pleasures of tobacco use were laid bare.

Images of beautiful smoking created an aesthetic attraction for tobacco use, which transcended the physical sensation to make smoking an art.[81] Beautiful smoking became cultured smoking in the figure of the dandy, and the smoking dandy breathed youth into the habit by connecting the art of smoking to current trends. The poster advertising A. Viktor and Son cartridges exemplified the look (figure 3.11). A slick gentleman of flamboyant mien and moustache stared slyly at the viewer while exhaling a thin stream of smoke. One manicured hand delicately flaunted a long papirosa while the other nonchalantly pointed to the products arrayed in front of him. Along with the careful grooming of hair, brow, moustache, and chin puff, the gentleman displayed an impressively composed outfit. His cufflinks held a hint of rose that complimented his boutonniere, cravat, and the buttons on his tweed vest. The height and stiffness of his collar gave a still more grand quality to the look as he suffered to look magnificent. Such a tall, starched collar would demand a demeanor so still as to be at odds with the

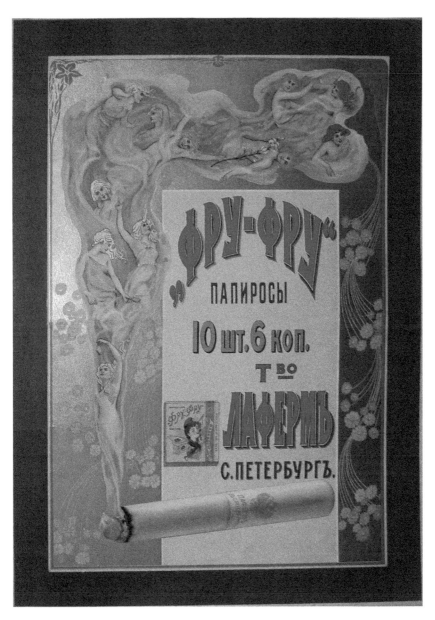

Figure 3.10 *Fru-fru* poster. 1904. Collection of Russian State Library, Moscow.

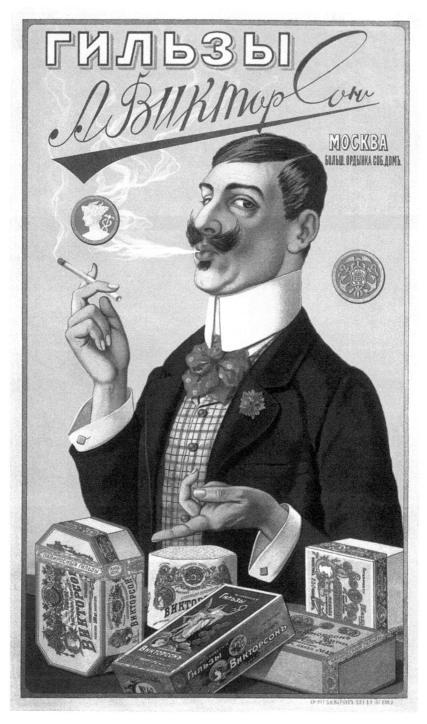

Figure 3.11 *A. Viktor and Son gilzy* poster. Prerevolutionary. Collection of Russian State Library, Moscow.

breakneck pace of the city, implying a hint of the gentleman of leisure, but perhaps also a bit of a comic figure, drawing in the smoker by encouraging him to be part of the joke and not feel like the butt of it.

The 1909 poster for Kolobov and Bobrov's *Diushes* (duchess) played with the dandy, too; it featured a pair of men, one sensibly dressed and the other flamboyantly smoking, implying a twist on the advertising stalwart of the before and after comparison (figure 3.12).[82] On the left, a young but stolid man in bowler and trench coat held a box of *Diushes*, one of the lower-priced tobaccos. When rolled they cost six kopeck for twenty. The poster advertised the even cheaper loose tobacco at little under a quarter pound for forty kopeck. His hand tentatively picked out a papirosa from the box even as he nervously darted his eyes to the left. The man to his right, however, already enjoying his inhalation of the "New! Miraculous" *Diushes*, showed none of the bowler-hatted bourgeois man's reticence. In the narrative of the poster, the boring businessman transformed through smoking to the fashionable lad—or at the very least, the comradely arm draped over his shoulder implied that he was now welcome in the community of smokers. The man at right, outfitted in high starched collar, extravagantly large boutonniere, watch chain, spats, and cane, exemplified the ostentatious yet joyful look of a dandy. The tobacco transformed him both inside and out in its promised "miraculous" fashion. A confident connoisseur, he greeted the modern world in a fully accessorized vision that included tobacco as part of the ensemble.

Fashionable smoking and celebrity genealogies gave smoking cultural capital, but the habit also gained adherents social advantages. In homosexual subcultures, tobacco etiquette signaled membership, while in memoirs and literary contemplations of wartime smoking, tobacco became shorthand for the camaraderie of the lines or the valor of individual actions.[83] For nihilistic youth, a style as well as an intellectual movement, smoking low-quality papirosy showed their rejection of convention and went hand in hand with the flouting of tradition, the triumph of utility, and the coarsening of manners in imitation of what they presumed to be working-class style.[84] A female revolutionary of the era remembered that her comrades smoked the cheap *Trezvon*, the odor of which was so pungent she had to leave the room.[85] Smoking became a ready symbol of the radical intelligentsia's quest for modern, worker-oriented, and anti-traditional behaviors in literary works from the 1860s forward. The transition in smoking styles can be seen in the landscape of radical literature as well as production figures. By 1877, progressive characters in Turgenev's novel *Virgin Soil* used only papirosy, as did those in works from Aleksei Pisemsky (1821–81), Dostoevsky, and Nikolai Leskov (1831–95).[86]

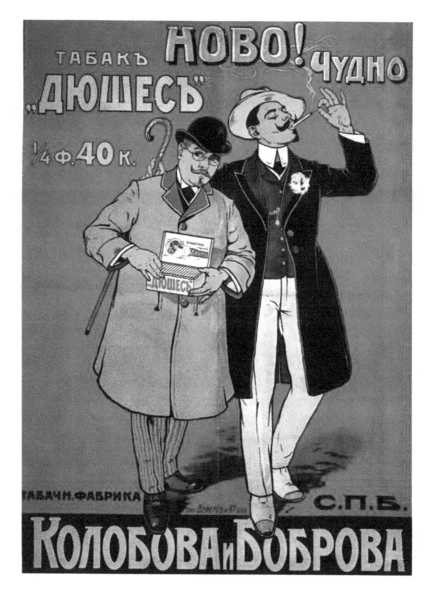

Figure 3.12   *Diushes* poster. 1909. Collection of Russian State Library, Moscow.

Sophisticated tobacco intake required accessories as well as thorough knowledge of the history, *terroir*, style profile, and production of a brand. The fashionable accouterment of tobacco changed with the method of intake. "The eighteenth century can be called the century of the snuff box," enthused a 1913 overview of the porcelain collections of the Hermitage.[87]

The same publication claimed that "the best and richest collection of snuff boxes in the world" lay in the halls of the famed museum because no other country had such widespread use of the delicate tobacco cases. Exquisite, ornate cases became a means of showing and conferring status.[88] The appearance of snuff and porcelain production coincided in Russia, leading to a run on the delicate cases, and in its early years Russia's premier porcelain factory produced little else. For the well to do, "every outfit, and almost every event in life, demanded its own snuffbox."[89] Accessories allowed for display of further class distinction in their price, number, and quality. Like the aristocratic snuff taker, the respectable smoker had the right tools of the best quality to show to others his discernment as a consumer of both material goods and tobacco.

Pipes, both water pipes (the *nargyl*) and carved pipes, enjoyed popularity in Russia in the early nineteenth century, and large collections became a material proof of respectable smoking.[90] Aleksandr Pushkin (1799–1837) had a particularly elaborate carved pipe in his collection, now on display at his house museum, and Tolstoy had his fictional protagonists smoke from the Turkish pipe in *War and Peace*. By the late nineteenth century, the papirosy case became an accessory with cross-class appeal. For the military men of the Russo-Turkish war, the silver papirosy case was an expected addition.[91] In the worker P. Timofeev's diary of his factory life, when the men of his shop struggled to find a gift for the foreman, their thoughts turned to perhaps a watch or a papirosy case.[92] Both carried an air of respectability and luxury, making them an ideal gift for the boss. Higher-end brands, with higher prices, differentiated themselves through elaborate artwork or sturdier materials for their packs, which might have been an option for those who could not purchase a silver gewgaw.[93] *Vazhnyia* for example, advertised its *portcigar* style pack (figure 1.7). Because of brand differentiation and price variation, packs themselves denoted status. Those who could not afford a full ten or twenty papirosy often bought their smokes "loose," thus to be able to purchase a full pack indicated economic power.

Ashtrays looking like slippers, shells, or other whimsical objects proved another extra where price could further separate users.[94] At times ashtrays took on more racy styles, such as one from the collections of Catherine's palace, which could be opened to show a woman nude beneath the porcelain shawl that preserved her modesty.[95] Perfumeries gifted ashtrays as part of their promotions.[96] The crossover between perfumeries and tobacco products suggested a connection between the two. Perhaps perfume was an expected necessity of the smoker to cover the scent of tobacco, or perhaps those who enjoyed tobacco's scent were expected to enjoy that of cologne as well. Maybe the ashtray became a gift for the husband and the perfume for the wife. Whatever the case, tobacco's fripperies apparently made perfect gifts for men and women. The poster for *Zvezda* included an ashtray on the desk as part of the smoking room of a guardsman, as did the setting for Fedotov's dandy (figures 1.5 and 3.6). The cover of the anti-tobacco tract, *Tabak—Iad* (Tobacco—poison), showed a fully curated table of accessories for the well-to-do smoker, apparently including a pack of tobacco, rolling papers, a pipe stand, a lighter or match case, and an ashtray (figure 4.1).

The fine mouthpiece, or holder, could be purchased to add to a smoker's sophistication, as well as a leather pouch for holding loose tobacco and a full collection of pipes.[97] The mouthpiece might have indicated concern by the user for the dangers of their habit, as some believed that distancing the burning papirosa from the face lessened harm. For those unable to afford a holder or disinclined to use one, packing the hollow tube of the papirosa with fibers might be used to filter smoke, or some even simply pinched the end of the papirosa in an accordion style. The crushing of the papirosa end allowed for the easier clench of it in the mouth while working, but also showed individualistic tendencies of the smoker as to how many times and in what ways they achieved their personal "filter." No pinch, one pinch, or three, each brought with it meaning for others to understand even as it changed the experience of the individual smoker.

Style distinguished one smoker from another according to the author's notes of a short play from 1904, "How They Quit Smoking." Every one of the seven characters in the play smoked, including the four women, and the author noted that care should be taken in their staging, as "for every smoker there is a manner of smoking in terms of how they light and snuff out a match, how they smoke a papirosa, how they hold it in their mouths, drag on it, and let out smoke, etc." In addition to showing a deft understanding of how the style of smoking might distinguish smokers, the author placed, in a conversation between his main character, the attorney Lozhbinov, and Lozhbinov's assistant Korinkin, his understanding of the intimate relationship between smoking and identity:

Lozhbinov: I cannot imagine myself without a papirosa. Me without a papirosa, that would be something . . . it would be like I was without pants!"
Korinkin: You were born without a papirosa, weren't you?
Lozhbino: I don't remember, friend. It was a long time ago! You'll need to ask the midwife.

Lozhbinov, a smoker of immense appetites, noted that he had tried to cut down and now smoked just forty papirosy a day.[98]

For those who could afford it, the trappings of cultured smoking included special clothing and dedicated spaces. The smoking jacket, an overcoat of thick brocade, protected the clothing underneath from residue of ash, odor, and loose leaf.[99] Fedotov's dandy sported the typical heavy robe and Turkish cap to protect the hair, and the smoker of the cover of *Tabak—Iad* had a thick coat as part of his outfit (figures 3.6 and 4.1) The smoking ensemble served multiple meanings in tobacco culture, feeding into imperial aspects of tobacco, displaying economic differentiation, and serving to repel scent so that others, perhaps a wife, might not smell or be repelled by the odor later.[100]

Not only clothes took on the residue. Smoke washed over furnishings to mark places as well as people. The smoking room developed in the architectural style of nineteenth-century Europe as a companion to the bedroom, where the greater the separation of the smoking space the higher the class of the smoker.[101] From early on, Russian smokers practiced a division of smoking and nonsmoking spaces by dedicating a particular room to the habit so they might indulge behind closed doors.[102] These rooms then functioned as a gendered space, a place where men retired after dinner for high-minded discussion, further reinforcing the association of tobacco with liberal, public, modern ideology.[103]

With the dedication of smoking spaces, etiquette required that a cultured smoker practice control to foreswear tobacco use in places and spaces where it was not welcome. A 1906 history of the Russian tobacco business asked for courtesy from smokers, noting that "nowadays smoking of cigars and papirosy in particular is allowed everywhere, though the well-bred and good-mannered person does not permit himself in another's house, even in a simple stand or store, to smoke a *papirosa* without the permission of the host."[104] Good manners demanded smokers consider spaces, company, and urban decorum. Where one did not smoke became as important as what and how one did smoke.

Collections of smoking accessories and specialized spaces for smoking in the home allowed users to display their economic status and distinguish themselves from other smokers of low means. Hospitality that involved tobacco showcased these objects and spaces as well as serving as a ritual honoring a guest. For example, the elite, formidable Russian dinner ended with tobacco. As one guest recalled of the celebration of the anniversary of the Battle of Plevna with Grand Duke Nicholas, "The dinner was a purely Russian one, made to suit the Russian palate, and certainly unacceptable to any other." After a full menu of appetizers, drinks, wine, sturgeon, suckling pig, champagne, kvass, roman punch, and game, the meal concluded with a "sort of pudding, sweetmeats, coffee, and cigarettes."[105] Tobacco heralded the closure of a hospitable evening.

In the home, offering a guest a smoke, and a light, became a standard for genteel sociability. The names of certain papirosy implied a specialized market for smokes for hosts to have on hand for guests, such as *Vizitnyia* (calling card) or *Kabinetnyia* (cabinet). The advertising copy for *Vizitnyia* even suggested it would be a surprise to the ladies to substitute the papirosy for candies, implying this was a standard courtesy.[106] The language of brand names and accessories indicated regularity to the process and a set of expectations. Like drinks or food, tobacco formed part of the ritual of entertaining in nineteenth-century Russia at both the highest and lowest levels, a habit that "soften[ed] the manners," according to one contemporary, and made for easier conversation.[107] To further facilitate the hosting of smoking, the "smoking candle" stood ready for the guest to allow easy lighting, though some considered the candle bad manners.[108] Not surprisingly, manners also dictated how the guest was to respond, a point that especially irked antismoking advocates. The archpriest Evgenii Popov railed against the centrality of smoking to hospitality: "You hardly have managed to sit in the chair and they ask you 'Smoke?' . . . If you refuse to smoke, it is taken as an insult to the host and forces him to smoke alone."[109] In the highly charged atmosphere of marking class and displaying gentility in the late nineteenth century, smoking eased social interactions and served as an invitation to greater intimacy, allowing for rewards far removed from nicotine's jolt.[110]

Cordiality required offerings of tobacco, ashtrays, a light, and space, though when not all were available the ritual was still observed as best the host could manage. In his memoir of the Russo-Turkish war of 1877–78, F. V. Greene detailed how in even the most humble settings, when all the necessary space and etiquette issues could not be met, Russians still included tobacco as a mark of their famed extensive hospitality. This service was not only about the guest but also the host's attempts to display respectability, minimize other deprivations, and hide any weaknesses. On the campaign Greene overnighted with a captain in the artillery, and he was overwhelmed by the generosity of his host:

> He occupied one room of a little hut. . . . His reception was in unison with that which I invariably received from every one of his class, and the open-hearted warmth of which I was often puzzled to account for. He spoke but a few words of French and German, barely more than the few phrases of Russian which I had by that time acquired, but it was enough for him to understand that I was an American. Everything was immediately placed at my disposal: my horses had the best stalls in the wretched little stable, and plenty of forage

to eat: the *samovar* was immediately set boiling for tea; whatever meat he had was at once put to cooking; his little flask of brandy was half drained to warm my chilled stomach; his chest was opened to take out the one or two delicacies which he possessed in the way of food; his one knife and fork were cleaned for my use; his servant was called a fool and a blockhead for not being quicker with the supper; his few St. Petersburg cigarettes were forced upon me; and when it was time to go to bed he insisted long and urgently, though I would not yield, that I should sleep on his camp-bed while he took the mud floor.[111]

Warm, expansive Russian hospitality decreed the provision of the best to a guest, no matter the difficulty of providing it nor the linguistic barriers to offering it. The provision of tobacco featured here as an expected part of the hospitable reception, a seal of the host's generosity and proof of his gentility. The type of tobacco further indicated the respect shown the guest—prized papirosy from the capital. In war, to be able to provide not just rudimentary but top-notch supplies signaled the status, foresight, and influence of the host.

In his memoir of a 1902 trip through Russia, Henri Troyat remarked on the full, if overpowering, nature of Russian hospitality in which tobacco played its role in differentiating each place he visited as either pleasant or fetid. After a family party, where he felt as if he were "choking with an abundance of alcohol and food," he was pleased in the last portion—a Russian papirosa "with a long cardboard mouthpiece. The tobacco had a sweet oriental flavor. Even the ladies smoked." He contrasted the civility and comfort of the evening meal among a family with his visit to a prison, where the air was "foul with the smell of boots and Makhorka" and where "smoke obscured the light of a petrol-lamp standing in the corner." The stench of rot, latrines, and vermin joined his description of the notes of scent that layered the space. Tobacco-drenched nights at the merchants club and among the Moscow students hinted at the full range of spaces, people, and activities that the smoke of the "cardboard-ended cigarettes" adorned during his trip. Troyat's remarks highlighted tobacco's taste, and especially its scent, as able to repulse or please, yet always as a marker of place and class.[112]

A gentleman did not smoke without permission of the host, and in spaces where men and women mixed, a man of higher social status asked before smoking because of the way that the smell of smoke settled not just in clothes but also in hair.[113] Tobacco's residue in a woman's hair and clothing, or at least that of cheap tobacco, might indicate that she kept company with ill-bred men or frequented public areas where smoking was allowed—the theater, the tavern, or the buffet. In the West, these scenarios indicated a woman's respectability and pushed women from the public into the private sphere, to protect their honor from threatening scents. In Canada, representatives of the Women's Christian Temperance Union argued that removing smoking from public spaces protected women's respectability, though a male backlash indicated that men saw women themselves as a type of contamination of public space. In Canada, men argued that transport gave them one of their few times for relaxation and smoking after the new, more exacting work discipline of the city.[114] In spite of the great concern from men for etiquette, Russian women seemed more accepting of smoke from guests and more prone to smoking themselves than women in much of the West, perhaps more evidence of the broad Russian hospitality.[115]

The restrictions on gentlemen's smoking were to avoid disturbing women. For working-class smokers, restrictions were imposed to avoid disturbing work. The effects on the shop floor led to smoking being fined. In *Pravda*, an account of a complaint by Barsov, a watchman who "fine[d] passing workers for smoking near goods" but regularly himself smoked all over the factory, indicated how smoking spaces could be as much a question of hierarchy as protection of goods.[116] The fine for smoking, according to another article, was the same as that for being five minutes late (ten kopek), perhaps a sign that management considering smoking work loss.[117] In addition to smoking at work being a matter of time, it could also be a problem of place. A *Pravda* article of 1912 listed smoking in "illicit places" as one of a number of "silly" fines that together totaled over 605,314 rubles in 1911.[118] Like workers, students risked fines and other disciplinary measures for smoking. One clergyman recalled how seminarians in the 1860s would endure the awful "hygienic conditions" of the privy for hours just for the chance at a quick smoke, which "symbolized their autonomy from the seminary authorities."[119]

The time or space for smoking could be limited by age, work, or income, but clubs or taverns provided both a point of sale and space for leisurely and relatively respectable use for those unable to afford smoking rooms or adorn oriental caps.[120] Beginning in 1842, tobacco could be sold in inns with food, and from 1860 onward it could be purchased and used in drinking establishments.[121] Taverns and inns were popular not just for the drink, food, and tobacco they peddled but also because they provided a place with warmth, lighting, and sociability, all at a premium in the city.[122]

The reputation of the tavern as a place of nearly impenetrable smoke, thick with masculine meaning, established itself quickly.[123] The metalworker S. I. Kanatchikov recalled in his memoir, *From the Story of My Life,* the centrality of the tavern and smoking to worker leisure, society, and culture:

> The tavern was stuffy, full of smoke, and noisy. But this was all drowned out by the powerful, ringing metallic sounds of the "orchestrion"—the so-called music machine. . . . After we had finished the vodka, Rezvov bought a pack of cigarettes and treated us to a smoke. At the time I still did not smoke, but for the company's sake I did not refuse the cigarettes and I began to puff courageously. This excessive mixing of alcohols, in combination with the cigarettes, had a stupefying effect on an "inexperienced" youth like me. I still cannot recall what we talked about at the table, under what circumstances we separated, or how I left the tavern.[124]

Kantchikov's story underscored not just the centrality of the tavern to worker sociability, but also the pressure to smoke to belong.

Be it as a guest in a home or a guest in a pub, politeness dictated that one should share tobacco "for company's sake," no matter the "stupefying effect." The pressures of sociability pushed many into smoking. According to a survey of St. Petersburg Mining Institute students published in 1902, of the 192 respondents who gave their reasons for smoking, the majority pointed to social reasons, with answers that cast this as a positive—"to be among the smokers"—and as a negative—"not being comfortable in social situations and the desire to have something in my hand." Over half answered that they began smoking for some reason corresponding to social pressure.[125] The high number of smokers reported in Russia likely contributed to social pressures that brought in new users and kept others from leaving, but there were also pushes against tobacco use. Smoking in public spaces aside from the club and tavern met resistance in Russia, just as it did in American and England, where smoking in public was forbidden in many circumstances.[126] Initial disquiet over smoking in public related to the fires that plagued the wooden structures of old Russia; later issues revolved around the smell. Alexander II officially legalized smoking in the streets of Petersburg only in 1865, and certain spaces, like the sidewalks around the Hermitage, remained smoke-free zones even after 1865.[127] Trains and steamships designated smoking cars for passengers.[128]

These earlier attacks on tobacco had been leveled when the number of smokers was still quite small, and while some, like smoking on the street, were abandoned, in other sectors anger intensified as the number of smokers rose. The rapid urbanization of the late nineteenth century, combined with greater scrutiny of malodor, the rising use of papirosy, and even, perhaps, the more pungent odor of papirosy versus pipes and cigars to create a new challenge to the order of odor.[129] Anger over the public smoker subsumed worries over contamination, class chaos, and the modern city. Upper-class smokers donned special clothing to allow them to escape these scent markers, but for lower-class smokers no such space in the home was available and no such clothing protected them. Smoke—because it wafted through the air, transgressed boundaries, clung to others, and could not be repelled—caused especial disquiet. No special clothing could protect a person from the secondhand odor of tobacco on the street, the railway, or in other public spaces.

Enticing perfumes were also important at the turn of the century. Musk deer, long prized for their glandular contributions to the Western perfume industry, thrived in Eurasia, and Russian musk earned more for its weight in trade than gold. Russia itself housed the largest perfume factory in Europe before 1914, and Russian concoctions received highest honors at world trade exhibitions.[130] Russia's advertising industry spent much time with toiletries and showed great invention in their promotion.[131] Indeed, powders and pomades were often enlivened by scent, and in central Moscow the largest pharmacy in the world produced its own line of delicate, aromatic cosmetics and soaps. As noted above, perfumeries gifted ashtrays as premiums, but further interconnections between tobacco and perfume existed. The perfumer's art surfaced in the tasks of the tobacconist, who flavored his blends of tobaccos with flowers, liquors, fruits, nuts, sweets, and savories. Scent tempered the taste of tobaccos by bringing odor to bear on the flow of sensation through mouth and nose.[132] Taste buds assess simple flavors; it was the nose that gave nuance and body to tobacco. Brand names like *Sladkiia* (sweetness), *Krema* (cream), and *Desert* (dessert) attested to the flavors of honey, sugar, cinnamon, sassafras, anise, or clove associated with certain brands.[133]

Once the smell of smoke penetrated the clothing and hair to make it noticeable to bystanders, the sensing of it meant diverse things for different classes and genders. For men, the smell of tobacco on their person indicated their social standing no matter the quality of the tobacco they consumed, because it showed they had not the means for dedicated spaces or clothing to avoid the smell of tobacco. Variations in the intensity of that scent could magnify disgust. The distinctively pungent scent of makhorka was recognizable and indicated the economic as well as social status of a smoker. In the writings of novelist Aleksei Bibik (1878–1976), workers who had progressed to the status of worker intelligentsia found themselves now disgusted by the odors in their homes, including the tobacco smells.[134] The conveniences of smoking room and jacket were not available to the worker. For those unable to launder their clothing or with a limited wardrobe the smell of tobacco could be further strengthened by unwashed apparel saturated with smoke and nicotine-infused sweat.[135]

Lingering tobacco on clothing and body occasioned disgust from non-smokers. The odor of tobacco from those around, complained one author, caused him to experience stupefaction, pains in the head and chest, and to cough. Turning the language of liberalism into a unique corner he asked, "By what right are they allowed to bring me harm?"[136] The protests against assaults on the citizen's senses mirrored arguments for protecting bodily integrity against capital punishment, torture, and other violations of the individual. Foul scent had further implications in the nineteenth century for political order and societal health. Since public smoking often came with a connotation of lower-class status, these commentaries on secondhand smoke became attacks on lower-class users from upper-class individuals. Although the smells of Russia's cities probably did not change appreciably over the century, the attention paid them, as well as the articulation of disgust, was modulated by political, social, and cultural circumstances. When Catherinian policies focused on the backwardness of the lower classes, stench became a marker of their social danger. As the century progressed and the well-ordered police state became more embedded and entrusted, this perception of the malodorous city was tempered, until the debacle of the Crimean War reanimated concerns.[137] Makhorka and its scent became therefore the smell of lower-class chaos, and the penetration of social spaces by bodies scented with its malodor a disrespect to hierarchy.

Respect for time—especially the imposition of work hours on lower-class smokers—carried its own restrictions. The *perekur* (the smoking break) became part of the lexicon in this period. The origins of this, like the machismo vision of smoking itself, came from the military. For men in uniform, the smoking break held special attractions as a respite from action and a cure for boredom.[138] The smoking break, an accepted way to gain time away from toil, translated into civilian life as a respite from the shop floor. Kanatchikov recalled how he would "slip into the lavatory" for a smoke while at work.[139] Certain shops held a strong reputation for smoking. One author alleged that fully 90 percent of typesetters smoked.[140] Time for smoking thus became a marker of respectability in the leisured class, who need not justify their breaks, while for the worker it showed their inclusion in the collective and respect for their rights.

Among the middle class, the papirosa became a companion in times of loneliness, and smoking allowed for thinking to be productive rather than boring.[141] Boredom, a word coined in the nineteenth century for an emotional state, became an increasingly problematic concept and troubled the European middle classes because of its shadings of despair and ennui. It was a problem projected onto problematic and unproductive others— women or aristocrats.[142] Smoking, often termed a cure for boredom, thus became a way to make leisure time productive either by making the break from work something more than just a break or by being associated with a spur to mental productivity and labor. Consumer culture as well became a way to triumph over boredom by presenting the unusual, thus papirosy advertisements that crowed of a "new" product or new attributes to an old product spoke to the curing of boredom by creating an original experience for the established smoker.[143]

Posters and advertisements reinforced the idea of where and when respectable smoking could take place.[144] Advertisements for Laferm connected smoking to cultured, elite leisure by placing their smokers in tuxedoes and top hats. The 1912 advertisement for *No. 6* papirosy used the already well-established trope of the monocled man of means, but this time presented him in a graphically arresting tuxedo of black and white (figure 3.13). More mature than the typical dandies, he exemplified respectability and cultured consumption. The raconteurs of the *Iar* (ravine)

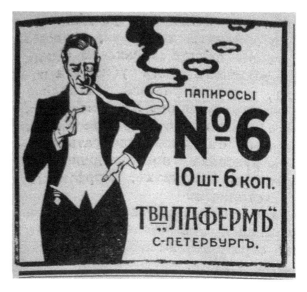

Figure 3.13   *No. 6* advertisement. *Restorannoe Delo*, 1912. Collection of Russian State Library, Moscow.

papirosy advertisement, also of 1912, were a bit more playful and indicative of a decidedly public venue (figure 3.14). All three dapper gentlemen appeared in a wide-legged, confident stance, and two stared directly at the viewer. They all donned top hats, indicating that they were outside, enjoying their mid-priced papirosy in evening dress for nighttime leisure. The public nature of the smoking showed that the correct way to indulge in respectable consumption was to be rich. The name *Iar* called to mind a popular high-end restaurant in Moscow famous for its infamous patrons—like Grigorii Rasputin—and for its mirror-lined dining room.[145] Given the placement of the advertisement in *Restorannoe delo* (Restaurant affairs), readers likely made this connection.

Tobacco use created communities, signified taste, denoted political affiliations, delineated space, and intimated status; these culturally fashioned meanings created incentives for others to take up the habit. Peasants, workers, children, and women all saw in tobacco a means to inclusion, whether it be in the public sphere, the adult world, the propertied elite, or the

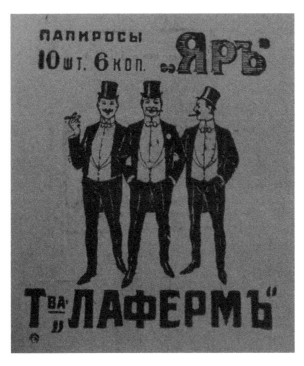

Figure 3.14 *Iar* advertisement. *Restorannoe Delo*, 1912. Collection of Russian State Library, Moscow.

sophisticated urban milieu. The city was an alienating space for newly arrived migrants. Even those who had been in the city saw a rapidly changing landscape of new buildings, technologies, transport, and ever increasing numbers of people. The city was confusing spatially, culturally, and socially. Tobacco use promised inclusion in the tavern, at work, and on the railway. An ever increasing number of newspapers, advertisements, pamphlets, and posters revealed the secret unwritten rules of how to behave and belong through direct advice on what to buy, where to purchase, and how to use. Advertisements often served as a type of urban etiquette manual for new arrivals. While advertisements clearly articulated the primacy of urban over rural ways, they also offered clues on how to create urban personae for those recently out of the village and its more collective society. Peasants entering factory life abandoned their old styles in preference for city looks by purchasing toiletries and clothing that distinguished them from the countryside they left behind and showcased their placement within the industrial and urban hierarchy.

Advertisers envisaged workers as barely removed from the village in their pitches, often using nostalgic appeals, brand names with rural themes, folk names, popular ditties, or country humor.[146] Workers, however, created in smoking their own rules for inclusion on the shop floor and in the culture of the tavern. The transition from smoking of self-rolled makhorka smokes to factory-made papirosy signified this shift. Because tobacco could indicate a generational shift as well as a geographic one, child workers displayed their transition from the countryside to the city in ways parallel to adult trajectories.[147] For Russian males, as in other cultures, smoking indicated the transition to manhood.[148] Thus smoking became for young males a way to show themselves as both urban and adult. Nineteenth-century social changes were evidenced in modified expectations for masculine behavior. Changing labor practices, the growth of capitalism, and the development of a radical intelligentsia prioritized different, sometimes conflicting character traits for the ideal man such as braininess and neurasthenic weakness or brawniness and healthful vigor. Tobacco bridged the gap in this confusing menu of manliness with scent and visual cues of either a gentleman lost in thought or a laborer taking a break, thus creating a simple yet multivalent manly marker for just kopeks a stick.[149]

Many authors attributed boys' smoking to the desire to appear manly.[150] In his 1913 essay *K psikhologii kureniia* (On the psychology of smoking), the neurologist I. A. Birshtein (b. 1876) attributed his son's smoking to his example and the boy's desire for "abstract qualities of adulthood, manliness, strength, and so on."[151] A cartoon in *Damskii mir* (Women's world) from 1909 poked fun at this idea of smoking with a discussion between a well-dressed girl and boy. According to the caption, the boy, in a fit of pique, upbraided the girl, saying: "How can you say I'm not a big boy . . . I'm not a big boy? I'm already a young man!" to which she calmly responded, "That's not true. In the first place you do not even smell of tobacco."[152] In addition to the dismissal of children's smoking as something humorous or even expected, the cartoon underscored the recognized connection of scent, masculinity, and maturity for Russian identity.

Smoking boys appeared in memoirs and cartoons but also in advertisements, indicating that this concept was humorous rather than horrifying for contemporaries. The papirosa-stealing scamp of the *Kapriz* advertisement was but one of many smoking boys sold as cute with a habit that was dismissible (figure 1.2). Shaposhnikov produced one of the most salient examples of this genre in a poster that advertised four of their papirosy brands including *Smirna, Evropeiskiia, Kabinetnyia,* and *Al'dona* (figure 3.15). The first two were in the highest price range, the last two in the middle. In the poster a youngster of perhaps eight clenched a papirosa in his teeth and prepared to light it from the box of matches in his hand. Dressed in peaked cap, jacket, vest, and pants to indicate a respectable stratum of the working class, he gave no furtive glance or skulking air to imply that he thought what he was doing was wrong or that he was worried about punishment. He smiled gently in anticipation of his first inhalation. The nonchalant way in which the coat draped on his shoulders, and the clothing itself, made it seem like he was imitating not just the smoking habit of his elders but also their styling. While children were not likely the intended audience, the visual would probably have appealed to them as well as adults. To make the case for adults, the date of the factory's founding, a seal from a major trade competition, and a slogan assuring "Papirosy of the highest quality" appeared on the right border.

Advertisements for many Russian products featured children, from cocoa and tea to confections and galoshes, indicating that cute children sold many goods, and they appeared frequently in tobacco advertisements. A series of advertisements for *Katyk* cartridges took the unexpected step of encouraging parents to purchase brands that would be less harmful when the children inevitably got hold of them. One advertisement from the series advised parents, "If your children smoke, and you cannot teach them not to with requests or punishment, then advise them, at the very least to smoke *only Katyk cartridges.* Remember that *Katyk cartridges* are produced without the touch of hands and *Katyk cartridges are the most hygienic.*"[153] *Katyk* had other rather crass advertisements, such as the newspaper appeal that

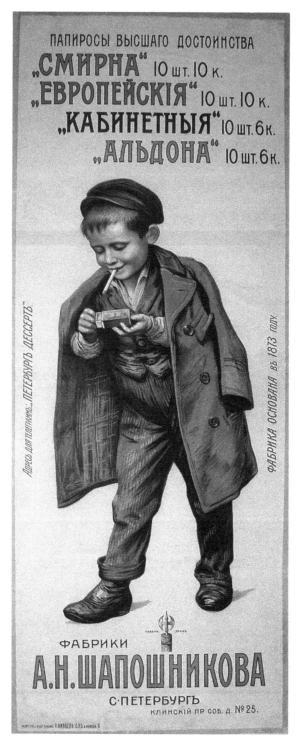

Figure 3.15 *Smirna* poster. 1900s. Collection of Russian State Library, Moscow.

featured a woman without arms to highlight the new "hands-free" machinery of the factory, but the marketers likely did not wish to be so offensive as to turn away users.[154] The appeal probably attempted to straddle the line between shocking and humorous. The dismissive attitude toward children's smoking as an unwanted yet amusing reality, along with the suggestion that the paper surrounding tobacco might be the major health concern when choosing a papirosa, indicated the relative lack of concern for this issue at the time. Instead of being a problem, smoking by boys was considered an essential step in their maturation.

Like young boys, workers, and peasants, women labored to be included in the ranks of cultured consumers and in the public spaces delineated by the smell of smoke. Although some sources reported that few women workers smoked, this did not hold true for women across class.[155] Literary works, memoir accounts, and advertising suggested that Russia had an unusually large, very active group of smoking women at the turn of the century.[156] Their numbers grew even as tobacco habits changed. Snuff had been popular among aristocratic women from the period of Catherine the Great. Russian manufacturers produced women's snuffboxes, perhaps with a mirror on the underside of the lid, for the domestic market from the late eighteenth century.[157] In the nineteenth century, the smoking of papirosy or slimmer, more effeminate *pakhitosy* gained a following among women and entered their own fashion.[158]

The painting *Girl with a Papirosa* by P. E. Zabolotskii (1803–66) was one of the earliest depicting the new style of tobacco use, and not coincidentally it showed the papirosa in the hands of a woman rather than a man (figure 3.16). Zabolotskii worked especially in the genre of romantic portraiture and played with the gently glowing, rosy tones of women's skin lit by the gentle radiance of fires of various sorts, such as *Girls Sleeping before a Candle*, although his portrait of Lermontov became perhaps his most well known work.[159] *Girl with a Papirosa*, from some time in the 1830s, indicated the relative acceptance of women's smoking at a very early point in Russia. The papirosa had barely been introduced, and yet here it served as a benign accessory to a romantic portrait of blooming womanhood. The beauty, health, and femininity of the figure were the highlights of the portrait, while the tobacco did nothing to detract from her beauty and barely merited comment it was so quotidian. Indeed, the glow of the match as the girl lit the papirosa became an enticement as it highlighted her luminous skin, the golden sheen of her hair, and her round, flushed cheeks and even hinted at her narrow waist and generous bosom.

Around the world, female smoking in the late nineteenth century was associated with the image of the New Woman, to varying receptions.[160] In

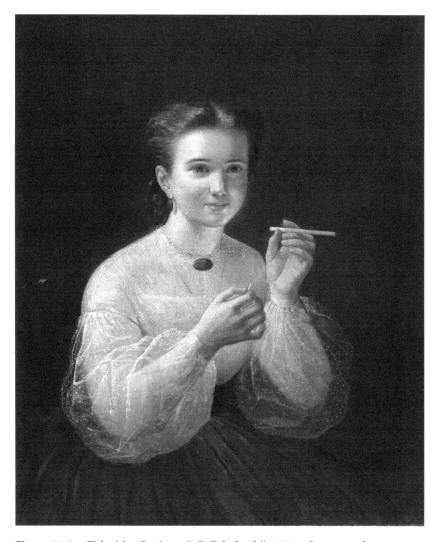

Figure 3.16   *Girl with a Papirosa.* P. E. Zabolotskii, 1830s. Courtesy of Ekaterinburg Museum of Fine Art.

the United States, public female smoking led to legislation and even arrest.[161] In China, many women smoked, but social and cultural changes marked public smoking by women as inappropriate and led to declining numbers of female tobacco users.[162] In Russia, women's smoking emerged as a political statement with the women's movement and radical politics of the 1860s.[163] Women of the nihilist movement adopted smoking along with unconventional dress and public independence to show their disregard for convention and in what was considered a denial of their femininity.[164]

Literary portrayals of smoking women fully realized the symbolic potential, where tobacco use served as an outward sign of political, social, and sexual liberation. In *Anna Karenina* (1873–77), several of the women smoke, with the evocatively named Sappho Shtolz even choosing the true papirosa over the effeminate *pakhitosa*. Leskov's *Nowhere* (1864) depicted smoking as prevalent among both genders in the young, featuring a pair of young noblewomen recently returned from Moscow who smoked as indication of their independence and their urbanity.[165] In Chernyshevsky's *What is to be Done* (1863), the smoking of the nihilist woman Evdoksiya Kukshina was but one more affectation for a political female ridiculed as shallow and silly.[166] In short fiction and stories, women similarly used tobacco as a sign of their revolutionary outlooks, youthful enthusiasm, and disdain for traditional women's roles.[167] The connection between sexual freedom and tobacco took a more sinister turn in police reports, where smoking on the street became associated with prostitutes.[168]

Fedotov, whose aristocrat breakfasting on black bread had shown the papirosa as accessory to the fashionable young man, featured the female smoker in his 1849 painting *The Modern Wife (Lioness)* (figure 3.17). Both paintings showcased the unstable status of the Russian male—in this case the wife dispensed with the many salespeople that have come to the door as the husband and child both clamored for attention. The upside down nature of the relationship—spoken in the subtitle of "the Lioness" and shown in the female negligently handling the bills while the forgotten child languished on the floor, squalling and playing with scissors—was brought to a point with the posture and actions of the wife, who gritted her teeth around a papirosa even as she leaned in most unladylike fashion, with one knee on a chair, and jutted her chin out menacingly. Fedotov's portrait of the smoking woman held none of the romantic allure of that of Zabolotskii.

In his memoir of Russian travels, Henry Sutherland Edwards witnessed the spread of Russian smoking for both men and women, arguing that it was the papirosa that allowed this, as "the delicate odour of a really fine *cigarette* is agreeable to most women," and that the "*cigarette* appears to have been adopted as a compromise between cigar-smoking, which to a certain extent excludes those who practise it from ladies' society, and no smoking at all, which is not pleasant. . . . All I wish is, to point out the fact that *cigarette*-smoking is gaining ground in England, and that, in every country where it has become general, ladies smoke."[169] Edwards correctly noted the spread of the tobacco habit to both men and women in Russia,

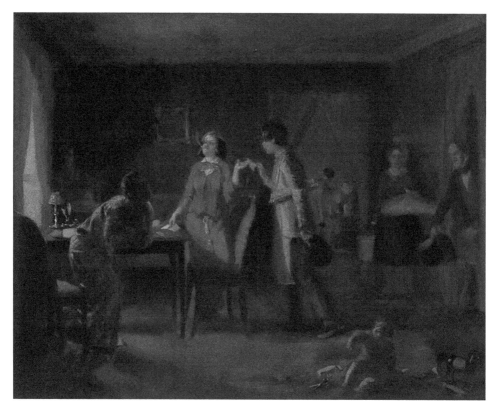

Figure 3.17   *The Modern Wife (Lioness)*. P. A. Fedotov, 1849. Courtesy of the State Tretyakov Gallery, Moscow.

and the habit did not limit itself to only the progressive and the fashionable. Despite the waggish remark from one author that to see a woman smoke was "like seeing a man knitting socks or embroidering on canvas," Russian women smoked with increasing frequency in the late nineteenth century and at a level far above their counterparts in Europe and the United States, if marketing, personal accounts, literary imagery, and general complacency about the habit can be given as indication of prevalence.[170] As one antitobacco advocate opined in 1889: "Russian women as a whole love to imitate foreigners, but in the case of smoking they have exceeded the motherly German, the elegant Frenchwoman, and the stiff Englishwoman."[171] He added, "In Russia the smoking of tobacco among women is seen as a full right of citizenship. Old women smoke, married women smoke, and unmarried women, the educated women, the uneducated women, the completely illiterate. Baronesses smoke as do their servants—the cooks, the laundresses, and the maids. In a word, all smoke—grandmothers, mothers, daughters, and granddaughters."[172] The author grumbled that elsewhere well-bred men did not smoke among women and young women did not smoke at all, but in Russia no qualms tempered the tobacco impulse.

The influence of the foreign, and especially fashionable foreigners, likely affected smoking habits for Russian women. An article in the women's fashion magazine *Modnyi svet'* (The fashionable world) highlighted the many royal women of Europe who smoked. The article "Znatnyia kuril'shchitsy" (Famous female smokers) told of the Austrian empress who smoked thirty to forty papirosy a day and her special silver case that she kept beside her bed. The Italian Princess Margarita also featured in the piece, as did a Serbian princess and the Queen of Spain. The article did note that Queen Victoria not only did not smoke, but did not like to be in the presence of smokers.[173] The stories of famed female smokers served the same purpose for women as they did for male connoisseurs—giving them both fashionable examples and a higher stratum of people to whom they could attach their behaviors. Not surprisingly, the magazine also advertised high-class papirosy from Egypt and Havana in the front and back of the same issue.

The British travel author Annette M. B. Meaken reported of smoking among Russian women as she journeyed across Russia on the Trans-Siberian Railway in the early 1900s. She recalled:

> In Russia smoking does not, however, seem to have done much harm to the women or to their children, yet the Russian woman is quite as much at home with a cigarette as her husband and brother. There are very few professional women in Russia who do not smoke The medical woman and the school teacher smoke quite as much as those who have no regular occupation. I have seen a Russian lady of means put a cigarette into her mouth as she sauntered into a fashionable shop for the purchase of ribbons and laces. The very woman who takes the greatest care of her appearance and wishes to enhance in every possible way her feminine charms is often the one most attached to smoking. I do not say, however, that even in Russia there are not to be found ladies who still cherish the old English ideas with regard to the propriety of this pastime for women.

From Meaken's description can be gleaned a vision of smoking as entrée to professional life and in no ways an obliteration of feminine charms.[174] Another British visitor, Lord Randolph Churchill, not only commented on the smoking of Russian women in the 1880s, but also noted that there was a special reception room dedicated to the practice.[175] One Russian author joked that so many professional women smoked that soon female students would be awarded port cigar cases when they graduated.[176]

The extent of societal acceptance of women's smoking by the late nineteenth century can be deduced from the widespread images of women in tobacco advertisements in Russia. These women did not appear as bait for the male smoker, as did the odalisque, but rather in imagery that underscored personal, rational enjoyment of tobacco for female smokers. Perhaps this reflected not just the more ready acceptance of women's smoking, but also the unique placement of women in the industry as owners and producers and the socioeconomic strength of women in the empire as property owners, as well as the developing women's press and the high number of women in newspapers and in journalism.[177] Perhaps in a state where all were oppressed and response ranged from armed insurrection to assassination, the danger to patriarchy of a woman smoking held less danger. Women's voting, a far more potent challenge, was similarly an early arrival to the Russian empire.[178]

The centrality of women in positive, active roles in Russian tobacco posters stood in stark contrast to tobacco marketing policies elsewhere. Advertisers in the United States and Britain did not pitch directly to women until after World War I because it was considered unseemly. American tobacco art featured either distant exotic females or, when white women were shown smoking in cards or posters, they were marginalized—actresses, prostitutes, or caricatured suffragettes.[179] Tobacco cards and packs might depict beautiful women, but these were temptations to male viewers. Occasionally, women were shown smoking, such as French advertisements for Job tobacco papers, but these art nouveau beauties in stylized labyrinths seemed more personifications of lady nicotine or lures for the gaze of men than inducements for female smoking.[180] Russian advertisers displayed no such hesitation in showing women smoking in appeals that pushed products directly toward female buyers.

In order to entice even more women to take tobacco, marketers pushed certain brands as especially appealing to female smokers. The names and copy indicated that these were blends that were sweeter. *Sladkiia* (sweetness) brand from Shaposhnikov implied a tasty blend of their papirosy with imagery directed to women (figure 3.18). The poster, which featured a beautiful young woman dolled up in feathers, flowers, and finery, implied a sweetness in the user as well as the blend. Unlike advertisements in other markets of the world, which would only feature active female smokers much later, this image showed a woman holding a papirosa and exhaling

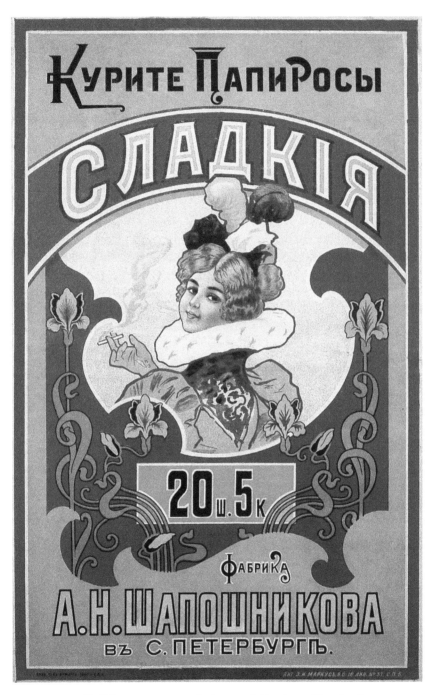

Figure 3.18 *Sladkiia* poster. Prerevolutionary. Collection of Russian State Library, Moscow.

smoke without any shame or even overtly lascivious messaging. No décolletage, unsavory companions, or questionable settings gave any hints of anything besides respectable female smoking. Not only did she smoke without societal approbation, the lilies pictured around the edges, combined with the name of the brand, and the look of the woman herself, implied none of the repulsive sensory experiences associated with tobacco in other venues. She smoked, and she smoked beautifully.

Marketers peddled the same respectable smoking to women that they did to men. Even Uncle Mikey made an appearance in a 1914 advertisement from *Put' pravdy* (The path of truth) for Shaposhnikov products (figure 3.19). With tongue firmly lodged in cheek, Uncle Mikey made an appeal to women similar to his earlier history of smoking under the tsars. Beginning with a call "to the daughters of the Scythian Kings (from a bas-relief from the excavations in Southern Russia)," he detailed the long history of women's smoking from the Scythians through the Amazonians, noting along the way that the Scythian army smoked only "Tary Bary" because of "their strength and exceptional quality" and that Herodotus established that the Scythians smoked only papirosy from the Shaposhnikov factory. Although the lineage he established was fanciful, the reference to the concurrent excavations, classical learning, and Amazonian warriors flattered

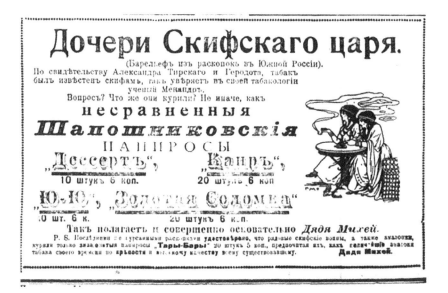

Figure 3.19 "Docheri Skifskago tsaria," *Put' pravdy*, 1914. Collection of Russian State Library, Moscow.

the female smoker's knowledge, bravery, and taste, allowing her to become part of the group of cultivated smokers and even, cheekily, the warrior smokers of the southern empire. The image of the two elegant women to the right, enjoying tobacco together, cemented the cultivated qualities of Shaposhnikov's female user. Even the social bonding pitched to men appeared here.[181] The smoking Amazon became a fitting companion to tobacco's other defender—the *bogatyr*.

The respectable female smoker of the home formed the centerpiece of a lovely 1901 advertisement for rolling papers of G. V. Frenkel of Odessa (figure 3.20). Featuring a woman in the act of smoking, this image was distinctive. A middle-aged woman with sophisticated coiffure, exquisite lace trimmed dress and petticoat, elegant hair comb, and stylish bracelets mirrored the carefully constructed look of the male connoisseur, including rational appeals to quality construction, indications of the intellectual liberation attendant to smoking, and an ode to the divine weed as both companion and beloved. At bottom, the slogan "of highest quality" assured women that they had purchased a worthy product and therefore intimated that women were capable of controlled, educated consumption. The woman's dreamy gaze communicated languor, but not sexual accessibility. She was not there for sexual objectification. Instead, her contemplative look suggested a level of intellectual engagement. The winged cupid indicated a possible focus for this wistful meditation—the divine nature of tobacco itself. In reveries of the male connoisseur, tobacco became the beloved companion, a stand-in for the spouse.[182] In this poster, the conflation of love for tobacco with actual ardor was made even more clearly by the cupid's presentation of the product. Instead of arrows to pierce the heart of the female smoker, the cupid brought papirosy.

Like men, women did not limit their smoking to the domestic sphere. Advertisers showed women out and about with papirosy, and memoirs indicated this was indeed the case. A traveler's account published in 1868 related the tale of a woman chain-smoking her way to Nizhnyi Novgorod on the train, indicating that women smoked in real life as well as fancy. Her traveling companion, who smoked cigars, joined her in a steady diet of tea and tobacco: an evening smoke at ten, another in the middle of the night, and a steady succession of them from the moment they rose until they reached their destination at ten the next morning. The observer remarked, "I thought this pretty fair work for a young lady."[183] A Laferm advertisement for Papirosa No. 7 from 1914 showed a woman not just smoking—she smoked while driving, alone, a carriage across the background of the poster.[184]

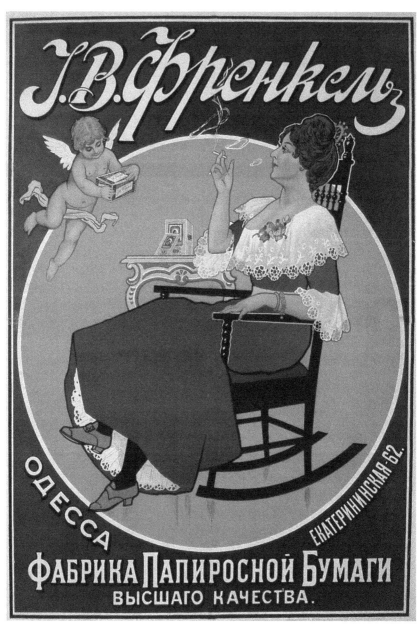

Figure 3.20 *Frenkel* poster. 1901. Collection of Russian State Library, Moscow.

Others expressed admiration for smoking women less for their stamina and more for their bravado. As one gentleman recommended, "Among the ladies there are many lovers of this pleasant poison. Therefore, if we want to be equitable, then we must acknowledge that a small, thin papirosa is far from a distraction to the beautiful ladies' lips, but gives them more readily a unique charge."[185] The frisson from women's progressive, if not trans-gressive and sexually suggestive, actions sprang from the challenge to con-temporary morality and politics that it implied. Even as it became more acceptable for some segments of society, it seemed to still be frowned on in others.

While *Sladkiia* seemed targeted directly at women, other manufacturers marketed the same brand to both men and women. In 1910 Shaposhnikov simply substituted a female for the male in their long-running newspaper advertisements for *Eva* brand. Copy and price remained the same. Only the user changed.[186] A similar switch of male and female central figures, while the composition remained essentially the same, appeared in the poster ad-vertisements of Isadzhanov in Moscow (figures 3.21 and 3.22). The striking similarity of these two posters, even down to the pose and copy, implied a normalcy for women's smoking missing elsewhere in the world. In these ad-vertising campaigns, women's smoking was the same as men's, and it might be assumed that if they did not reflect an opinion shared across society, at the very least it hit the marketers as not overly shocking an idea.

The woman smoking Isadzhanov seemed a fitting companion to *Peri*'s cockerel with her full appropriation of cultured consumption on the eve of the First World War (figure 3.22). In the poster for Isadzhanov brand cartridges of Moscow, a woman stood confidently, and publicly, on the edge of a horse paddock. Her figure, complexion, hair, outfit, and haberdashery were impeccable, and her assurance almost palpable. Unlike the odalisque, she gazed not out to invite the viewer in or ask their approval, but instead a different companion, one with whom she seemed completely satisfied, commanded her attention. With the bemused yet evaluative gaze of the connoisseur she contemplated the smoldering end of her preferred papi-rosa, which the copy assured her was made of quality paper that "will not rip in the mouth."

Like our lonely cockerel, the Isadzhanov beauty stood alone in the frame. Her social disjuncture, however, was belied by her fashionable ensemble, implied activity, and placement next to the white-fenced paddock. Her out-fit indicated that she had either just completed or was about to undertake a ride on horseback. Riding was an activity fraught with meaning in the late imperial period—from the undulating, supposedly arousing movement of

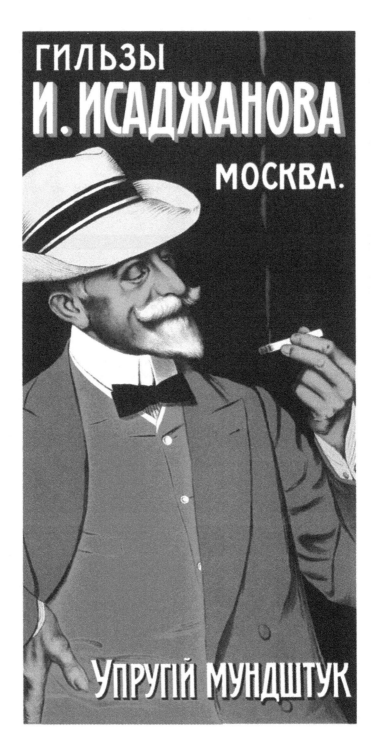

Figure 3.21 *Isadzhanov* poster. 1910s. Collection of Russian State Library, Moscow.

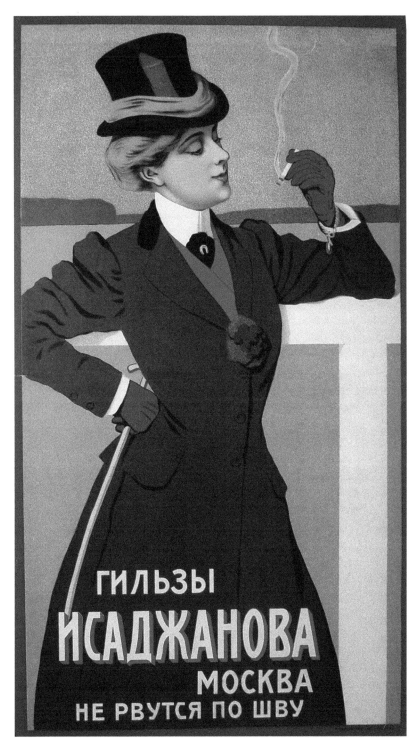

Figure 3.22 *Isadzhanov* poster. 1910s. Collection of Russian State Library, Moscow.

the horse to the freedom of movement and liberty from oversight that it implied. Not only did she smoke, she engaged in an activity outside male oversight and even, perhaps, substituting for the touch of a male. Any implications for female health were countered by her healthful figure, vigorous activities, and gorgeous complexion. Her setting and outfit—outside and in a male-style haberdashery—all implied equality to smoking women. Confident, beautiful, sexually satisfied, and socially accepted, she served as a compelling reason for women to take up the habit. Indeed, she seemed even more confident, comfortable, and integrated within society than the rooster of *Peri*. If consumption of a rationally chosen commodity conducted in public space signaled membership in the community of smokers of distinction, then the modern "Amazonian," the beloved of advertising mavens, had truly arrived in twentieth-century Russia.[187]

THE PERIOD of the rise of the papirosa witnessed rapid urbanization, mass industrialization, and the expansion of consumer culture. Smoking, which marked space, people, and political affiliation, became a means of identity creation and individuation, even as it seemed becoming part of the crowd might allow new urbanites to belong. The social dislocation of Russia's rapidly expanding, increasingly chaotic, and crowded urban setting made such appeals especially attractive. Even as tobacco offered inclusion, distinctions of taste, smell, and feel, along with behavioral expectations of where to smoke, with whom, and in what fashion, distinguished quality users and products from those who did not have good taste, proper etiquette, or fashionable habits. Manuals, fiction, art, advertisements, and examples from others showed the bourgeois male how to consume rationally, responsibly, and in an elite way. History, fame, modernity, and devotion all mixed in the appeal of the papirosa.

The etiquette of cultured smoking created both boundaries and incentives for outsiders to take up the habit. Peasants, workers, children, and women all saw in tobacco a means to inclusion, whether it be in the public sphere, the adult world, the world of the propertied elite, or the sophisticated urban milieu. Sensory impacts from smoking held central importance in the creation of boundaries and groups. Connoisseurs understood and appreciated the taste and smell of good tobacco for themselves and in others, while bad taste could be visible in packs, evident in quality of ash, smelled in the smoke, and vicariously tasted and judged. Where and how a person smoked, with whom, and why all became evidence to be used in the anonymous urban arena for discerning respectable spaces, decent people, or fashionable behaviors.

The social instability of the time created opportunities for such identity creation as well as reasons to do so. For those already in elite positions, displays of taste allowed them to shore up their recently won status in presentations of commodities and acquired habits. Excluding others for not knowing or understanding became a way to feel more secure. Decisions of what to smoke, when, and where held implications for respectability, legitimacy, and inclusion that varied according to gender, constructing political identities as well as social ones.[188] These identities, built by individuals according to their own aspirations, undermined the tsarist state's attempts to immobilize social change.[189]

Ironically, freedom supposedly came with tobacco even as the user became enslaved to the habit. The sensory and the social are both intimately linked to addictive behavior today, and the situations, tastes, smells, spaces, and social groups outlined in this chapter created situations for increasing the number of smokers, reinforcing the behaviors of those already hooked and limiting the ability of those who wanted to quit to do so. The Russian city was a maze of traps in the forms of temptations, social situations, and etiquette rules pushing them always toward smoking. Social and cultural cues worked as an addictive force akin to nicotine, and the Russian city was alive with influences.

4 : CONDEMNED

Social Danger and Neurasthenic Decline

In 1890 Tolstoy identified a series of "stupefying" substances capable of emboldening wickedness—"wine, vodka, beer, hashish, opium . . . ether, morphine, mushrooms"—and condemned them for their power to blur the distinction between the two contradictory drives of human consciousness, the "blind and sensual" and the "sighted and spiritual." Tolstoy argued that the physical, animal side of humanity and the spiritual conscience of individuals worked independently and that "all of man's life, one can say, consists in only these two activities: (1) the aligning of one's actions in agreement with conscience and (2) concealing from oneself the revelations of one's conscience so as to live one's life as before." Tolstoy acknowledged the difficulty of bringing morality and deed together, as it required full enlightenment. But the second path, doing as one wished and then finding a way to live past without tremors of conscience, could be accomplished either by distracting oneself with "external" activities or by "clouding one's conscience [zatemnenii samoi sovesti] . . . by poisoning the brain with stupefying substances."[1]

Of all intoxicants available for confusing the spiritual aspect of consciousness, of all the stupefying substances outlined in the piece, Tolstoy vilified one as "everywhere" and "probably the most generally used and most harmful," and he awarded it alone among the condemned a section entirely to itself. This third division of Tolstoy's polemic against illicit substances built at length his case against the modern scourge—tobacco.[2]

The greatest temptation, Tolstoy recalled, came to him at those moments

> when I particularly wanted to not remember that which I remembered; when
> I wanted to forget, or not to think. I would sit alone, doing nothing, knowing

that I needed to be at work and not wanting to—I smoked and continued to sit. I promised someone to meet with them at 5:00 and went to a different place; I remembered that I was late, but wished to avoid it—and I smoked. I was irritated and spoke unpleasantness to a person, and I knew that I was behaving poorly and saw that I needed to stop, but I wanted an outlet for my irritation,—and I smoked and continued to be irritated. I played cards and lost more than I wanted to—I smoked. I left myself in an unpleasant situation, I acted poorly, mistakenly, and I needed to recognize my situation to escape it but I did not wish to—I accused others and smoked. I wrote and was not happy with what I had written. I needed to throw it away but I wanted to write what I conceived of—I smoked. I argued and saw that my opponent did not understand and we could not understand one another, but I wanted to talk out my thoughts—I continued to talk and I smoked.[3]

Tolstoy depicted a thousand little cuts to consciousness that a thousand little papirosy could plaster over, allowing life to continue but never allowing for a soul that was whole.

While some might call tobacco the lesser evil compared to wine, Tolstoy said they were mistaken. He argued that tobacco not only similarly degraded morals, but in fact was even more damaging. As evidence, he pointed to a murderer of whom he knew, who had found that drink could not help him carry out his grisly task, but after smoking a papirosa "he sensed in himself the strength to return to the bedroom, slaughter the old lady, and rifle through her things." He advised, "If you wish to do something untoward, smoke a papirosa to stupefy yourself as much as necessary so as to then do that which should not be done."[4] Tolstoy depicted the desire as something beyond amusement, a habit so unnatural and so intense as to supplant hunger. His admonitions mixed physical, moral, and developmental warnings as he noted that interest in tobacco arose in boys as "they lost their childish innocence" at a point of dangerous liminality.[5]

Not just a problem for the individual's moral standing and mental abilities, tobacco use presented problems for all of society. Tolstoy pointed out that tobacco differed from other drugs because it was more intoxicating yet considered harmless. It was highly portable but did not inspire horror if consumed openly. This portability allowed tobacco products to be everywhere, and used by everyone, revealing yet another strain on the conscience from smoking. Smokers did not pay attention to the comfort of others—especially women and children. Although Tolstoy had considered tobacco a helpmate to thought when he smoked, he argued that he now understood this was not the case. Rather than inspiring thought, the profusion of ideas observable while smoking Tolstoy attributed to a lack of control. The resulting thoughts might be many, but their quality, he said, was lesser.[6]

Tolstoy's aversion to tobacco emerged later in life. As Tolstoy's son noted in a 1939 essay, his father had been like most fathers early on and ate meat, drank, and "smoked the whole day long."[7] In the 1880s, however, the elder Tolstoy came to an epiphany to eschew meat, alcohol, tobacco, and sex and embrace an abstemious lifestyle. Of all the pleasures of the flesh, tobacco proved the most rooted. As his son noted, "What was most difficult for my father to give up was smoking, and many times he came back to his old habit. It was a real need for him to smoke while writing. But in the end he succeeded in overcoming even that weakness."[8] Tolstoy's personal struggle explained his focus on tobacco as the most dangerous of all.

Tolstoy did not just preach a life of abstention, nor did he just write essays on his choices, or serve as an example for others; he also advocated for the publication of antitobacco and antialcohol tracts and formed an organization to fight for temperance—the Union against Drunkenness (Soglasie protiv p'ianstva).[9] While only about a thousand ever joined his group, its impact and the influence of others like it was much larger. Tsarist authorities regarded independent organizations with suspicion, and because of the taxes raised from manufacture of both alcohol and tobacco, temperance groups were doubly dangerous. Tolstoy's stance against stupefying substances brought him into conflict with the state, which profited handsomely from the vodka monopoly begun in 1894 and to a far lesser extent from tobacco excise taxes. In 1901, in the aftermath of his continued disputes with state and church on a variety of issues, including the divinity of Christ and the authority of Church and State generally, the Russian Orthodox Church excommunicated Tolstoy.[10]

Others before Tolstoy decried tobacco's dangers to man and morals, but Tolstoy's admonitions came at a crucial time. The uptick in tobacco production and consumption and increasing visibility of the habit in the burgeoning urban areas coincided with rising concerns for popular health, a developing medical profession, an increasingly literate population, and a flourishing boulevard press. The newspapers, journals, pamphlets and books left a ready record of the anxiety surrounding tobacco consumption. Although some authors were motivated from a religious standpoint to borrow Tolstoy's words or those of certain spiritual leaders, others came to their antipathy for tobacco from the fields of medicine, criminology, sociology, or psychiatry, part of a rising tide of professionals dedicated to medicine and the human sciences.[11]

Shared condemnation created strange combinations of comrades in cessation. Medical experts drew material from moral reformers. Statisticians dipped into case histories and anecdotal speculations. Moralists employed commentary on etiquette and style. Russian Orthodox authors mentioned with approval the antitobacco stance of Old Believers. As in other countries, no single approach dominated antitobacco literature, but common themes united the works—the danger of smoking to the social fabric, to the individual body, and to the future of the race. In pamphlets, lectures, and articles, moralists and medical experts worried over what they considered the rude, asocial behavior of smokers, the poison of nicotine for nerves and the brain, the neurasthenic complications of autointoxication, and the racial degradation sure to follow.[12]

A consensus emerged in antitobacco works in the late nineteenth century that tobacco use endangered contemporary society and the future through a poisonous process triggered by nicotine that passed the moral and physical weaknesses of one generation on to the next. In their attacks on tobacco, antitobacco advocates expressed their anxieties over the future of Russia, the behavior of youth, the emancipation of women, the decline of patriarchal control, and the direction of the country generally. Neurasthenia, a nervous disorder that endangered men and women's nerves, minds, and procreative abilities, emerged in antismoking works from religious and moral authorities as well as medical and psychological figures. These interdisciplinary tracts spoke also to international connections by revealing the relationship of Russian commentators to the primary bogeyman of contemporary Western social criticism: national degeneracy. As social disturbance intensified in the early twentieth century, such language became increasingly prominent, and the language of degeneracy, slippery and adaptable, allowed for diagnoses that applied to many ills, caught public attention, mirrored a popular mood, and gave rising professionals an eye-catching platform.[13] The same strategies used by advocates and marketers to push for tobacco use as a symbol of imperial domination, masculine power, and sexual strength revealed themselves in antitobacco tracts as worries over tobacco-induced weakness, flaccidity, and social disruption. The foundations of condemnation lay on the same stones as those of advocacy.

IN THE DECADES before the outbreak of World War I, a flood of popular literature swept through Russia and met a ready audience of new urbanites, many barely removed from the village but emboldened by the economic and social mobility afforded by the emancipation of 1861 and the opportunities of industrialization and urbanization.[14] Growing literacy, increasing incomes, new technologies, and entrepreneurial hunger for novel markets and endeavors spurred the rise in reading material. While rural literacy rates remained low, urban rates reached as high as 70 percent in some regions by the eve of World War I. Literacy functioned as a tool for social mobility for middle- and lower-class immigrants to the city, but not all pursued a purely utilitarian reading list. A flourishing press of light fiction spread messages that resonated with the population and reflected a "consumer sovereignty" rather than only a top-down approach. A profusion of chapbooks, thin journals, and newspapers made their way into the greedy hands of voracious urban readers.[15]

Popular fiction catered to mass tastes with detective stories, fantasies, and war stories, while works of a more didactic nature appeared in the form of popular science and medical advice, moral commentaries, and behavior manuals—works that helped the newly urban to negotiate written and unwritten rules of class, etiquette, and urban life.[16] The publishing firm Intermediary (Posrednik), started in 1884 by Tolstoy in cooperation with his colleague V. Chertkov and publisher I. D. Sytin, was one of the most successful at wedding paternalist impulses to popular tastes. In its first four years it published more than twelve million copies of works and distributed treatises by other presses for a total reach of twenty million volumes through the empire.[17] Tolstoy urged the press to produce titles that promised not esoteric or scientific knowledge, but instead gave concrete answers to how to live according to these messages of sobriety. Starting in 1888, the firm issued pamphlets with mixes of science and morality alongside abstinence in titles like "Be Sober!" or "Stop Smoking!"[18]

Religious groups put out pamphlets against smoking as part of their general moral mission. Mount Athos's St. Panteleimon Monastery published brochures throughout the 1890s and early 1900s, including the 1896 *Kakoi vred prinosit cheloveku tabak?* (What danger does tobacco bring a man?) and the 1901 epic *O p'ianstve i drugikh bogoprotivnykh privychkakh kurenii tabaka, skvernoslovii, penii mirskikh pesen, igrishchakh, kataniiakh, sueverii i bozhbe* (On drinking and other offensive unto God habits—smoking tobacco, cursing, singing sea shanties, games, rolling, superstition, and oath making).[19] Religious authorities were not the only ones to jump into the publication of antitobacco tracts. Experts in medical and psychological diseases authored their own polemics. The famous clinician S. P. Botkin offered *Vrednyie posledstviia ot kureniia tabaku* (The dangerous effects of smoking tobacco), which appeared to be mainly a pasting together of materials from two pamphlets by other authors to which he loaned his name and reputation.[20] These works echoed those of popular fiction writers, who lionized the scientific, medical, and technological triumphs of the age.[21]

The publication of brochures and articles on tobacco did not necessarily mean that people bought them, read them, or followed their prescriptions, but the steady appearance of antitobacco titles and articles over the years suggested that the topic retained a strong market or at least consistent visibility and interest. Multiple editions of certain works, like the nine versions of P. K. Komisarenko's *Pagubnoe privychka* (The ruinous habit), perhaps indicated a solid audience for particular messages.[22] Additionally, the spread of these ideas into other venues, including posters and public lectures, revealed the reach if not its reception.[23] The title page of the 1890 pamphlet by the female doctor M. Valitskaia, who followed the health of factory women, identified the publication as emerging from a presentation she had previously given at a Pedagogical Museum in St. Petersburg.[24] S. A. Beliakov's pamphlet noted that he had given the material as a lecture in 1904 at the People's House in Samara.[25] Other publications showed a message aimed at readers as well as live audiences at urban and rural assemblies.[26]

While there was some change over time in the science of pamphlets, for example in the inclusion of bacteriology, there remained a remarkable consistency in the rhetorical styles. From the 1845 work by Dr. Bussiron, *O vlianii tabaku kuritel'nogo, niukhal'nogo i tsigar, na zdorov'e, nravstvennost' i um cheloveka* (On the effect of smoking, snuff, and cigar tobacco on the health, morality, and mind of man), to the misleadingly titled 1888 cessationist tract, *Tabak: Sredstvo izbavit'sia ot mnogikh boleznei* (Tobacco: A method to escape many diseases), which remained in print all the way up until 1910, the points and style of the argument stayed steady.[27] References to, and liberal borrowings from, other works appeared frequently, sometimes without attribution, but most often the referenced work was praised at length, with the name of the author featured prominently. Valitskaia's studies on the health of factory workers, Dr. Il'inskii's data on tobacco's effects on individual bodies, and Metropolitan Filaret's (Drozdov, d. 1867) and Tolstoy's diatribes against tobacco as moral corruption all made it into multiple works across the period, lending continuity to the message across pages and through decades.[28]

An essay by Dr. A. L. Mendel'son (1865–1940) typified the antitobacco argument, and its easy slippages between medical expertise, popular appeal, public health initiative, and spiritual campaign. A lecture he gave in the late 1890s took on a second life as an article in the *Zhurnal Russkago obshchestva okhraneniia narodnogo zdraviia* (Journal of the Russian Society for the Protection of Public Health) in September 1897. Not just an author and a public speaker, Mendel'son's professional standing assured that his voice resonated beyond the speaker's hall and the journal's pages.[29] A doctor of medicine and specialist in nervous disorders, he rose within a decade to be the leading physician for the cure of alcoholism for the St. Petersburg

Guardianship of National Sobriety publishing widely on neurasthenia, sobriety, and psychological disorders.

Mendel'son followed a common style for antitobacco activists, relying on a mixture of foreign expertise and Russian statistical studies to condemn tobacco as a poison to youth and nation. Statistical analyses held powerful authority in the late nineteenth century even when samples were small and methodology sloppy.[30] An 1883 statistical study of students in St. Petersburg formed the center of Mendel'son's lecture and provided the foundation for his conclusions. A survey of 1,071 students—556 medical and 515 technical—found 54.66 percent of medical students smoked, averaging about 19.64 papirosy per day. The survey found that 47.18 percent of technical students smoked an average of 22.88 papirosy per day.[31] This compared favorably with the military, where Mendel'son noted an 1891 study had found 68.1 percent of soldiers and officers smoked.[32]

While in other contexts, authors decried smokers as frivolous or immature in their habits, for medical students Mendel'son held some sympathy as he attributed their smoking to "the necessity of working in practical anatomy in malodorous fumes that cause many to run for the papirosa as the tobacco smoke might drown out the smell of rotting corpses." In this case, a benefit to tobacco often forgotten—the cover provided by the smell to other more unpleasant odors, or the lingering belief that malodorous fumes might trigger disease and tobacco could counter that—became a permissible reason for smoking. Mendel'son posited that the first-year anatomy course recruited many to the habit, which they abandoned after leaving the dissection theater.[33] This was an argument made elsewhere for the prevalence of smoking among doctors and contained a class-based dispensation as well as one for professional courtesy.[34]

Mendel'son jumped from arguments based on consumption statistics to data on illness, identifying three major health consequences from smoking: problems with breathing, eating, and both eating and drinking together. Confronted with greater illness among the medical students than among the technical students, who consumed more tobacco, Mendel'son suggested environmental and social reasons. Technical students had a better cafeteria, hence they were healthier. Additionally, they were more likely from the provinces or were "realists" instead of "classical academics," and thus less likely to suffer from exhaustion, a coded term for neurasthenia.[35] While he connected the poison from tobacco to chronic catarrh because of the irritation of throat, nose, and lungs (the result of swallowing tobacco infused saliva), he also pointed to digestive problems (dyspepsia, constitution, and flatulence), and possibly tuberculosis, as coming from tobacco.

By far Mendel'son's greatest concern came in worries over tobacco's impact on neurasthenics, especially those upper class sufferers who were seen as most susceptible—"the intelligent workers, government officials and all kinds of employees in the public and commercial institutions." To combat this pressing issue, he urged the population to stand up against smoking, especially among children. If smokers quit, which only sixty-one of the 547 smoking students had managed to do, Mendel'son's statistical analysis assured them that their medical problems would stop and all would be well.[36]

Mendel'son joined moral and religious appeals to his numbers and scientific references, such as an epigraph from Metropolitan Filaret: "Is it not strange that people devised for themselves a new type of hunger, which nature did not know, and a new type of food, of which she had not conceived? By means of this habit [*privychka*] they have left themselves to its unnatural whims and multiplied their number of needs, making necessities of the superfluous."[37] The words of a religious figure on the sinful, unnatural essence of tobacco use began Mendel'son's pamphlet, setting the stage for a scientific discussion of a public health problem with an ethical commentary. This mixture of messages—from moral to medical—reflected the jumble of ideas in antitobacco works as a whole. While clearly different camps participated in the campaign, they borrowed weapons from their comrades in arms.

Case histories, often copied from European scholarship that was available in translation or had been used by others, figured heavily in Russian antitobacco tracts from both medical authorities and religious pundits.[38] The story of an infant sent into convulsions after his head was slathered with a tobacco ointment was part of works by others in 1845, 1871, and again in 1906.[39] The anecdotal case of two brothers who smoked, respectively, seventeen and eighteen pipes in a row and then both keeled over first emerged in a journal in 1859 and later found its way into the 1887 multiedition pamphlet of Archpriest Popov and then scores of others by doctors and religious authors for the next several decades.[40] Another popular tale from an 1868 *Moskovskaia meditsinskaia gazeta* (Moscow Medical Gazette) that showed up all the way into the 1900s followed a woman who fell asleep on a pile of tobacco leaves, never to awaken again.[41] The fantastical nature of many of the anecdotes undercut the serious message that the pamphlets tried to impart. The military officer who became unconscious when chewing tobacco for a toothache, the smoker who spontaneously lost his sight and then was stricken with paralysis, the forty-four-year-old man who smoked four cigars in four hours and became comatose, or the gentle soul who died having entered an overly smoky room—all seemed more myth than science.⁴² The stories read like reverse miracles for the age—a type of spontaneous magic medical death. When readers saw so many around them who went through the exact same situation and did not experience such fantastical effects, the strength of the argument paled.

Serious comment and scholarly detachment suffered in the service of anecdotal allure. Dr. V. I. Zasidatel'-Krzheminskii, the house surgeon for the Clinic for Nervous Ailments at the University of St. Vladimir, recounted two case histories of smoking-related illness. After doing so, the doctor admitted that he indeed was the source of the second case because he had once suffered from tobacco, but his pains had completely disappeared when he quit smoking.⁴³ In the 1891 *Ne kuri, ne niukhai i ne zhui tabaku (Pis'mo uchenogo i opytnogo vracha)* (Don't smoke, don't snuff, and don't chew tobacco [A letter from a learned and experienced doctor]), the author confessed that because of smoking, "I was already almost deaf and blind and coughed up blood!" When advised to quit, he sought a second opinion from a well-known doctor and pharmacist, whose letter of reply concentrating on the toxic nature of nicotine and the benefits of quitting became the bulk of the pamphlet.⁴⁴

While many works combined scientific, statistical, moral, personal, and medical rhetoric, the specific points brought against tobacco varied. Historical precedent anchored numerous antitobacco tracts to lists of historical figures who resisted tobacco. Attempting to borrow legitimacy from history for their contemporary antipathy to tobacco, authors recounted the long, broad narrative of antitobacco forces. Heroes to the cause were King James I of England/James VI of Scotland (d. 1625), with his *Counterblaste to Tobacco* (1604), Sultan Murad IV of the Ottoman Empire (r. 1623–40), infamous for his executions of tobacco users, and Tsar Aleksei Mikhailovich (r. 1645–76), who meted out beatings and flayed nostrils for those who used or traded tobacco.⁴⁵ Professor I. M. Dogel of the University of Kazan detailed a full history from ancient Mexico to France, England, and Spain in his published speech on the dangers of tobacco.⁴⁶ Dr. Rokau began his 1885 diatribe with a thorough history of tobacco's introduction to the world and the response of governments and authorities, as did Dr. Bek in his 1902 book.⁴⁷ Dr. F. A. Udintsev included the familiar list of antismoking historical figures—kings and popes and sultans—in his 1913 *O vrede kureniia (Nauchno-populiarnyi ocherk)* (On the danger of smoking [A popular-science essay]).⁴⁸

The prohibitions against tobacco enacted by the first Romanovs earned the most play both within Russia and outside it as foreigners saw the brutality as proof of Russia's barbarism, and Russians saw the early and lengthy ban as evidence of their foresight.[49] In 1634 Mikhail Fedorovich Romanov (r. 1613–45) issued a decree forbidding possession, use, buying, and selling of tobacco, giving rise to draconian punishment for infractions.[50] Bek and Rokau both carefully noted that the law resulted from the patriarch's disgust over the smell of tobacco and the tsar's worries over its role in fires.[51] Bek explained the overturning of the ban by Peter the Great in 1697 as a craven, money-making ploy that then opened up Russia to her current status where smoking poisoned the population alongside alcohol, and everyone—young and old, male and female, rich and poor—smoked more and more.

Antitobacco enthusiasts compiled lists of other famous figures who decried tobacco—Johan Wolfgang van Goethe (1749–1832), Victor Hugo (1802–85), Honoré de Balzac (1799–1850), and Alexandre Dumas (1802–70)—creating a type of reverse celebrity endorsement.[52] Others testified from beyond the grave tobacco had dug for them. The pamphlet *Bros'te kurit'* revealed that America's Ulysses S. Grant (1822–85) died from smoking cigars.[53] In 1912, Dr. Tregubov added Mark Twain (1835–1910) alongside Grant.[54] A French author died from a glass of wine poisoned by nicotine, warned several other pamphlets.[55] Bodily disturbance centered the tale of the American president William McKinley (1843–1901), who became constipated when quitting tobacco and experienced a "copious bowel movement" a half hour after smoking a cigar on a doctor's recommendation, though the merit or detriment of tobacco remained unclear in this example.[56]

An argument against tobacco uniting Tsar Mikhail, Botkin the clinician, and religious commentators was the danger of tobacco use sparking fires in the countryside and the city.[57] One of the more colorful denunciations of the smoker as accidental arsonist came from the 1904 pamphlet of I. V. Ponomarev, who railed that smokers started fires "on the street and in the yard, in the hayloft and the stable, in a word everywhere; even on the smoker himself flames shoot up, as can be seen on almost all their over-clothes with holes or a shirt singed by papirosy. If they cannot protect themselves, can we think that they could be careful with a flame, especially when not sober?"[58] Prohibitions on smoking supposedly emerged from concerns over fires in Russia's largely wooden cities, and well into the twentieth century reports regularly blamed poorly discarded papirosy for fires in the city and the countryside.[59] The moral opprobrium of Ponomarev paled in comparison to that of Popov, who lamented in a footnote that "the main thing is these arsonists are unpunished because it is hard to convict them. Their judgment will be the terrible judgment of Christ."[60]

Many pamphlets began with historical figures and arguments, but moved into modern ideas regarding economy, social obligation, and the role of the citizen. The waste of the state's resources thumped a steady drumbeat of derision for tobacco from both medical and moral authorities. Dr. Preis, a hygiene instructor in Kharkhov to children, workers, and tradesmen, lamented that cultivation and manufacture of tobacco exhausted the best land of the empire on the banks of Crimea.[61] A similar cry to save the land echoed in the religious appeal of Popov.[62] The 1906 Old Believer pamphlet, *Neskol'ko slov o tabake i ego upotreblenii* (A few words on tobacco and its use), bemoaned the misuse of agricultural fields, resources, and labor.[63] In a call that resonated for nation and health, Dr. D. P. Nikol'skii wrote that tobacco cultivation was not just hard on the land but it made it unsuitable for growing grains for bread. A decade later, A. Appolov lamented that tobacco had "begun to replace bread" among Russians, whereas if the harvest in tobacco were a harvest in grain it could feed 150,000 people.[64]

While the tax on tobacco might be helpful to the coffers of the state, the monks of Mount Athos maintained that costs, in terms of the health of the population and the decline in their morals and strength, more than outweighed the revenue.[65] Others made a similar calculus.[66] The preference for tobacco over bread in the family budget anchored appeals just as economic arguments of wasted farmland.[67] The logic came straight from antialcohol rhetoric. As Rokau argued, "The drunkard denies his family bread in favor of drink. The smoker denies himself bread in favor of smoke."[68] Pamphlets informed readers that the yearly expenditures on tobacco could purchase a home or a library.[69] Not surprisingly, reformers regarded this exchange as especially irresponsible and shameful in the poor.[70]

Authors identified time as another thing lost to smoking, though not just the time of the smoker but also the time of manufacturers that could be used elsewhere or the time of others, such as the customers waiting on a clerk who took a smoke break.[71] In the new industrial age, arguments based on wasted time and money held particular resonance, but such advice had appeared earlier and elsewhere. In eighteenth-century China, the Confucians decried tobacco as a waste of land.[72] In the twentieth-century United States, businessmen like Henry Ford said they would not hire smokers because their habit was a drag on productivity. Ford publicized the problem of the smoking worker in his volume, *The Case Against the Little White Slaver*.[73]

The social failings of the smoker enlivened pamphlet attacks, directing a litany of complaints against the character of users like "all smokers and drinkers are irritable, bleak, contemplative, and constantly feel frustration if the one does not smoke or the other does not drink."[74] Archpriest V. Mikhailovskii detailed the many ways that smokers inconvenienced their fellows, including the disgust nonsmokers suffered from being near a smoker with their filthy teeth and the danger to clothes and furniture as smokers scattered their ash everywhere, in his multiedition tract, *Tabak i vrednoe vliianie ego na cheloveka* (Tobacco and its dangerous effect on man). He elaborated on the many unpleasant behaviors associated with smoking as smokers begged papirosy off others and erupted into moody tempers over bad leaves or poor papers. He moaned that smokers created an unpleasant society for all around them.[75] Archpriest Arsenii pointed with disgust at the papirosy butts that littered the streets, as did Tolstoy.[76] *O kurenii tabaku* (On smoking tobacco), another multiedition pamphlet, highlighted the unpleasant nature of the smoker who railed against his lack of tobacco.[77]

Popov denounced the untoward effects on civil exchange from smoking, where smoking began "for want of conversation" and then continued until smoking became a part of every conversation. A serious discussion was impossible with a smoking youth: "Notice how his attention quickly slackens: He—and here is the deal—he quickly turns to look elsewhere at his tobacco or he takes from his own pocket a papirosa. In a word this person becomes shallow if in his eyes or in his hand there is tobacco."[78] Smokers disturbed others most seriously with their smoke. "Especially dangerous is the effect of tobacco smoke on those who do not smoke," cautioned Nikol'skii.[79] Another author concluded, "On the smoker there lies a huge moral reckoning for the evil which he has brought to others forcing them to breath in the smoke of his papirosa."[80]

Smoke contaminated the entirety of the city's public spaces with its disgusting odor, according to Popov: "In a word, there is almost nowhere that you can escape the smell of tobacco. Tobacco pours over you on the sidewalks of the roads. You meet tobacco and it accompanies you in service and public areas (banks, council, and other offices). But what of sacred places? Inside church walls? There the impatient smoker, leaving the church, often right away lights up, or during the time of service runs to the entryway or bell area so as to smoke, so that the smell of tobacco often flows onto the church porch."[81] Adolf Fedorovich Grinevskii concluded in his multiedition pamphlet, *Bros'te kurit'!* (Stop smoking!), that the cities were already awful in terms of living space and air, so why add "voluntary and conscious systematic self-poisoning!"[82]

E. S. Krymskii echoed the lament over the pernicious, floating menace that flowed from the smoker: "Look at the people walking around the city streets. How many of them have a cigar or papirosa in their mouth! Almost everyone smokes. Go to the railroad station in the wagon of the train, in the buffet of the theaters—in these areas it is hard to breathe and for those unaccustomed to smoke, it is absolutely detrimental. How the air is spoiled![83] For Krymskii, smoking in public seemed both omnipresent and particularly objectionable.

Of the many urban spaces tainted by smoking, one of the most discussed and regulated was the railroad wagon. The railroad became a battleground for smoking rights in Europe, America, and Canada, and a similarly charged atmosphere existed in Russia in the late nineteenth century, perhaps made more heated by the more prominent place of smoking in the environment.[84] One foreigner observed that because earlier regulations forbade smoking in the streets, the railway became a refuge for smokers. After his 1861 visit he remarked, "It was curious, after passing through the narrow thoroughfares of the capital and not meeting with a vestige of tobacco, to find at the first station . . . the last place where we should expect to find them in England—a multitude of smokers; in fact, the whole body of travellers, women as well as men, inhaling and exhaling the fumes of the fragrant *papirosses*."[85] Other regions of the world outlawed street smoking. Boston forbade smoking in the streets in the 1840s.[86] Some prohibitions came out of fear for fires, others out of distaste for the smell and litter.

A quarter of a century later, the rampant railway smoking of Russians would come under scrutiny. In 1886, the Railway Ministry called for special nonsmoking wagons, but regulation did not mean compliance, and a 1911 clarification from the railway industry for the full meaning of "no smoking wagon" revealed the ways in which laws were sometimes unable to dictate behaviors and how the passengers might have been circumventing previous strictures. The ministry specified that no smoking would be allowed in the corridors or bathrooms of a nonsmoking car and, most amusingly, that "in wagons and spaces set aside for nonsmokers, the smoking of tobacco is not permitted even if a general vote is held of those in the wagon or it is approved by the conductor."[87] Posters adorned railway cars asking smokers to more carefully discard their butts because of fire hazards.[88]

The waste, inconvenience, danger, and rudeness of smokers joined in a vision of a group who cost society rather than improved it, who imposed on others rather than contributing to their welfare, and who pushed fellow citizens from the very public spaces that allowed civil exchange. As citizenship became a marker of membership in the modern political community and urban environment, and advertisers promoted social inclusion as a feature of tobacco purchase, antismoking advocates displayed a different vision of smoking as antisocial, uncivil, and a threat to liberal values. Preis summed up this sentiment: "People who drink and smoke waste their free money and not a little time on the buying of tobacco and wine. They are rude to the people around them (ash, cinders, spit), people dirty the air of rooms (smoke, wine steam), and smokers in an inebriated frame set fire to homes, the countryside, and even people. In the end how much land and bread is lost in the production of tobacco, wine, vodka, and beer."[89] These problems, unlike smoke itself, did not dissipate. In an undated wartime pamphlet, Dr. A. F. Gamalei lamented that usually one would shun a room with "an unusual smoke, unpleasant odor, and dust," but the acceptance of smoking meant that "we quietly live with this day after day." He described the epic span of the problem and the lack of empathy from smokers

> at home, at the train station, in the wagon, and the passages, in the restaurants, clubs, etc. The smokers respond to nothing—not the natural protests of the child's organism, the protests of good will from non-smokers, or the posters on smoking. Nor domestic comments of the filth of tobacco, ash, and butts . . . not the pumping of smoke into the apartment, hair, and clothing of themselves and others. . . . Smokers respond with laughter to any comment and simply force all to breathe their disgusting exhalations. Even on the streets, there is no safety from tobacco and cigar smoke and often . . . smoke wafts into the eyes while walking or even riding in a [horse] carriage.

He noted that makhorka made it all infinitely worse, bringing class connotations to his social commentary.[90] Makhorka, with its lower cost and stronger smell, echoed in tobacco form the vision from the upper class of the masses as coarse, vulgar, and far too present in the city.[91] The fears over the wafting scent of their vile habits betrayed a disgust with the urban necessity of sharing spaces with those of lower rank and ranker odor.

By harnessing appeals to civil discourse, etiquette, history, and fiscal responsibility, antitobacco authors created a picture of the smoker as anticitizen, antisocial, and anticonnoisseur. The 1911 cover for Dr. E. Meier's *Tabak—Iad* visually presented the inversion of respectable smoking (figure 4.1). At left, a botanist's drawing of a tobacco plant borrowed the authority of scientific observation for the contents of the pamphlet. The titled expertise of Meier elevated the pamphlet over minor speculation. At center, the respectable man, smoking in a private space, well appointed with accessories, and in proper attire, indicated both the intended audience and the responsible party. Interestingly for an antismoking pamphlet, the featured man actively smoked, rather than being a healthy nonsmoker, or

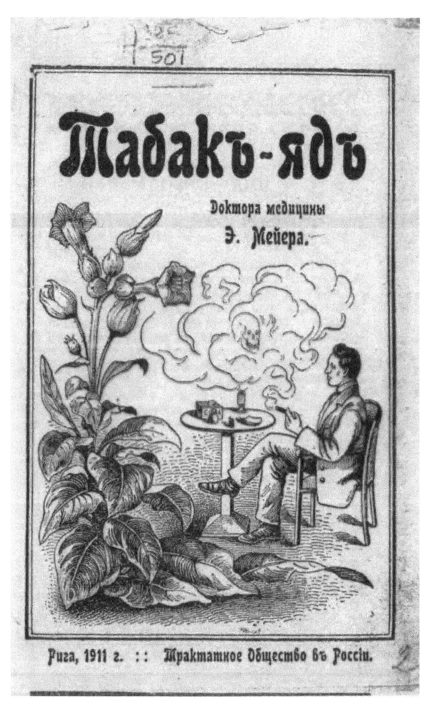

Figure 4.1 Cover, Dr. E. Meier, *Tabak—Iad*, 1911. Collection of Russian State Library, Moscow

even presented in contrast with someone who had quit. The hidden, future danger of tobacco to even a healthy smoker, however, hovered in the air above in the form of a jeering skull.

In addition to highlighting the danger to the social fabric from smoking, antitobacco authors agreed on the individual effects from tobacco. Although authors detailed many toxins that emerged in the smoke of tobacco, they focused, from the 1840s to the late tsarist period, on nicotine. The alkaloid, discovered in the early nineteenth century, became in all sources the primary danger of smoking to one's health.[92] The rhetoric did not center on the addictive qualities of nicotine or its status as a carcinogen, points that now focus research, but instead on its poisonous qualities.[93] A funeral procession of animals—frogs, rabbits, cats, dogs, and horses—proved nicotine's poisonous effects in lectures, labs, live demonstrations, and pamphlet descriptions.[94] Religious tracts included the physical poisoning of nicotine as part of their attacks alongside moral considerations.[95] While a capful could kill most animals, a favorite statistic was the amount that an average smoker (twenty papirosy a day) would ingest in a lifetime—about two pounds of pure nicotine.[96] While other methods of tobacco use occasioned concern, authors joined in a belief that "the greatest chance for nicotine poisoning is through smoking tobacco."[97]

From the first drag, the poison of nicotine began to work on the system.[98] As the popular pamphlet from Preis outlined, nicotine "first strikes the brain—inducing headache, blurry vision, dizziness, in a word, the destruction of full awareness," followed by convulsion, paralysis, or tremors. It then moved on through arteries where it "chilled" the blood and brought a drop in body temperature, and finally to the heart where it slowed the pulse.[99] His description of tobacco's effects on the system countered earlier medicinal understanding of tobacco from the humeral scholars who argued that tobacco constituted a hot dry substance that warmed and invigorated, yet in the language of cooling, slowing, and blood, Preis continued to work in the idiom of the humors, displaying the crossover of concepts of bodily health.

Another pamphlet gave an evocative description of the onset of tobacco poisoning: "From the ingestion of the poison the face goes white as a sheet. On the brow there is a cold sweat. A strong weakness comes over the person and the legs crumple. The poisoned one sickens and throws up. The heart begins to beat more frequently. Breathing is wheezy. The head spins and the eyes dim. The poisoned one is tortured and miserable. Convulsions begin, and in the end he slips into unconsciousness and dies with foam on the lips."[100] Anecdotal warnings of the dangers of direct contact with tobacco leaves and the quick onset of nicotine poisoning that resulted from such carelessness became standards for antitobacco tracts. Applying a dampened tobacco leaf to the skin would bring on poisoning, according to Dr. Il'inskii's 1888 pamphlet.[101]

The emphasis on the quick and deadly effects of nicotine on the system left authors to explain how smokers continued to live at all. Most relied on an explanation of "slow suicide"—the gradual poisoning of the system by small doses of nicotine. This language tapped into a turn-of-the century fascination with suicide as a signal of societal decline as well as a Russian antiurbanism that portrayed progress as sickening society and the city as a site for moral breakdown, degradation, and decadence.[102] This might be misdiagnosed, explained Aleksandr Zybin in a pamphlet of 1907, but all smokers eventually had the poison catch hold of them.[103]

A 1906 pamphlet outlined the dismaying array of symptoms resulting from nicotine poisoning: "headaches, dizziness, sleepiness, weakness . . . and sometimes even sight and hearing difficulties, loss of consciousness or memory, difficulty moving or breathing, strong cramps, hoarse voice, irritation of the throat, cough, dandruff, hemoptysis, anemia, nausea, vomiting, tinnitus, at times diarrhea, poor pallor, and sweating, trembling of hands and legs, even fainting, burning or dryness in throat, especially in the morning, loss of taste and appetite."[104] Variations of the effects of tobacco came from differences among individual bodies. As the multi-edition pamphlet *O preduprezhdenii kureniia tabaku v detskom vozraste: Populiarno-nauchnyi ocherk dlia roditelei i vospitatelei* (On the prevention of tobacco smoking among children: A popular-scientific essay for parents and educators) pointed out, "People of strong constitutions and a correct way of life may *long not notice* the harmful effects of tobacco smoking, but it is *not as if they are not there*. . . . Its effects may be in some cases stronger and in others weaker . . . only the degree of danger from tobacco might change, but the danger is always there.[105] Variation existed for the organs themselves, so that nicotine attacked the weakest, thus "the danger of smoking appears first of all in that organ, the normal working of which, without smoking, is already slightly disturbed by something (for example, overexertion)."[106] Il'inskii argued in this vein for tobacco's connection to "illnesses of the lips, tongue, stomach, salivary glands . . . no one has shown it, but on the other hand, it is apparent that more often than not the chosen illnesses strike those who have zealously used tobacco."[107]

Tobacco simultaneously made the smoker sensitive to all outside stimuli and yet dead to the cues of their own body. The long list of symptoms was a commonality of most antitobacco works, aligned with an emphasis on nervous disorder and sensory vulnerability. In 1859 I. Buial'skii warned of how tobacco acted on the brain and nerves as well as on mental capacity, sensory perception, and motor skills.[108] Two decades later Rokau reaffirmed that nicotine poisoned nerves.[109] In 1911, the pamphlet *Tobachnoe otravlenie* (Tobacco Poisoning) reiterated the same point of tobacco's primary effects on the nerves, detailing from clinical examination tobacco's progress through the nervous system from "tobacco heart," to sight disorders, and finally to poor workings of the sex organs.[110] Even V. E. Ignatiev's positive entry in the 1896 Brokgauz encyclopedia conceded the harm possible with smoking, remarking, "Those who are irritable, weak subjects, of young age in the period of development when the nervous system is under enhanced demand, withstand smoking relatively poorly."[111] The author implied that tobacco for an adult male of strong constitution was fine, but those already considered feeble risked great harm.

Krymskii argued that nicotine produced an "abnormal stimulation," which ended with "profound enervation" as a reaction. This process had drastic consequences: "The constant excitement and weakening of the nervous system by tobacco smoke draws to itself a change of the nerve matter."[112] The stress produced mass effects for the body as a whole: "Almost every smoker of tobacco after a larger or shorter progression of time, will become ill: cough, dyspnea [labored breathing], catarrh, bronchitis, chronic inflammation of mucous membranes of the mouth, fauces of the larynx [the arched openings at the back of the mouth] and the wind pipe."[113] An author of a 1905 pamphlet conceded that not every smoker would develop every listed complication, "but tobacco serves as an impulse to their appearance."[114] Tobacco irritated the system in ways doctors believed caused further complications.

In an inversion of smoking's celebrated pleasures, antitobacco advocates argued that the heavy tobacco user eventually lost sensory perception. Smokers endangered all senses in pursuit of their habit. Beliakov and Nikol'skii cautioned that smokers might either lose hearing or become overly sensitive to even the smallest sound.[115] Tobacco blindness—*amblyopia nicotiana*—erupted in the heavy smoker as well as conjunctivitis and trachoma according to Il'inskii.[116] Petr Ivanovich Poliakov cautioned that tobacco's danger to sight came because "tobacco fires up your tears, the old folks told me, and they clean your eyes."[117] The experiments of M. O. Tsitovich connected smoking to damage of the auditory nerve.[118] Ignatiev described damage to the membranes of the nose and loss of smell.[119] Nikol'skii warned of the smoker's loss of the sense of the taste.[120] An 1887 *Vrach* two-part article bundled together sensory and sexual difficulties as part of the full slate of nervous disorders brought on by tobacco.[121] Another implicated nicotine in this attack.[122] Antitobacco advocates dismissed the arguments of smokers that they did not display any symptoms with the explanation: "The poison silences for a time your sensitivity."[123]

Perhaps drawing on the knowledge of German medical authorities, who posited that overburdening of the senses led to neurasthenic complications, Russian authors pointed out the disturbing evidence of mental disorder that came from the exhaustion of the system through smoking.[124] In 1845 Bussiron described the general mental defect of the smoker and his "inability to grasp concepts, dulling of the senses, insensibility, being in a dreamlike state when awake and not sleeping well."[125] Tobacco's deleterious effects on the mind came out, according to another pamphlet, in the reaction of the smoker to the first papirosa of the day, with "clouding of the head, dizziness, and weakness over the entire body."[126] Dullness revealed itself most fully in memory loss attributed to smoking.[127] While smoking advocates painted it as the helpmate of intellectual endeavor and philosophical contemplation, antitobacco tracts countered: "Don't delude yourself! . . . your brain is weakened by excessive smoking. . . . The mind of the tobacco user needs incitement, to whip it up, just as an aged person with a weakened stomach needs something to awaken the appetite (a glass of wine)."[128] Such incitement, the author implied, was unnatural and unhealthy. Even as authorities depicted tobacco as connected to the modern disease of neurasthenia, they also brought it together with the social and cultural fissures they saw as plaguing Russia as a whole. Leonid Alekseevich Zolotarev, author of numerous pamphlets on children's sexual development, onanism, and healthy marriages, suggested in his book on tobacco that it was a companion of modern life, "as a diversion or for the calming of the over stimulated brain," but he cautioned that it carried with it far too much danger compared to other means of relaxation, such as walking or labor.[129]

Botkin attributed the smoker's decreased appetite to a nervous effect of nicotine as it "paralyzed the feeling of hunger" but like opium did not nourish.[130] This grew from early European theorists' contention that tobacco entered the body through the stomach, not the lungs.[131] Another author argued that, rather than being a boon, this disrupted the digestive system and led to serious complications.[132] Bek held that the appetite diminished, but the body suffered from constant hunger.[133] Thus smokers developed catarrh of the stomach according to Preis, who quoted the research of a London doctor as his support.[134] Nikol'skii argued this led to environmentally or racially specific problems so that smokers of the north might die of edema or dropsy, while Russians died of emaciation or stomach cancer.[135] The symptoms of these maladies came in the form of coughs, bitter saliva, and bad breath.[136] Authors did not depict the appetite-suppressing aspects of tobacco as a positive attribute for health but instead a symptom of the unnatural appetite fed by smoking and the detrimental effects on digestion, of primary importance in the conception of the body as a closed system that could be depleted or invigorated according to lifestyle.

Popov considered the juices of tobacco that trickled down the throat to be the source of stomach problems.[137] Il'inski argued that tobacco lessened the output of saliva and therefore "food [came] to the stomach less worked over and prepared."[138] The smoker's attempts to "build up the desire" to eat caused further troubles. "He drinks vodka, eats salted and smoked foods, horseradish, onion, garlic, mustard, pepper, and other spicy condiments." These foods induced hunger but "at the same time weaken[ed] the ability of the stomach to digest food." He concluded, "This is why it is so rare to meet a person of good digestion in our time."[139] Mikhailovskii echoed the medical tracts, arguing that tobacco suppressed the appetite and cautioning that meals should not be prepared in smoky atmospheres.[140]

Tobacco's harm to the digestive tract manifested in changes to breath, teeth, and lips. According to Il'inskii's 1898 *Tri iada: Tabak, alkogol' (vodka), i sifilis* (Three poisons: Tobacco, alcohol [vodka], and syphilis), the heat of tobacco weakened tooth enamel, making it more prone to cavities, and dried the lips, leading to cancer.[141] Popov remarked on the disgusting yellow teeth and repulsive whitened tongue of the smoker as well as the danger of cancer on the lip.[142] The cautions about discolored teeth featured across decades and from religious and medical authors.[143] While Nikol'skii acknowledged that toothache happened to smokers and non-smokers, there was "one difference that for nonsmokers teeth are cleaner and prettier."[144] The references to smokers' yellow teeth as marring their appearance acknowledged a growing interest in surface as well as inner beauty, yet also signaled an internal, hidden danger made manifest in surface changes.

Religious tracts focused on the dampening of hunger by tobacco just as medical authorities did, but added a disgust with the unnatural, even sinful, nature of this. A 1905 pamphlet from Mt. Athos railed that tobacco displaced hunger yet "*[did] not feed the organism but instead suffocate[d] the organism*" [emphasis in original].[145] Another compared the passion for tobacco to gluttony—evidence of excessive desire rather than its satiety.[146] Metropolitan Filaret likened the craving for tobacco to a manmade hunger.[147] Perhaps in a religious tradition where fasting showed proof of devotion, the lessening of appetite through artificial means held special danger. By defining tobacco-enabled abstention as a medical debility, religious authorities countered the image of the divine weed.

Moral dangers occupied the antitobacco activists of the United States, but in the Russian case, these were but one of many problems from the habit, and not the primary concern.[148] Depicting the ramifications of smoking as primarily to the nerves, Russian antitobacco activists of the late nineteenth century connected the habit to the spectrum of diseases associated with neurasthenia rather than lung problems or heart issues. If tobacco connoisseurs celebrated the sensory banquet of tobacco, antismoking authors warned that their habit would bring no satisfaction. With degeneracy as a touchstone, links were made between smoking, madness, and sensory deadening, tied together with an internal logic that posited poison as the primary danger of smoking and neurasthenic complications the leading manifestation.

Neurasthenia's elastic nature as a diagnosis allowed association with a massive number of symptoms. As articulated by the American Dr. George M. Beard in 1869, neurasthenia could present in over fifty different ways, from nervous sensitivity to insensitivity, so that smokers might be overly irritable and lacking sensitivity at the same time. A popular theory of the source of neurasthenic disorder was that improper waste excretion allowed for the buildup of poisons in the system and the onset of "autointoxication."[149] In light of the emphasis on internalized toxins on the system, the attention to the poisonous qualities of nicotine makes an easy transition.

Despite its late arrival to the ranks of the industrialized and urban world, Russia readily took to the diagnosis of neurasthenia.[150] Discussions of neurasthenia occupied the professional classes, who visualized an epidemic of degenerative disorders brought on by the rapid industrialization and urbanization of Russia.[151] Russians concentrated on neurasthenia as an urban problem, either dormant and triggered, or created and induced, by the pace of modern life, which produced exhaustion and weakness.[152] Life in the city could cause the disease, as could consumption (alcohol, coffee, or tobacco), modern entertainments, or vice.[153] An 1887 article from the journal *Vrach* gave an expansive listing of what constituted the neurasthenic disorders associated with smoking, including "diseases of lung, heart, stomach and intestines."[154] The lumping of tobacco use together with neurasthenic disorder was in keeping with a global understanding of both as modern maladies of industrial peoples in urban environments. In addition to being a cause of neurasthenia, tobacco use was depicted by experts as emerging from the increasingly exhausting political atmosphere, which led Russians to embrace tobacco or other artificial stimulants to offset constitutions weakened by the stressful environment.[155]

Be it from the city, the crowd, or habits, physicians thought most Russians had some type of neurosis. In addition to the more general diagnosis of neurasthenia, psychiatrists, rising in number in the late tsarist period, also latched onto hysteria as presented in females as a space for discussion of both the value of psychiatry and the problems in Russian society. Hysteria, presenting in pain and complications in the abdomen as well as nervous problems, anxiety, and emotional instability, allowed specialized diagnosis of women's physical problems and the gendered injustices of tsarist society, while connecting these problems to neurasthenia.[156]

The omnipresence of tobacco made it the worst of modern habits and the greatest danger to nerves and the future. Like Tolstoy, who saw in tobacco the most hazardous intoxicant, Il'inskii concluded in 1898:

> *Tobacco cachexy* . . . is still worse than that of drinking because many use tobacco more and the number of smokers is ten to twenty times greater than the number of people in alcoholic excess; the poison of tobacco—nicotine— is more dangerous than alcohol. This explains the great number of nerve and other illnesses where the patient and even the doctor and no one on the world can diagnose the cause of the illness. Realistically if we do not bring tobacco poisoning up, not the ill, nor their companions, nor his doctor will be able to diagnose the illness or all the conditions. . . . It is impossible to decide from where the illness came and sometimes they fall ill suddenly and without visible symptoms.[157]

If tobacco users were indeed "twenty times" more prevalent than alcoholics in Russia, and tobacco was considered a leading cause of nervous disorder, smoking then became the most prevalent cause of an omnipresent, elusive, and dreaded disease.

The language of neurasthenia brought Russian tobacco problems to a world of medical and psychiatric literature on degeneracy. Degeneracy became a dominant explanation for a perceived social and biological decline documented in many fields of the late nineteenth century, including the natural and social sciences.[158] Europeans attributed the prevalence of the disease to the inevitable degeneration of races, borrowing in particular from the French psychiatrist Benedict Morel (1809–73), who emphasized the poisoning of the system with alcohol, tobacco, and other drugs as part of the physical, intellectual, and moral degeneration of humanity. They depicted certain groups as more prone to degeneracy—among these the Slavs and Jews—lending immediacy to these questions for Russian theorists.[159]

While degeneracy showed the decline of society, theorists claimed it only became apparent in highly civilized nations. Thus the disease marked decline as a sign of achievement.[160] For Russians, neurasthenia displayed alternatively progress or decline, and contemporaries deployed it as a reason to have hope for Russia's path toward cosmopolitan development or a desire to turn away from Western habits. The literature of the late nineteenth century suggested that Russians considered themselves as prone to neurasthenia as any other nation, and in the antitobacco discourse, neurasthenic terminology as well as degeneracy cautions figured prominently.[161]

Europeans considered the documentation of increasing insanity as a sign of tobacco's aftermath, neurasthenia's outcome, and degeneracy's progress.[162] All drugs were implicated in racial deterioration, but Russian antitobacco activists connected tobacco use to fears of madness and neurasthenia explicitly and degeneracy obliquely in their critiques of smoking.[163] In his 1904 work, Beliakov mentioned the work of the Moscow University professor of mental illness Sergei Sergeivich Korsakov as support for his contention that "*mental instability may develop as a consequence of smoking tobacco*" [italics his].[164] The symptoms of this instability—tremors, memory lapses, or mental difficulties—could come from fifteen cigars or fifty to one hundred papirosy a day, a quite prodigious amount that he depicted as typical. The first indications of illness emerged in exhaustion, progressing into silence and feelings of depression and concluding in suicide. For others, insomnia, hearing voices, violent behaviors, paranoia, and hallucinations occurred.[165] Ignatiev found that "smokers are typically irritable and hot-tempered, dissatisfied with their lives and their acquaintances." He documented further mental instability, and even insanity, in some, though when smokers quit such issues fully disappeared.[166] Beliakov connected the most severe of these manifestations to smokers who were also syphilitics and alcoholics. In these sufferers, smoking led to the complete collapse of the nervous system in paralysis.[167] Ignatiev mentioned the problems of the nervous system for those of weak constitution or the young, noting that their organisms, already under enhanced demands, could not withstand the additional stresses of tobacco.[168]

Degeneracy dominated as a disease frame for tobacco, leaving absent other ailments that modern observers might expect to see, particularly tuberculosis and cancer, and taking sensory debility, mental illness, and lung, genital, and heart problems from tobacco as signs of nervous effect from nicotine.[169] Tuberculosis, or consumption, appeared rarely in antitobacco tracts. Il'inskii argued smoking was the "source for all future consumption," but only if done by youth in "the age of the expansion of the chest organs (that is between ages seventeen and twenty)," thus making consumption, an acknowledged mass problem, a sign of the neurasthenic complications of smoking.[170] Popov noted that smoking was especially bad for those with already compromised lungs.[171] Antitobacco activists depicted smoking as a trigger for degeneracy, rather than a specific cause of issues of the lungs.

Instead, authors blamed tobacco for other problems. For example, three quarters of those with typhus and diphtheria were smokers, according to Il'inskii.[172] Cancer, too, was an innate condition triggered by tobacco, though Il'inskii concluded, "And who of us knows if he is susceptible or not to that illness [cancer]?"[173] Only lip cancer from cigar use was accepted as a problem directly attributed to cigar smoking, appearing in literature as early as the 1880s.[174] Lung cancer would only be tentatively linked to smoking in 1898, with the first statistical evidence appearing from Germany in 1929 and the first epidemiological study from Germany in 1939.[175]

While antismoking advocates railed against smoking in general, their most pointed attacks concerned tobacco use by two groups in particular—youth and women. They considered both to be particularly susceptible to developing neurasthenia and especially vulnerable to the exhaustion brought on by tobacco's poisons, youth because they were at a point where bodily energies, conceived in a closed economy, needed to be focused on development, and women because they were naturally weak.[176] Both groups began smoking with increasing intensity in the late nineteenth century. Researchers upheld the idea that children were smoking at high rates. In an 1889 article in the journal *Vrach,* the author alleged that in a study of 262 school-age youth, 31.29% drank and 45.41% smoked. A breakdown by age displayed the largest numbers of smokers were in the groups of eleven to fifteen years old.[177]

This concern over women and children's smoking may have been simply a perception raised by patriarchal concerns for lost authority—a moral panic. Certainly, there was a great deal of worry over drinking by women and children. At the turn of the century, the perception of increasing alcoholism among women, especially in the city, led to targeting by temperance groups.[178] In the case of tobacco, it may have indeed been the case that there were more female and young users because inhaling lighter blends of flue-cured tobacco was easier and might have lured new smokers; it may have been based in some real increase in smoking by these two groups.[179] Cigarettes and safety matches also allowed for easier use than pipes and tinder.[180] Perhaps, too, new conceptualizations of childhood as a time apart intensified feelings of children's vulnerability, while rising feminist agitation lent immediacy to fears of female disorder. Most definitely, concepts borrowed from degeneracy and from campaigns against the smoking boy carried out abroad deepened interest in youth and women as the future of the race.[181] In the United States, activists widely decried nicotine as a "race poison" that was visiting disastrous eugenic consequences.[182]

The danger of the smoking boy appeared in his immediate health as "polluted" blood poisoned the entire body.[183] From this autointoxication a host of problems followed, including "irregular heartbeat, circulatory disorders, difficulty with digestion, slowness at mental tasks and larger or smaller propensity [*sklonnost'*] to hard liquor, and for one child there was lung consumption. Several struggled with significant nose bleeds and their blood was completely spoiled."[184] Priklonskii noticed additionally low weight and poor growth.[185]

By far the most often repeated charges against youthful smoking were those regarding tobacco's harmful effect on student's abilities. In 1902, Bek deployed the statistical analysis of a Dr. Fisk to note that of smoking students only 20 percent enjoyed good success, while of those doing poorly 57 percent were smokers.[186] Earlier, I. Buialskii backed the anti–youth smoking conclusions of his 1859 *O vrede ot izlishchniago kureniia tabaka* (On the threat of excessive tobacco smoking) with research from Dublin and France that documented the low exam scores of smokers.[187] The study was elsewhere identified as an 1855 investigation by a Dr. Bertil'on of Paris. As another pamphlet noted, "Doctors long have pointed out that for children of school age smoking above all weakens memory. That which their non-smoking students are able to remember with ease becomes a great difficulty for those smoking comrades, even though earlier (until smoking) they both studied with similar success. The failing of memory is especially strongly seen in the study of chronology, cities (in geography), words (in the study of language), and so on. In addition under the influence of smoking the attention is weakened and quick-wittedness dulled."[188] An 1887 article in the journal *Vrach* repeated these conclusions, noting the "lack of stability in work, irritable psyche, and poor memory" of smoking students.[189] Such arguments doubled as concerns for parents and warnings for children.

An 1888 pamphlet skipped any supportive material, instead asking the readers to consult their own experience as evidence:

> It is easy to know a smoking child from the first look: it is the puny, ill, pale, exhausted one, with the tenderness lost in the face. Their growth is stunted. They struggle with eating problems and nervous disorders and from these are anemic and emaciated. The well-known folk saying is that only in a healthy body can there be a healthy mind, but in the body strained by tobacco there cannot be a healthy mind and therefore, all smoking children

are distinguished by their dullness [*tupoumiem*] and inability to do mental work. They soon tire and have trouble committing to memory that which they have been given to learn by heart. . . . It is especially strange that they do not remember proper names. Beyond that it is well known that a student starting to smoke goes from good to poor.[190]

The same effects authors identified in adult males intensified for the developing body, bringing new problems. Mikhailovskii commented on the detrimental outcomes of smoking on the voice of youth and the distressing lack of tenors this occasioned.[191] Elsewhere Popov repeated this unusual caution, arguing that youth smoking could "take away the beautiful tone of their singing voice."[192] The dearth of tenors or the damaging of tenderness in students functioned as a shorthand for the loss of innocence attributed to early smoking, which betrayed concerns over early maturity and especially sexual awakening. The language echoed comments regarding masturbation and other precocious behaviors.

Tobacco became a gateway to further problems of the will and morals, an area of increasing concern for contemporaries.[193] An 1887 essay argued tobacco made youth "disrespectful of their elders."[194] A 1906 pamphlet baldly stated that smoking children simply had "no desire to study."[195] Preis condemned youth who smoked, as they would "become inaccurate and prone to slovenliness." As they were forced to steal papirosy to keep smoking, they would "become accustomed to deceit and lies."[196] Smoking youth soon turned into drinking youth, according to several authors, as tobacco brought forth a burning thirst.[197] The connection of the two vices spoke more to moral understandings than to medical reflections on comorbidity. The focus on adolescents in multiple forums—smoking, drinking, masturbation, sex, and loss of innocence—revealed anxiety over a perceived coarsening of society as well as a concern for increasing loss of patriarchal authority and parental or communal oversight frayed by the opportunities and anonymity of the urban environment.

Smoking took children from being productive members of society to mental degeneracy and, according to even more dire voices, into criminality. A 1906 pamphlet quoted "many doctors" as concluding that more than half of children who become mad or incarcerated began smoking early.[198] The basis for this mental instability was the nervous irritation of tobacco, which made for peevish and unstable adults. Nikol'skii expressed some skepticism that the statistical correlations would allow for one "to certainly conclude that smoking tobacco awakens the criminal desire and leads to madness." He argued that the link was such that "it makes one think."[199]

Experts, however, considered the connection of smoking and criminality among adults well established. Udintsev said in 1913 that this was because smoking "may help to weaken the moral feelings of a criminal at a crucial moment."[200] Priklonskii made a similar case, pointing out that 79 percent of recidivists were smokers.[201] For Russian progressive intellectuals, especially those in the human sciences, legal, and medical professions, theories of social ills emerging from individual deviance held great sway.[202]

Youths encountered antitobacco materials directly during public lectures held at schools and delivered by medical professionals like the one from Preis. At times, the lecture later materialized in the form of a pamphlet.[203] Youth smoking, defined by one pamphlet as smoking at any point "up to the moment of full physical development (no less than twenty five years for men)," held the potential for "great danger."[204] Pamphlets warned that smoking stunted growth and development of the heart and the breathing organs. In a word it was "the death of youth."[205] More dangerously, among youth who had smoked anywhere from a few weeks to a few years, "half of them had heart palpitations . . . in a quarter were noted anxious sleep and frequent nose bleeds."[206] Botkin cited the research of American doctors into the changes of red blood cells among child smokers.[207] Girls who smoked stopped menstruating.[208] In addition to the physical effects of smoking, mental and moral lapses became apparent as smoking by children "awakened a desire for the use of strong spirits."[209] Botkin alleged, "Tobacco destroys youth morally and physically."[210]

The cover for Grinevskii's 1889 pamphlet *Bros'te kurit'!* (Quit smoking!) depicted the anxiety surrounding youth and women's smoking in two visuals set diagonally from one another (figure 4.2). On top left, a young woman smoked while reading in the garden. At bottom right, two youth shared a papirosa near a garden wall. In both images, a furtive air surrounded the figures, hinting at the illicit nature of smoking. The worries of boys and young women defying authority in hidden places outside the oversight of parents and teachers revealed fears that Russian patriarchal authority had lost its power. Such anxiety appeared not just in visuals but also in discussions of boys smoking in washrooms, children sneaking tobacco from their parents, or women hiding their habit. Neurasthenia provided a scientific language to articulate fears of declining masculinity, waning patriarchal control, and concerns for women and youth grown wild. If nervous disorder became the medical perspective for anxieties of societal chaos and male inadequacy, then the smoking boy and woman became physical embodiments of emasculation. The authoritarian state's revocation of basic rights of citizenship to Russian males already feminized men in the late tsarist

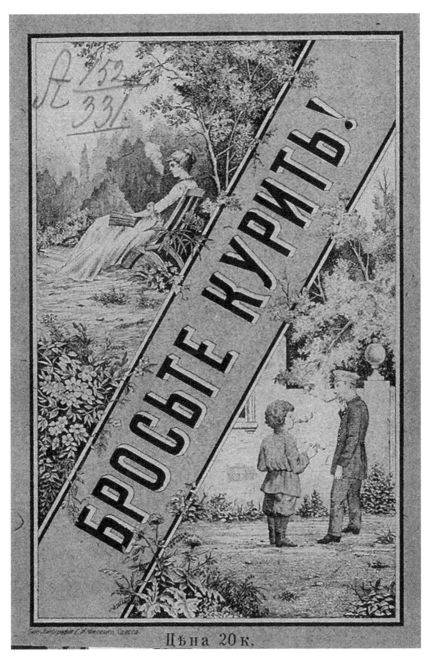

Figure 4.2 Cover, Dr. Grinevskii, *Bros'te kurit'!* 1889. Collection of Russian State Library, Moscow

period, and tobacco became a way to channel those fears into biological, social, and pedagogic frames.

On the cover, the young woman sat outside in a park or garden, an area lacking the same oversight of the home. With a papirosa stuck between her teeth like a sprig of grass rather than held in her hand or even guided in the act of inhalation, the woman in the image conveyed neither eroticism nor elegance. Instead, her profile looked hard and her slumped posture unladylike. The boys appeared to be in a relationship of tutelage, with the older one demonstrating the habit as the younger watched in awe. Both images implied the moral and physical effects of tobacco on women and children. Women became more mannish and children looked to the wrong role models for behavior cues.

The stakes for youth smoking might have been a manifestation of male fears of inadequacy, but they emerged in cautionary tales for all of society. The smoking youth tumbled down a slippery slope from tobacco use to mental and physical problems and finally to poor citizenship as "boys, beginning to smoke tobacco, [would] become capricious, irritable, and upset. They [would], without any reason, disturb discipline and disrupt the correct pace of class. All of this [came] because of their nervous conditions born of their smoking tobacco."[211] From this, "the poor success of students" who smoked came as no surprise.[212] Arsenii commented on how the tobacco "stupefied" the child: "His nerves are overexcited; it affects him poorly on the sexual side and spoils his character. From a nice, open, and pleasant child he becomes sly and bold."[213] Priklonskii connected early smoking with criminality, mental illness, and prison populations. He conceded, "All this, of course, does not yet show that smoking tobacco brings people to commit crimes or go insane, but in the most minor case, even when not evident, tobacco shows its influence, and we need to think about that."[214] Popov saw the inception of criminality in the way in which children first took up the habit, when they stole the tobacco or the money for it from their parents, lied about it, skipped lessons to smoke, or even did so "in the outhouse amid the stench and filth."[215] All signified the sinfulness of the habit and for some the general degradation and "lack of manners among cultured society."[216] The papirosa offered a ready, material answer to what was wrong with kids today, and unlike so many other things, seemed easily fixed with admonition, cessation, or prohibition.

Surveys in medical literature contributed to a picture of widespread smoking by youth and the vulnerability of adolescents to the allure of tobacco. A survey of students at St. Petersburg Mining Institute found that 91.6 percent of students had tried tobacco at some point. The author contrasted these figures with those of medical students (54.6 percent) and technical students (47.2 percent), noting that medical and merchant students smoked more while those of the nobility, petite bourgeois, clergy, and peasant background smoked less.[217] The survey found the critical age for starting to smoke was sixteen to eighteen.[218]

If smoking endangered youth because of their developing constitutions, it visited havoc on woman, because as Grinevskii advised in 1889, women were "from nature more nervous with a weaker constitution." He concluded, "Incidentally, female smoking is widespread among us."[219] Popov's anti–youth smoking pamphlet contained an extensive section on women's smoking. He noted that, if anything, smoking was worse for women and girls: "The effect of tobacco on girls is even more detrimental and destructive because in the female sex the nervous system is significantly susceptible and in general the nature of women is more able to become accustomed to passion."[220] Weak of moral will, women were more susceptible to tobacco's allures and suffered more from its effects; as Preis noted, "Smoking is dangerous for all people, but especially for women."[221]

Which women smoked seemed a point of contention. In the idiosyncratic 1907 pamphlet *Kurenie tabaka* (Smoking tobacco), A. Virenius suggested a general shift in tastes that marked both men and women, tracking their movement from enjoying spicy items and chocolate as youths to consuming tea and coffee as adults. After that, men moved on to "a strong desire for spirits, tobacco, the most piquant, spicy items," while only women workers similarly desired spirits and smoking.[222] Virenius noted a taste for tobacco only among working class women, but Preis bemoaned the fact that "smoking women are for the most part educated and cultivated." While one would expect their characters to be "reasonably good" by virtue of education and cultivation, this was not the case. "Education does nothing to change them and their soul takes on the desire to do evil. Thus there can be no discussion of the perfect and eternal good of the soul of women," because a smoking woman threatened the health and moral standing of all around her.[223] The Eve of the modern age threatened to take down the world by taking up tobacco rather than an apple.

Antismoking authors saw female smoking as "exceedingly widespread" and a national disgrace.[224] Women painted it as their "full right of citizenship," moaned Krymskii. He dismissed the smoking of the old women, because "for them there is nothing that can harm them." Women in the prime of life, however, were "weaker, more tender, and more graceful." For such vessels to smoke led to even greater harm, as "women are more nervous than men and more susceptible to the poisonous effects of nicotine."[225] Krymskii argued that while women might consider tobacco a political right, smoking wreaked havoc on women of childbearing age.

Antitobacco activists depicted a woman's smoking as injurious to her attractiveness. In an 1889 pamphlet the author described the assault of tobacco on the beauty and sensual attractions of a woman he saw on the train. He lamented that, from smoking, "her face is yellow and teeth are black. Her eyes are feverish with fleeting brilliance." More than just skin deep, her allures as a companion were lessened as she appeared "dense [*tupoi*] and she cough[ed] frequently displaying shortness of breath." The similar display of a woman at a stylish salon forced her guests to leave from disgust. The inhospitable atmosphere resulting from the smoke and the unpleasant vision of the female smoker repulsed.[226] A 1907 commentary from a clergyman glorified women as the embodiment of virtues—"cleanliness, modesty, humility, purity, gentleness, and beauty." But "tobacco destroys all of these." He wrapped together the moral, physical, and aesthetic effects of tobacco, warning that "it corrupts morals and dangerously effects health." He concluded that women smoked without reason, without restraint, and without modesty.[227] Internationally, such depictions of the smoking woman as loose, dangerous, and even criminal frequently made it into medical, psychological, sociological, and criminal classifications of deviant femininity.[228]

Another author commented that while watching women smoke might be erotic to some, as blowing smoke rings could "bring on reveries to man," this could not hold true for all. The sensory disgust brought on by the smell of smoke, the sound of coughing, and the ugliness of spitting destroyed any beauty, so that "the entire scene [was] completely unpleasant."[229] Preis gave a detailed account of the visual decline of the female smoker: "If you see a woman sucking on a papirosa, the unavoidable consequence is the awful odor from the throat, black and sooty teeth, and smoky fingers. A smoking woman falls unavoidably from aesthetic quality without which in my opinion, a woman cannot exist. . . . Beyond that must I remind you that the papirosa is the first step towards moral laxity?"[230] Preis argued that women's use of tobacco so soiled her appearance—her teeth and hands; so engendered repugnance—the foul stench from her mouth—that she no longer existed as a woman. From there, her moral decline seemed an incidental issue

Smoking brought changes more than skin deep as antitobacco activists argued that smoking attacked women by disrupting menstruation, inducing miscarriage, and tainting breast milk with nicotine.[231] As an anonymous author stated in 1904, children suffer from a mother smoking.[232] Another author went so far as to suggest that a smoking mother showed no love to her children, terming women's tobacco use a type of child abuse.[233] Arsenii further maligned the smoking woman as not just sexually unattractive but also unsexed, becoming physically unable to gestate or nurture. The smoking mother poisoned her milk and the air of her home, and thus "it [was] not surprising if [her] children [would] grow up weak, nervous, with poor capabilities and susceptible to disease." Not only did this mother endanger the health of her child, her presumed innate, nurturing feminine instincts were corrupted and her protestations for her child unbelievable: "That same mother, in the face of a serious illness of her child, is prepared to cry and wail, but the tears of such mothers have little value. Such a mother does not inspire complete sympathy. How we want to tell her, are not you the one to blame for the weak health of your child for the bad stomach and thinness. Do not poison your organism with tobacco poison, the organism that bore the child onto the earth. Do not poison the air he breathes, and he would be for you healthier and fresher. Now you reap the fruits of your lust (*strast*)."[234] According to Arsenii's estimation, the smoking mother was beyond human sympathy, beyond Christian charity, beyond understanding.

The dangers to women's sexual function echoed in warnings over tobacco's danger to male potency. An 1887 essay mentioned research connecting tobacco use to rabbit sterility as well as bringing up a proposal by a Frenchman that tobacco so disrupted sexual function that smoking should be encouraged in single-sex educational establishments because it would diminish masturbation.[235] In 1904, Beliakov detailed, at length, the sexual debility brought on by tobacco smoking, with a candid comment that smoking caused pain with "erection." Beliakov's study included references to the newly popular glandular explanations of sex and noted that tobacco caused degeneration of the testicles and ovaries in experiments on dogs and rabbits. He backed up his discussion with two anecdotal case histories. In one case, a husband and wife had a childless union until they both stopped smoking and produced a son. Another example detailed five youth who smoked and all suffered from "sexual weakness."[236] Pamphlets in 1914 and 1915 reiterated the problems for both sexes, citing research on roosters and rabbits where tobacco caused smaller testicles, sterility in females, and a general weakening of "sexual strength and sexual attraction."[237] Increasing diagnosis of sexual weakness, a symptom of overcivilization and developing degeneracy, signaled Russia's arrival in the pantheon of modern nations subject to modern diseases.

In 1909, Priklonskii argued that while some wags might claim that tobacco poisoning was a death that took a hundred years, men were no longer strong enough to enjoy such trials. Contrasting the smoking man of the present with the valiant, frontier-defending soldiers of the past, Prik-lonskii wrote, "Are there many such *bogatyr* in our nervous, ill century? And *bogatyr* do not always survive excess without punishment."[238] The consequences of smoking to the looks of men merited their own detailed disgust. Their eyes, ears, and lips suffered, while their face was "unclean and pale." The mouth, always hot, held a "dirty" tongue, yellowed teeth, and some teeth even blackened.[239] Another author pointed out how smoking destroyed attractiveness: "Not only the skin of the face, which yellows and wrinkles (premature aging), but also the whites of the eyes get murky and yellow, the blush disappears in the cheeks, the lips often crack and the mouth emits the smell of tobacco smoke."[240]

The male smoker's physical attractions, his virility, and his sensory perceptions all came under attack. In a 1911 pamphlet filled with anxieties of sexual and racial danger, Meier detailed the perils of syphilis for smokers. His rant was particularly aimed at cigar smokers because factory workers sealed the smokes with their saliva. Even worse, Meier noted, "Havanna cigars infect one even more easily (as there have been cases), because the negroes [*negry*] in America roll the cigars on their bare thighs."[241] Similar charges emerged in the United States, where fears of racial contagion and sexual danger took the guise of hygienic prescription.[242] Other health pamphlets warned of the danger of transferring syphilis through shared papirosy.[243]

Fears of male and female sexual impotency tapped directly into the ongoing fervor over nervous diseases, neurasthenic decline, and national competition. One author posited tobacco as the base for all neurasthenic problems and the creation of "the nervous man": "Already several times tobacco poison has been found to provoke nervous disorders, whereas nerves are, in our times, almost the public property of all mankind. In many cases of neurasthenia, the disease is blamed completely unfairly on other causes not on tobacco poisons."[244] By the start of World War I, the links between tobacco, nervous disorder, sensory degradation, and sexual debility made explicit from the 1880s came into further relief as tobacco use increased, neurasthenia became a more popular diagnosis for both males and females, especially of the middle and upper class, and social and political anxieties intensified in the wake of 1905.[245]

The rise of concern over the degeneracy brought on by tobacco, the disrespectful behavior of youth, the deteriorating attractiveness of women, and the declining sexual potency of males brought anxieties about Russian tobacco's dangers into direct conversation with concerns over Russia's place in the modern world. Since neurasthenia could indicate either the attainment of civilized progress or overdevelopment and a threat to existence, tobacco was implicated in the discussion of Russian progress. In attacks on tobacco lurked commentary regarding social and national standing and even humanity. Appolov noted that tobacco possessed the power to drown the conscience, dampen intelligence, and weaken those things that distinguished man from beast.[246] Even the tales of tobacco's arrival in Russia—from discounting it as a habit of "savages" to recounting at length the evil machinations of France's Catherine of Medici (r. 1560–74) and her connections to Jean Nicot (1530–1600)—were offered as proof of the wicked origins of the habit.[247]

Although not as explicitly linked to nervous disorder, neurasthenia, or degeneracy as other antitobacco arguments, discussions of the moral effects of tobacco engaged a widespread concern over the direction of imperial society. Religious authors featured moral arguments in their works taken directly from scripture: from Leviticus and Corinthians; from St. Paul, the rock of the church; from St. Michael, the patron of Moscow; or from Metropolitan Filaret.[248] Despite the religious trappings, they did not shy away from using medical cases.[249] Popov utilized the diagnostic points of neurasthenia in his pamphlet, arguing that the effects of smoking progressed inexorably from the nervous system to "somnolence, disinclination to serious studies, and laziness." From there it simply spiraled out of control: "In the end smoking a lot will impart to you an irritable character and at the same time an irregular character so that you will be jolly but will appear despondent and ill."[250] The reverse also occurred, as with the work by Mendel'son and Botkin, who detailed the efforts of seminaries to end smoking among students.[251]

Unlike alcoholism, which the church increasingly considered a disease in the early twentieth century, carefully distinguishing the habit from dissolute behavior, which was sinful, no such division tempered the depiction of smoking.[252] Tobacco became not just a danger but a sin akin to gluttony and the gradual poisoning by nicotine a slow suicide and offense against God.[253] Others decried it as either the substitute for devotion among believers, who awoke to smoke rather than to say their prayers, or as the opposite of incense, carrying "dreams of the devil . . . of laziness and lusts" rather than conveying prayers to the heavens.[254] Not only was it wicked, but also it was distressingly common. According to Priest Vvedenskii's multiedition pamphlet, "Modern people have many bad habits, but among these almost of the first place is the habit of smoking tobacco. Tobacco smoking is a much more widespread vice than drinking, foul language, or card playing."[255] Isidor Cherniaev told the tale of tobacco as not just sinful but a trick of Satan, as did the modernist writer Aleksei Remizov (1877–1957) in a fantastical, and lewd, story of 1908.[256]

Schismatics considered smoking a habit brought by the devil and vocally opposed tobacco along with alcohol.[257] One legend of tobacco was that Satan introduced it to cause the fall of man.[258] Another claimed that tobacco was sprouted on the unholy ground on which were buried the children of Jezebel. Other religious groups similarly opposed tobacco and urged abstention on their followers. The sect led by the charismatic "Brother" Ivan Churikov pledged abstention from drinking, smoking, and swearing. They numbered some fifty thousand members in 1908. The *Skoptsy* added sex and meat to their list of forbidden pleasures, alongside drink and tobacco.[259] The Old Believers, Baptists, and Tolstoyans all provided strong support for antitobacco work and produced pamphlets in the period.[260] The interesting spectacle of Russian Orthodox figures opposing tobacco on the grounds that its use offended the sensibilities of a sect the government and church opposed showed the strange bedfellows of antismoking activism.[261] Appolov bristled at the suggestion that Old Believers were better because they did not smoke. In so doing, he went off-message in his antitobacco pamphlet by noting that some smokers could be good, just as some nonsmokers were bad.[262]

Ioann of Kronstadt (1829–1908), a charismatic leader of a popular religious movement, drew a compelling picture of tobacco's moral and religious dangers: "Along with the fragrance of the censer in the church, the world has invented its own fragrance—tobacco—and zealously, greedily smokes it up, almost eating and swallowing it and breathing it in, thus blackening their insides and their homes. This breeds an aversion to the fragrance of the censor and many become fearful to enter the church."[263] In Ioann's vision, tobacco offended God and sullied the body, and like an evil fiend pushed people away from the church. He described in detail how demonic impulses emerged in tobacco: "Many constantly burn the tobacco censer to the demon that lives in the flesh. Their soul has slyly turned their lives to smoking and their mouths, destined to thank and glorify God, have become the means of a pedestrian passion."[264] Deriding man for creating a sinful habit that even an animal would not stoop to, he compared tobacco to a graven idol worshipped by man.[265]

In Ioann's message, tobacco use became but one symptom of the complete destruction of the senses, the body, and in the end, the soul. He despaired: "Look at how perverted is the delight of feeling. . . . For the sense of smell and taste . . . burns almost incessantly an acrid, odorous smoke . . . infecting the air of their home with this smoke and the air outside, but above all ruining themselves with this evil." The smoke was both foul and evil, and as it penetrated the body and the senses it soiled the soul, "ruining [the] senses and [the] heart swallowing continually that smoke . . . which imparts with it fleshly desires, rudeness, and sensuality."[266]

Medical men similarly shuffled between tobacco's physical and moral effects. In 1888, Il'inskii argued that the slow poisoning of tobacco, which eventually brought illness and death, destroyed the organs, nerves, and eventually the brain, the receptacle of the soul.[267] Tregubov called on medical authority when cautioning consumers about the moral failings of the tobacco addict, noting, "In the opinion of learned men and a few doctors smoking tobacco affects not just the bodily health of the smoker, but also the mental abilities and the standing of his soul."[268] Bussiron charged that tobacco made burdens harder to bear, be they hunger, poverty, boredom, or sadness; he concluded, "The drug is often worse than the disease."[269] Even for the user who perhaps had the force of character to practice moderation, the torments of the "demon tobacco" would overcome his rational choices.[270] The best of men, Bussiron argued, would be unable to quit once they started.

Contemporaries debated the effects of tobacco but focused on certain targets. Perhaps because dedicated smokers were considered incorrigible, or alternatively because authors considered it easier to stop smoking at the start, onset was a target. Conceivably because youth and women were seen as more suggestible, or because threatened males saw in the further subjugation of women and children a way to prop up their fragile masculinity—for one or a combination of these reasons, antitobacco authors focused their attention on remonstrance to youth and female smokers. Set apart from smokers generally because of their greater vulnerability, women and children had not the will to be moderate, according to authors, and thus had to be discouraged. How to stop children and women from smoking took several forms.

Adults, especially smoking parents, received criticism for being horrible examples.[271] Preis called out teachers, doctors, and spiritual leaders who smoked as bad models and simply asked, "Can people who are involved in the upbringing of children smoke?"[272] Meier featured young males in his study and included a conversation he had with one boy addicted to nicotine; the boy reportedly commented, "My father also smokes. Everything my father does is good for me too."[273] By involving children—having them prepare a papirosa or find a tobacco case—parents introduced them to the habit. As Arsenii commented, "It is not surprising that after this, the child borrows their father's tobacco or imitates mother and smells of papirosy."[274]

Parents who smiled at a child handling tobacco because they deemed it a necessary passage to adulthood or those who helped their children smoke received a stony censure from individuals like Arsenii.[275]

In his 1914 pamphlet, Zolotarev noted that since smoking began in youth, it must be prevented at that point, and he put the onus on parents. Not only must they be good examples and not smoke—or if they did smoke, do so surreptitiously—they also needed to be mindful of the summer holidays, a time when children often took up papirosy. During the critical ages of twelve to seventeen, they had to ensure exercise, study, and "healthful and wise development." He hypothesized that physical exercises could stop youth from smoking, and he concluded, "In general it can be said that the more natural the way of life, that is the more they answer the natural calls of growth and development of the organism, the less chance for the beginning and taking on of the habit of smoking tobacco."[276]

Just as the parent led the child astray, "servants learn to smoke from their masters"—an accusation that revealed the paternalism of master-servant relationships and the prejudices against the lower classes.[277] A 1904 pamphlet charged, "Everybody smokes, even old women and young ladies learn to suck on papirosy from gentlemen. One starts to smoke and from her example another—and then the entire province is under a fog."[278] Not just masters were at fault. Workers and soldiers both were blamed for spreading the habit back to the countryside.[279] It seemed that even the village, at times depicted as the idyllic bastion of Russian values outside the pernicious influences of the modern city, could not withstand the taint of tobacco.

Some authors dismissed youth and women's smoking as frivolous. Young boys began smoking to seem older, as a prank, to flout the rules, or to gain friends. They then continued despite the unpleasant sensation and could not quit.[280] Women smoked as a "whim" or from "silliness."[281] Some women took it up "out of boredom and idleness, others began lightly falling in with those already fallen or others to be audacious," which was especially true of those women who "[did] not wish to set themselves apart from the males with whom they [felt] they [could] be seen as equal."[282] The appeal of smoking in the modern age entered into the arguments of Preis regarding women's smoking; he noted, "Even Russian women with their sensitive natures—feel the separation between life and conscience so strongly that they give themselves over to some type of narcotic."[283] Preis depicted tobacco as the weakling's method for dealing with modern ambiguities, except, unlike Tolstoy, he argued this sensitivity was a particularly feminine attribute.

Questions in surveys indicating the reasons students started smoking barely differed from the motives cited by antitobacco activists. The students of Mikhailovskii's study began for "comradery," "a prank," "bravado," "stupidity," "nerves," or "boredom." The enigmatic reason of "under the influence of living conditions" and the pathos-laden explanations of "grief" or starting out of "sorrow with the country" suggested more philosophical underpinnings for tobacco use with some.[284] The connection between modern urban life and smoking may not have been exactly that posited by antismoking authors, but the habit and its condemnation both tapped into a fascination with nerves, psychology, and disquiet floating across the urban landscape.

IF DOCTORS of the fifteenth century encountered tobacco through the lens of the humors, then it should not be surprising that nineteenth-century physicians understood tobacco through the diseases, problems, and technologies of their times. Antitobacco authors focused on problems for society and individuals, highlighting order, morality, and health while targeting women and children as the ones that most needed to stop. Their arguments grew out of an international and national conversation between social reformers, scientific authorities, church figures, and other progressive intellectuals. In their discussions of how to make society move forward and the many perceived dangers to progress they identified, this almost exclusively male group of authors revealed anxieties about the status of the Russian nation and their own authority. They displayed their concern across a growing body of reading materials for an increasingly literate population.

In their pamphlets, statistics, and scientific studies, reformers revealed the disquiet under the surface of smoking's image as manly and valorous and attempted to fashion an alternative idea of tobacco as a threat to moral standards, social interaction, civic norms, and the next generation. They articulated this threat as part of the large cluster of ailments termed neurasthenia. Neurasthenia served as an appropriate frame for antismoking advocates not just because it conveniently countered tobacco marketing. The diagnosis was fashionable, flexible, and pertinent. Gender, class, age, and paternalistic assumptions all swayed the ways in which antitobacco activists confronted the problem. In their moralizing and disgust over the scent of tobacco from women, youth, servants, and the peasantry emerged concerns very similar to those of neurasthenia—for a loss of control, for emerging challenges to masculine authority, and for the seemingly rapid pace of change.

Urban smokers in the late tsarist period likely had heard of the many charges against tobacco. Frequent fires and regulations for smoke-free wagons on trains made antipathy to public smoking apparent. The religious admonitions, from the Metropolitan as well as from popular figures like Tolstoy and Ioann of Kronstadt, assured the resonance of antitobacco activists' moral concerns. The burgeoning popular press made the message available to a growing number of users, and the fervor of professional intellectuals translated into public events, lectures, and posters to introduce the public and students to tobacco danger. The influence of antitobacco advocates on behavior remained equivocal. The focus on poison led wags to speculate that if a capful of nicotine could kill a horse, smokers' ability to smoke and live proved their vigor. The invocation of neurasthenia—supposedly brought on by everything from masturbation to bicycling—both elevated tobacco use as a concern by tying it to a fashionable disease and diminished it by lumping it in with a host of other doomsaying about infractions that many found minor. At the very least, the growing numbers of smokers indicated that few took the cautions to heart.

5 ∶ CONTESTED

Medical Dispute and Public Disbelief

In 1890, the mysterious "V. V." published *Kurite skol'ko khotite: Istoriia upotreblenia tabaka, psikhologicheskiia osnovy etoi privychki, bezvrednost' i ee vazhneishie gigienicheskiia pravila kureniia* (Smoke as much as you like: The history of tobacco use, psychological foundations of desire, safety of it and the most important hygienic rules for smoking). The pamphlet, penned in language flagrantly antagonistic to cessationist forces, boldly outlined the author's agenda. V. V. alleged that antitobacco tracts misled readers by completely ignoring the important question of tobacco's attraction in favor of dismissing smoking as a dangerous habit. The pamphleteer reasoned that man only took on habits that "give him some type of positive use—be it favor, pleasure, or enjoyment." He claimed tobacco, especially the omnipresent habit of smoking, had an "insignificant" physical effect on adults; therefore nicotine must hold a psychological attraction. Because of this mental allure, smoking's popularity spread around the world and penetrated various levels of the social spectrum.[1]

To divine the psychological attractions of smoking, V. V. called on the "theory of boredom," describing the phenomenon as a modern affliction of people who possess an active character without enough practical occupation. He argued that industrial society created monotony: "The more complicated life becomes the more demanding is man. Now boredom has become in truth a chronic illness of civilized people. Doubts, uncertainty, and boredom are the three evils overpowering civilized man." The onset of what V. V. termed alternately *tosca*, ennui, or boredom was the result of modern civilization's discontents.[2] If ennui was the disease of the modern age, V. V. posited smoking as its cure because "not finding better satisfaction of their complicated needs in their surroundings, man turns to artificial means." He cautioned, however, that "to name these means as bad habits perceives this in an extremely narrow and pedantic fashion. Tobacco is an artificial means of satisfying the needs of our active souls." Looking to historical precedent, he noted that in the past singing, which was both physically active and pleasurable, had served as a remedy to tedium, and now smoking, which used similar muscles, could do the same duty, giving a workout to the lungs after meals or mental work or even providing a break during the workday. Thus argued V. V., tobacco combatted the stultifying aspects of modern life and served as "a medicine out of boredom."[3] For V. V., tobacco was a modern solution to a modern problem that held no moral connotations.

Smoking was not a cure V. V. offered to all people. Unsurprisingly, over-civilization and boredom were diseases not available outside the ranks of upper class European males. According to V. V., women need not smoke because they were "affective" personalities rather than "active" and therefore less likely to suffer from boredom. Youth were not yet physically developed and therefore unable to stand the rigors of smoking. V. V. dismissed as "laughable," however, the idea that smoking could hurt a healthy, grown man.[4] He wrote that, "contrary to popular opinion, smoking is completely without harm and at the same time an able weapon against boredom." To be able to smoke healthfully, one had to be of "a healthy and completely ripe organism" characteristic of males at a certain age, though smokers did have to moderate their behavior by employing shallow inhalations and indulging only in well-ventilated areas.[5]

V. V. wrapped up by ridiculing the case against smoking, judging its arguments not to be compelling, and offering up his own science to counter it. He mustered research by the Army Medical Academy to argue that discussions of the poisons in tobacco smoke meant little when other consumables like tea and coffee could also be dangerous if taken in large doses. He decided that no proof existed for the harm alleged by others, and summed up: "The use of tobacco, especially in the form of smoking, has a deep psychological foundation and cannot be called a stupid or bad habit, and even less an indulgence or luxury."[6] Instead, "the diseases attributed to tobacco are the fruits of the fantasy of biased doctors and popularizers."[7] Not only did V. V. see tobacco as a modern, morally neutral answer to the problems of the day, he dismissed as ridiculous any commentary on its physical dangers. He dismantled the condemnations and labeled detractors as fanatical and delusional.

Antismoking forces did not passively weather the attack; V. V.'s vision of tobacco as a companion of modern life received a fiery rebuttal in the 1891 *Vestnik vospitaniia* (Education gazette) from the pen of V. Portugalov. In over twenty pages, almost half the length of V.V.'s sixty-page publication, Portugalov railed against what he called a cheap marketing ploy by manufacturers or at the very least a "stupid brochure." He reiterated the case against tobacco with the standard condemnations, focusing on the threat of the "strangling and disgusting smell" from smoking, the damage to nerves, the dangers to workers, the anxiety of depopulation, the specter of sexual debility, the scourge of underage smoking, and the harm for "singers, actors, and orators."[8] Portugalov condemned smoking as injurious to almost every aspect of modern citizenship from sociability to productivity and from health to speech. Speech, an essential skill for liberal citizenship with its emphasis on giving witness and being a member of the public sphere, could not be impinged upon.[9]

V. V.'s case for the psychological necessity of tobacco to modern, civilized life as well as his belief in the utility of moderate smoking was but one of many arguments made for tobacco use as safe or even beneficial in the late imperial period. In journals, pamphlets, posters, and articles, medical authorities and connoisseurs made the case for healthy smoking through moderation, modes of use, types of leaf, quality of tobacco, or age and gender of the smoker. As V. V. alleged, the lack of a strong case against tobacco opened a space for such discussions, as did the flexibility of scientific and philosophical language and evidence. Crucial too was the lack of consensus on whether tobacco was addictive, and if so, whether the fault lay in the individual or existed as an inherent aspect of the product. Ironically, the case against tobacco crumbled even as papirosy picked up more and more adherents.

General indifference from temperance groups concerning the danger of tobacco and anxiety from government officials regarding the hazards of independent antitobacco and antialcohol groups hampered any efforts against smoking. Experts considered oppressive government actions to be ineffective or even counterproductive. Together with the widespread use of tobacco, this disbelief regarding the dangers of smoking and a general wariness of cessationist groups and policies sparked derision, disbelief, and mockery of the antitobacco arguments. Rather than winning adherents against smoking, antitobacco advocates became the means for fostering the habit, becoming humorous, ineffective scolds in popular literature and even finding their negative comments turned into incentives in tobacco marketing. Even when smokers were confronted with discussions of danger, in a period when tea, coffee, masturbation, bicycling, train riding, and excessive reading all were medicalized, implicated in nervous disorder, and decreed dangerous in excess or even deadly, tobacco commentaries likely did not rise above the general noise.

ALTHOUGH the monks of Mount Athos contended in 1896 that "science long ago concluded tobacco is dangerous in every way and situation," such a consensus had not yet been achieved by the eve of World War I.[10] Not even antitobacco advocates presented a united front. While some might have argued for complete destruction of tobacco culture, many tempered their commentaries against smoking with mentions of the safety of "moderate" or educated consumption or even recommended tobacco as beneficial. An 1887 essay from the journal *Vrach* noted, "The literature on the question is wide. In it, on one side, exists the foundational designation of tobacco's dangerous effects; on the other, there are essays in which tobacco is seriously lauded as a disinfectant and a protection against infectious diseases."[11] After an extensive, in-depth survey of the literature in English, French, German, and Russian, one 1906 pamphlet dismissed the majority of antitobacco works, remarking that smoking did not lead to most of what it was accused of, such as "nicotine psychosis." The author did caution against excessive consumption in the modern style of "alcohol, tobacco, abuse of coffee and tea, etc. etc.," which might lead to neurasthenic complications if unchecked, but the caution was equivocal.[12]

The history of tobacco's introduction into Europe and Russia undoubtedly contributed to the confusion. The French employed tobacco in a number of humeral remedies in the sixteenth and seventeenth centuries including use as a purgative, enema, and inhalant. They even termed it a panacea.[13] Europeans used tobacco as an antidote to poisons or a fumigating agent, even going so far as believe that London tobacconists had survived the plague because of their trade.[14]

Russian authors referenced this early history in works for and against tobacco. Russia received tobacco with a deep distrust for certain substances considered medicinal elsewhere but deemed sources of disorderly behavior by Russian authorities.[15] Professor Bek noted that when tobacco first came to Europe it was valued for its flowers and in time became a medicine for headache and toothache, colic, rheumatism, coughs, and wounds.[16] V. V. recorded, in his case for tobacco, the utilization of tobacco against skin diseases in topical application and "internally for cholera, dropsy, hydrophobia, persistent rashes, tetanus, and also as an antitoxin for poisoning with strychnine."[17] Homeopaths routinely employed poisonous substances in diluted forms in their remedies, and by using tobacco to heal, perhaps homeopaths blunted criticism of tobacco's ability to kill.

Antitobacco works referenced past medical use, but argued that those days had long passed. Dr. Beliakov wrote that the only current useful point of tobacco was as a pesticide.[18] Dr. L. S. Minor lamented that medical authorities irrationally latched on to tobacco: "As I said already in one of my lectures, in that way medicine is strongly like a one-year-old child: everything that falls in his hands—bread, sugar, matches, piece of broken glass—he without care puts into his mouth."[19] Minor attacked medicine even as he attempted to uphold "the scientific foundations" for antitobacco opinions, pulling the rug out from under himself as he stood on it.

Some antitobacco authors complained of the disinterest of doctors. One pamphlet included the observation that when Professor Dogel of Kazan University spoke to the Pirogov Physicians, a progressive medical group, at their second meeting in 1887 regarding the dangers of tobacco, the medical professionals were largely "indifferent" to the question.[20] Dr. Botkin explained the reticence in the medical community to take up the antismoking cause as emerging from the twin forces of disinterest and medical contention.[21] The author of the pamphlet *Ne kuri, ne niukhai i ne zhui tabaku* (Don't smoke, don't snuff, and don't chew tobacco) assured readers that while older doctors resisted antitobacco work, younger ones were better educated and more open. Counting on a mass generational shift, he argued, "After another twenty years we can strongly predict that there will not be one doctor who looks on tobacco in a way other than as an evil scourge of man's life and happiness."[22] The lag in medical opinion noted here was not simply hyperbole. Medical professionals went to school for only a few years before moving into practice. Their professors may have used the latest materials for some of their lectures, but they likely relied on a standard corpus of established materials for many. Once out of school, due to specialization or simply the pressures of practice, not all doctors would keep up to date. They might even have resisted new materials. If taught by a moribund professor and then unable to keep up themselves, a physician could be practicing with ideas twenty or even thirty years out of date. While certainly innovative technologies would be incorporated in some cases, the transition of technology and knowledge in medicine could be slow.

Antitobacco activists were disingenuous when they painted medical professionals as indifferent. Multiple works testified to the ongoing research into tobacco's dangers, but the ambiguous findings of these experiments would not conform to the case that antitobacco advocates wished to make.[23] A. A. Fal'kenberg investigated the question of whether tobacco use protected one from diseases, publishing his findings in *Vrach* and then as a pamphlet in 1892. Using tobacco smoke exhaled onto glass or wool and then cultured for bacteria, Fal'kenberg reported, "It may be concluded that it has a mildly beneficial effect on the organism, strengthening its resistance . . . to pathogenic bacteria's penetration of the body."[24] In his own antitobacco pamphlet, Dr. Udintsev conceded that smoking did lead to "the betterment of mental and mood standing," a trait especially valuable in the modern era when there was such "a great desire for mental and physical work."[25] Dr. P. P. Orlov concurred that tobacco helped with the brain and nerves, though he surmised that this was not an acceptable exchange given the problems it later caused.[26] In her survey of production-related health problems for tobacco factory workers, Dr. Valitskaia determined that she could not "prove any certain forms of disease" from her research, though she did admit to seeing many symptoms of illness.[27]

In the 1914 pamphlet *Nauchnye osnovy bor'by s kureniem tabaka* (The scientific foundations of the fight with tobacco smoking), a version of a talk given to the Obshchestvo nevropatalogov i psikhiatrov (Society of Neuropathologists and Psychiatrists) in Moscow in 1913, Minor took on the case against tobacco at length and concluded that it had no merit. Citing the literature on nicotine and the effects of tobacco use on the nervous system and the glands, he argued that while tobacco was frequently compared to alcohol and syphilis, this was an incorrect analogy. He pointed out that tobacco caused no social danger because the smoker did not harm others, maintained good work habits, and even used tobacco to enable night work. Indeed, "A papirosa or a cigar helps to banish boredom and lessen sorrow but does not degrade a person morally as does alcohol. Therefore the smoker—as far as it concerns smoking—stays a good member of society, especially if he generously invites others with his cigars or papirosy."[28] He conceded that, in excess, tobacco use could be bad for the nerves, arteries, and stomach, but that this was rare because smokers did not inhale all the smoke nor did they do so deeply or all at once. Thus they gradually became used to the poisons. Minor discounted any loss to male sexual function by using Orientalist arguments based on the presumed hedonism of the East. He noted that Asian males smoked excessively, yet remained "sexually active late into life and engage[d] in polygamy." It was only smoking women, prone to miscarriage, who had sexual debility from tobacco use.[29]

In addition to disputing depictions of tobacco as harmful, medical tracts often defined beneficial aspects. Dr. Rokau in his pamphlet of the 1880s noted that some doctors prescribed smoking, believing it excellent for "intestinal problems, asthma, incontinence, and ameliorating tetanus." Rokau did not agree that tobacco fought scurvy, arguing instead that it "sooner [brought] ill than use" and that drugs that were more effective could solve these conditions, but he did not fully condemn tobacco.[30] Folk healers reportedly also utilized tobacco in poultices, baths, or as snuff or chaw in their remedies for toothache, skin conditions, and as a general aid that "cleanse[d] the brain of phlegm, refreshe[d] sight, etc."[31] They also promised smoking could clear eyesight.[32]

The lack of consensus on tobacco among Russia's medical establishment, the educated public, and traditional healers was typical. In Britain, the first article in the *Lancet* about smoking appeared in 1843 and reported that with moderation there was no danger. A more extensive round of antitobacco literature hit the magazine in the 1850s, but continued to suggest moderation as safe, with the issue becoming relatively silent by the 1860s. By the end of the nineteenth century, antismoking commentary no longer made headway in Britain's premier medical journal.[33] American doctors dithered also.[34] British and American antitobacco campaigns found some success with the issue of youth smoking, but their hyperbole led medical professionals to pull away from arguments they found unreliable.[35] The Canadian medical establishment determined adult male smoking to be harmless and even speculated it might be beneficial in early stage tuberculosis and excellent for nervous asthma, though again women and children could not safely indulge.[36] Russian physicians and clinicians were well acquainted with foreign research, following its progress and using methods they found applicable, so these opinions likely made their way into Russian discussions.[37]

The calls for moderation were not restricted to connoisseurs and prosmoking groups. The title of Dr. Buialskii's pamphlet, *O vrede ot izlishchnego kureniia tabaka* (On the danger of excessive tobacco smoking), acknowledged the issue of immoderate intake.[38] The six-edition *Bros'te kurit'! O vrede kureniia tabake dlia zdorov'ia* (Stop smoking! On the danger of smoking tobacco for health), ironically determined, "A few papirosy per day, smoked after meals, cannot do a great deal of damage to a healthy person."[39] Dogel's speech at Kazan University noted that mild smokers could live long lives.[40] The definition of moderation seemed fairly expansive, as another author judged: "A person smoking twenty papirosy a day is considered a moderate smoker."[41] Minor recommended five to fifteen papirosy a day, or four to five cigars.[42] Dr. Preis, however, a prolific and vehemently antitobacco author, maintained that even moderate use—ten to fifteen papirosy per day—did nothing but incrementally slow the speedy march of smokers to their early deaths.[43] The debate over moderation echoed calls within the temperance community regarding drink, where some groups pushed back against total abstinence as impractical and unnecessary.[44]

Prescriptions for controlled smoking detailed not just the amount of tobacco but the type, processing, and style of intake.[45] Not surprisingly, the discerning smoking of expensive tobacco from the upper classes was depicted as healthier than the tasteless smoking of cheap tobacco from the lower classes. In 1889, E. S. Krymskii argued that the worst sorts of tobacco (makhorka) ran to 4–8% nicotine while the best contained only 2%.[46] In 1902, Bek similarly argued that better sorts of tobacco were less dangerous.[47] Dr. Keibel described in detail the problems of higher-nicotine tobaccos and noted that ammonia contributed to the strength of tobacco and thus higher-ammonia and higher-nicotine tobaccos were more dangerous than others.[48] In the encyclopedia of Brokgauz and Efron, detailed chemical entries from different varietals underscored the primacy of nicotine content to hygienic arguments. Additionally, the author put forward the idea that higher costs could lessen danger because quality tobacco held less of the poison. He also argued that scientific processing could decrease nicotine to an "undetectable" amount. To dismiss all worries for the connoisseur, he pointed out that in "storage of cigars over many years, the nicotine dissipates and at the same time, quality increases."[49]

Given the focus on gradual poisoning as the most deadly aspect of smoking and the higher nicotine of makhorka, none of this is surprising. Not all experts agreed on which leaf was least dangerous. An 1852 pamphlet on tobacco fabrication suggested that low sort Hungarian tobacco, because it was highly aromatic and required less manipulation and fewer additives, was "most tolerable for health."[50] Contention continued into the later period as some authorities decried the highly aromatic, cheap makhorka as the most hazardous with the highest nicotine while others deemed it "less dangerous than all those named Turkish tobacco."[51]

Modes of use also came into the discussion. In 1890 Keibel argued that the best way to take tobacco was snuff, as the nose could not distribute it as easily through the body, but that chewing immediately introduced nicotine to the digestive system. The 1882 pamphlet *Ne po nosu tabak: Russkaia skazka* (Do not put tobacco up your nose: A Russian tale) was not keen on the relative safety of snuff.[52] Observing that the countryside was healthier than the city and that pipes were more prevalent in the countryside, the author of this pamphlet concluded that pipes were the best.[53] A 1905 pamphlet argued that the more aromatic the tobacco, the more poisonous, not just because of the leaf but also because of the processing, which endangered smokers and workers.[54]

Another popular means proposed for safe tobacco use was filtration—either through the water pipe or batting. The 1852 production manual *O razvedenii i fabrikatsii tabaka* (On the cultivation and fabrication of tobacco) suggested, "When one smokes in the Turkish fashion, then the combustibles stay in the water and the mouth only takes in the gentle smoke and nicotine."[55] This advice echoed forward through to pamphlets in the late 1800s and early 1900s.[56] Even Bek's 1902 pamphlet for the journal *Narodnoe zdravie* (The people's health) suggested the safety of smoking with the water pipe and pipe because of the distance the smoke had to travel before entering the body as well as the lack of direct contact of skin with tobacco. He cautioned never to smoke a cigar to its end and to avoid the direct contact of the lips with either cigar or papirosa because this was the primary cause of tongue and lip cancer. He theorized that the nicotine gathered in "cool places," staying at the end of a cigar, or pipe reserve, and he recommended smoking in the open air with a mouthpiece, which kept the dangerous cigarette paper smoke from the eyes and mouth, a cause of catarrh.[57] Such connections between proximity to the smoke or leaf and danger entered into earlier recommendations for pipes.[58] The water pipe, immobile, expensive, and not as easy to use as papirosy, also took from smoking many of the qualities that made it available to lower classes.

Dr. Il'inskii, author of multiple antismoking packets, advocated filtered papirosy for safer smoking in his otherwise stridently antitobacco multiedition pamphlet *Tri iada: Tabak, alkogol' (vodka), i sifilis* (Three poisons: Tobacco, alcohol (vodka), and syphilis). He confided, "Smoking papirosy with filters is healthier than those set in mouthpieces because the smoke, which goes through the batting, is cleansed and leaves in the batting many burnt items or what is known as tobacco sauce, which falling into the lungs is much more strongly dangerous to them and brings forth nervous consequences."[59] For even safer smoking, he urged, "*the best method is to never inhale but simply to push the smoke out of the mouth before smoking*" [emphasis original]. He argued that this allowed enjoyment of the habit with much lessened danger, since the "chief pleasure of smoking is the feeling of smoke for the mucous membranes and not in the stupefaction of the body."[60] This was a sensual pleasure not mentioned in other sources, but may have been akin to modern discussions of burn quality. Minor recommended the following strategies for safer smoking: switch to lighter and higher-quality tobacco, which was "comparatively safe for health," especially when smoked in longer-length papirosy or with an extended holder. He told smokers to inhale less and, when smoking, to do so in fresh air and never in the bedroom. Finally, if possible, he cautioned users to find nicotine-free papirosy or to include in the mouthpiece iron trichloride (*polutorakhloristoe zhelezo*), which he cited as a way to fight the effects of nicotine.[61]

In 1913, Udintsev spoke out about filters as being useless, but he offered recommendations for safer smoking including smoking in open spaces and using holders.[62] Dr. Mendel'son compared the health among smokers who inhaled versus those who did not, with the conclusion that "smoking without inhalation brings significantly less danger."[63] The reasoning behind his support of filters—moderating inhalation and limiting nicotine intake—came from a different perspective than that of later arguments. Filtered papirosy and low-draw technologies became popular in the West in the 1950s in the wake of the evidence on the danger of tars. Studies later concluded that filters did not provide any clear health benefits and may have made smoking more deadly by encouraging deeper inhalations of smaller particles, which led to tumors deeper in the lungs.[64]

Manufacturers and entrepreneurs took advantage of the interest in safer smoking and the general belief in the beneficial effects of filters. The *bogatyr* of *Vazhnyia*'s poster enjoyed a filtered smoke (figure 1.7). Smokers in the Soviet period sometimes pinched the hollowed tubes of their papirosy in order to effect a filtered smoke, though when the practice began was not documented. Some brands chose not to filter but instead removed the poisons altogether. The mid-priced brand *Nora* was advertised as being without nicotine.[65] The Mir factory marketed several brands as "hygienic" without specifying how this was measured.[66] A. Lopato and Sons noted that their smokes were produced "under doctor's supervision."[67] A Dr. Kozha pitched his mouthpiece that "destroyed" the poison nicotine.[68] Nicotine-free options emerged in response to arguments regarding neurasthenic decline. Such options might have helped to decrease dependency, though no sales reports emerged to document this. When later American manufacturers attempted to decrease nicotine in cigarettes, however, they witnessed a dip in demand.[69]

An A. L. V. Khofman advertised his soon-to-be-patented system for safer smoking in a 1913 pamphlet, noting how it helped those without the "strength of will" to quit to not "over smoke." As he underlined, *Smoke judiciously and do not rush. Try not to swallow the smoke. With slow, careful smoking, the larger part of the nicotine in the tobacco can fly away. With such smoking you will feel better.*" His method required a modification of the cardboard mouthpiece of the papirosy by placing therein a small pinprick, so that "there was less smoke and it was lighter." This small adjustment, he promised, overcame all the dangers of overindulgence. "I smoke as I wish and do it as I want—if I want a strong papirosa or if I want a weak one. My good appetite has returned and I sleep better. My health has improved and it is as if I were reborn." The rest of his pamphlet was filled with similar testimonials from users on how to smoke as they wished but with less danger through use of his patented system, which would soon be up and producing papirosy for sale.[70]

The controversy swirling around the dangers of tobacco extended to debate over whether smokers used tobacco voluntarily. Understanding of what constituted an addiction, or dependency, as opposed to a chosen activity or habit bundled together a host of issues regarding will, sin, personal liberty, social responsibility, bodily integrity, and governmental reach.[71] Research into addictive substances had barely begun by the end of the nineteenth century and it moved forward without the sophisticated biochemical analysis at the cellular level that would later unlock answers as to the physical responses of bodies to dependency-producing substances, the nature of withdrawal symptoms, and the single-mindedness that could possess addicts.[72]

Discussion of smoking often centered around the same questions as those of drinking: did people use because they wanted to or had to, could they quit through strength of will or was it beyond their control, and did the source of addiction come from the substance or reside in the individual body?[73] The concept of excessive alcohol use as a disease arose in Europe in the preindustrial period and later in temperance literature, but the context of what disease meant, the parameters of what might be called a disease, and the place of the individual, the will, and sin fluctuated.[74] In the mix of moral, governmental, religious, and medical ideas, Enlightenment concepts butted up against older religious ideas and discussions of Westernization, autocracy, and modernity. An important early author on the place of tobacco within discussions of problem behaviors was Benjamin Rush (1746–1813), the American founding father, physician for the Continental Army, and credited "father of psychiatry." Rush, who wrote on alcohol use more extensively, condemned tobacco as a gateway to the abuse of drink and for its connections to idleness, even estimating that up to five work days a year were lost to snuff breaks.[75] The transition from condemnation of gluttonous use of alcohol as a sin to discussions of overuse of substances as a disease occurred over the course of the nineteenth century. Alcoholism, instead of drunkenness, manifested in symptoms that included a crisis of will that left the behavior out of the individual's control.[76]

Russian physicians and psychiatrists, highly influenced by the material school and that of physiology, investigated the nature of addiction, looking to identify material causes for mental problems and rooting psychological developments in the functions of the nervous system.[77] In the West, the work of René Descartes (1596–1650) led to rooting dependency in the mind (ideology), not brain (the material), begetting a therapeutic culture of blame and admonition rather than understanding and treatment.[78] Western theorists argued that addiction was a disease brought on by continued use from a psychological, not physical, weakness—what was termed "inebriety"—and that already weak or nervous types were more susceptible, although blame still leaked into discussions of the illness.[79]

Psychology was a relatively new discipline in Russia. The first Russian department of psychiatry was founded in 1857 in St. Petersburg and by the turn of the century the study had spread to most universities.[80] Clinics and sanatoria sprang up for psychotherapy and the ideas of psychiatry held popular resonance as authors including Dostoevsky and Tolstoy read widely in the field and dipped into its theories for their works.[81] Major theorists like Ivan Pavlov (1849–1936) and V. M. Bekhterev (1857–1927) moved the field forward, yet they held an uneasy relationship with the government and pushed forward with progressive political agendas that were often in opposition to the state.[82]

Russian authorities both medical and psychiatric debated the nature of addictive substances in the late nineteenth century with particular attention to alcoholism but also in connection with opium, hashish, coffee, tea, and tobacco. Theorists argued for alcoholism as an individual and social problem that must be fought with economic and cultural programs.[83] Alcoholism was acknowledged with a clinical term in Russian and regarded as being akin to a disease, though the concept was debated in a 1905 issue of the journal *Trezvaia zhizn'* (The sober life).[84] Organizers of the 1909–10 "first all-Russian congress on the struggle against drunkenness" (Pervyi vserossiiskii s"ezd po bor'be s p'ianstvom) in St. Petersburg consciously used the less clinical term in their title, over physicians' objections, because they thought the public would be more familiar with drunkenness than alcoholism.[85] In the same period, Metropolitan Vladimir (r. 1898–1918) argued that a drunkard was different from a dissolute person and that he could be cured with the correct application of culture and habit.[86]

While Vladimir expressed sympathy for alcohol dependency, no such empathy developed for depictions of smoking. Most religious authorities, following the words of Metropolitan Filaret, characterized smoking as a "new type of slavery."[87] Archpriest Popov used the popularity of the vice as its condemnation, noting that good habits spread slowly and less widely: "If smoking is a blameless habit, if it is not a sin . . . why does it so strongly hold in captivity such a large group of people of every age, sex, and profession? . . . So quickly and widely has spread the habit of smoking it clearly exposes its sinful, passionate properties."[88] In his 1914 anti-smoking pamphlet, the anonymous V. P. argued that those who served the church and smoked offended God with their breath and should be ashamed.[89] Even the distinguished Botkin did not eschew condemnation of the smoker, arguing that "often there is the desire among many smokers to quit, but after the desire comes the thought of the boredom without it, which completely destroys the desire, and the man under the beast's power becomes a dependable-unchanging slave of this ruler." As support for his argument, Botkin used not clinical exams or even anecdotal case histories but Gogol's Cossack hero Taras Bulba.[90] Russian psychiatrists often used literary figures as a basis for diagnosis of real-life medical problems—a reflection of the interest in psychology by famous authors.[91]

In Western discussions of temperance, the effects of compulsion and especially the point of losing control became central to identifying alcoholism as a disease. In the case of nicotine, a great many of the sources continued to depict smoking as a chosen habit rather than a passion outside the user's willpower.[92] Russians used a variety of terms to describe tobacco use, some borrowing from morality, others from psychology or alcohol studies. In the nineteenth and well into the twentieth century, "passion" (*pristrastie*) and other morally charged terms such as "evil use" (*zloupotreblenie*) and the category "evil habits" (*durnye privychki*) categorized smoking. To use the term "habit" downplayed the severity of cravings, as noted by the monks of Mt. Athos: if smoking is a habit, "is it possible that those habituated cannot in their power be unhabituated? . . . Nothing in the world that is a habit cannot be unlearned." They warned that, without care, the habit could progress, as "little by little a habit becomes a passion which then ruins people."[93] The monks dismissed as volitional and easily overturned the use of tobacco that came from habit, but warned of the moral danger of a "passion" for tobacco, when habit had turned to the point of becoming offensive and a sin. American antitobacco activists centered their critiques of smoking on the uncontrolled desire of the habituate that turned them into "cigarette fiends," but Russian admonitions tended to have greater faith that smokers could modulate use. Perhaps this reflected the much higher familiarity with smoking in Russia compared with the United States.[94]

Authors in favor of smoking, or those who advocated moderate use, typically employed the term "habit" (*privychka*) and seemed to have a rather high bar for abuse. Preis considered the immoderate user someone who smoked over ten to thirty papirosy a day. He used the term "nicotinized" (*nikotizirovannyi*) for the condition, which resulted in an unhealthy body in which, he argued, following the materialist line of logic, no healthy brain could be situated.[95] Il'inskii delineated progress from a habit to a passion (*pristrast'*), which brought with it "feebleness or hard smoking" (*tabachnyi khodosochii, tabachnyi zapoi*).[96] Other medical authorities responded that because of the progression of the habit to more intense levels with time, no amount of smoking was safe. Adolf Fedorovich Grinevskii clarified in 1889 that there needed to be a line between "use and abuse" (*balovstvom i zloupotrebleniem*, literally "evil use") and since smokers did not slow over time but instead tended to intensify their nicotine exposure, "one papirosa is already abuse."[97] In 1909, Dr. Priklonskii argued that most started smoking as youths and then developed a habit difficult to stop, even though they did not enjoy it when they began nor did they really savor it later in life.[98]

The definition of habit as a disease occupied the conclusions of Vitol'd Khmelevskii for his 1876 dissertation for the degree of doctor of medicine. Khmelevskii situated the problem of habit formation in the rhetoric of neurasthenia and autointoxication, arguing that nicotine poisoning struck the nervous system and that while the chronic, low-dose poisoning associated with smoking might explain the lack of symptoms, this might be itself a form of illness. "It is said that habit deadens the effects of narcotics; but in order for the nervous system to become inured to tobacco, does it not follow it must change? That is, that the physical status must move to ill, abnormal, and pathological?" If tobacco poisoning therefore changed the system, moving it into the domain of illness, then he concluded it must be akin to alcohol problems and thus "at the very least the after effects of them [were] similar—the destruction of health and the shortening of life."[99] Using the theory that tobacco and alcohol acted as similar neurasthenic poisons, he concluded that their health effects were comparable.

Discussions of tobacco and alcohol often joined the two in terms of danger, but while the vices were repeatedly paired and the dangers to morality and the body compared, the consequences of quitting the two were treated differently. As the anonymous author of the 1904 pamphlet *P'ianstvo i kurenie tabaku i ikh vrednye posledstviia* (On drunkenness and smoking tobacco and their dangerous outcomes) argued, "Chronic poisoning with nicotine is somewhat analogous with alcohol poisoning, but the change to the organism from these two items is different. . . . If today you smoke 100 papirosy and tomorrow not a one then . . . it will be great! Nothing bad will happen to you and no aftermath except a good one will occur."[100] The visible nature of alcohol withdrawal symptoms as well as their established place in the medical lexicon distinguished the commentary on alcohol and tobacco. The term alcoholism, coined in 1849 by Swedish physician Magnus Huss (1807–90), referred to the narrow set of symptoms of alcohol withdrawal. The modern concept of alcoholism as a disease that could strike the individual or society with affects psychological, social, or physical came from the ideas of E. M. Jellineck (1890–1963), the prominent scholar of alcohol related disorders, in the 1940s, not those of the nineteenth century. Authorities reached no consensus on causes or treatments for alcoholism, but clinics appeared as early as 1896 devoted to recovery for alcoholics.[101]

The symptoms of alcohol withdrawal, the delirium tremens, were well recognized in the nineteenth century and commented on in many medical journals. The markers of tobacco withdrawal, however, were not universally recognized or respected. Dismissive assessments led to trivializing smokers and their treatment. Dogel wrote extensively on alcohol and authored a popular multiedition pamphlet on tobacco.[102] In his discussions of alcohol, he derided those who would claim an "instinct" for alcohol, instead supporting an "environmental" understanding of use.[103] For tobacco, Dogel argued that there was no conceivable reason for people to smoke. If it were a question of fashion, he pointed out that the habit should have long fallen out of style. For those who called it tasty, he hypothesized that they could not judge it as wonderful as sugar, and those who called it aromatic he hoped they would not dare compare it to fine perfumes. If a smoker argued that it was a process leading to contemplation, he countered that the spitting, hacking, and horrible burning odors accompanying tobacco use hindered serious thought. Any reasoning that might be applied to tobacco use he summarily dismissed.[104] Dogel asked smokers when their preference began, reporting that many started smoking in imitation of others and out of curiosity and then "little by little" it became a habit as the body needed to continue the stimulation of tobacco. Despite his thorough and considered deconstruction of the reasons for smoking, Dogel did not completely condemn the practice. In keeping with other medical authorities of the day, he advocated safer consumption by means of water pipes and long-stemmed pipes

Like Dogel, Dr. D. P. Nikol'skii worked in antialcohol and antitobacco arenas, writing pamphlets such as his multiedition *O tabake i vrede ego kureniia* (On tobacco and the danger of smoking) and *O kurenii tabaka sredi uchashchikhsia* (On smoking tobacco among students). In his tobacco works, Nikol'skii argued for a strong connection with alcohol, calling smoking and drinking "two sisters."[105] In his alcohol work, Nikol'skii stressed the need for medical professionals to address the problem, as previous tracts were inadequate, being either anecdotal or moral. By emphasizing scientific approaches, Nikol'skii simultaneously shored up medicine as an important arm of social control and promoted himself and his profession.[106] With about three-quarters of doctors employed by the state in the late imperial period, the relationship between medical and governmental authority was more than just rhetorical.[107]

Despite his derision of moral arguments against alcohol, Nikol'skii emphasized these same arguments in his antitobacco polemic, noting that Metropolitan Filaret had spoken against the habit and that "even if tobacco was harmless, then it would still be a whimsy, lust, and passion that binds a human." In dismissing tobacco as a habit, Nikol'skii implied that quitting should be a condition of soul, not body; of mind, not brain: "From quitting tobacco no one has died or gone mad." He discounted both physical and mental effects as mild and quickly passing, since while "quitting smoking a person will experience at first a few unpleasant feelings, in the style of melancholy [*toski*], nervousness, headache, shakes, disinclination to study, etc., but all of that soon goes away and the person quickly feels better."[108] Therefore, he argued, it was best to quit immediately: "In the end, once a person understands that tobacco is dangerous, he can always take control of himself [*sdelat' nad soboi usilie*] and quit. The consciousness of smoking's danger engenders strength of character, which is of primary importance."[109] In his arguments, he depicted nicotine as easily quit. To not do so was folly.

By painting quitting as the logical choice, and rationality and character as the only needs for abandoning the habit, Nikol'skii belittled the smoker who struggled to quit and diminished the problems for cessation, a theme echoed by Popov, who scoffed, "But if you ask anyone, 'Why do you smoke'? Not one will give you a smart answer."[110] Bek similarly considered that it was "harder to find a habit more stupid and dangerous than the smoking of tobacco."[111] If the habit was senseless and irrational, with no physical compulsions, it should come as little surprise that self-possession was considered sufficient for quitting, even from doctors and neurological specialists.[112] Whereas St. Petersburg public health authorities discussed how best to combat alcoholism and theorized various causes for drinking from biological to social, no such nuanced, detailed, or in-depth understanding of tobacco's users was attempted or seemingly even merited.[113]

In the 1907 *Zagadka kureniia* (The mystery of smoking), S. Tormazov gave one of the most detailed understandings of tobacco use as a compulsion that strayed beyond mere preference, giving rise to an appetite that was grounded in the organism but that he still termed "a mystery." He argued that habit described smoking only to those who have never tried tobacco, whereas those who had become accustomed to nicotine felt for it "a commanding need." Tea, he posited, might become a habit, but "the need for smoking is acquired so quickly and instilled so firmly that to explain it as a habit is impossible." He further noted that use was not predicated simply on enjoyment, as a smoker unable to find good tobacco would make do with bad just to have it. He offered that "every smoker knows its reflexive [*mekhanicheskii*]" and that waiting for it became a "hunger . . . from both psychological and physical factors."[114]

Tormazov's conception of tobacco compulsion, however, held class connotations. The passion to tobacco came more readily to mental workers than to those of physical tasks. Indeed, he noted that physical laborers did not smoke with the same intensity as that of mental workers. As he observed, the need to tobacco came from psychological foundations:

> It rests upon the following: every time when the attention focuses on something at one point, the control of the will weakens on that which does not come into the sphere of attention, and thanks to that, the desire, at other times repressed and contained, does not meet obstruction and possesses the person; therefore the desire to smoke, generally restrained by the proper limits of the mind's control, takes power of the smoker, and in those instances when his will is paralyzed by the concentration of attention on some mental interest or emotional episode he smokes more commonly.[115]

But he countered those who would say tobacco use was fully psychological and reflexive with the listing of the actions associated with smoking—finding a light, getting papirosy, and so on, which were not simple enough to be reflective actions. Thus something else had to be at work.

Tormazov combined his discussion of the psychological pulls to smoking with a description of the actions of smoking that led to physiological reactions in the body, especially the "overexcitation" of the brain with blood. The body became conditioned to such stimulation, and if not repeated, the smoker turned agitated, impatient, and finally, angry. Thus "the smoker is nearly helpless against the desire to smoke because his brain is used to it and even if he does not know it, he feels it." At other times, the need for nicotine could be triggered by "mental disturbance" (*dushevnoe volnenie*), "in particular as the rise of anger, anxiousness or offense call before the regular smoker the rising desire for nicotine."

Tormazov gave one of the more nuanced portrayals of the difficulty of quitting. He posited that repetition of actions or intake of other substances might simulate tobacco's stimulation without dangerous aftereffects, but he conceded that there were both psychological and physiological barriers to quitting.[116] He recommended physical exercise, especially "physical labor, [which,] in opposition to mental labor, weakens the desire for smoking." Not just a physical remedy was necessary, however; the attack on tobacco must also be "a social battle" with controls on sales and access. As he reasoned, if opium were sold everywhere, everyone would be smoking opium. In opium's case, controls worked he argued, and he extended the logic to smoking. The battle had to move to the family, too, because smokers' children had "a large affinity to smoking and a lower protection against its dangerous effects. The danger of smoking multiplies in the offspring."[117]

With little consensus as to the effects of smoking on the body in terms of health or addiction, small wonder so many different approaches to smoking cessation emerged. Some argued that quitting was an issue of little concern. As I. Tregubov helpfully commented in his pamphlet committed to helping smokers stop their habit, *Normal'nyi sposob brosit' kurit'* (Normal method to stop smoking), "talk of not being able to give up is silliness."[118] Those who could not or did not quit became irrational and frivolous in their continued devotion to an easily abandoned whim. In his 1890 pamphlet, Keibel argued that quitting was difficult but must be undertaken before tobacco smoking had penetrated "to the core."[119] Similarly, some activists simply gave up on adult smokers and turned instead to children as the focus of their prophylactic message. Priklonskii recommended moderation and other mitigating steps for smokers, but argued that a focus on stopping youth from smoking would gradually decrease the number of smokers "because at a mature age, when people are more conscious of their habits, they rarely begin to smoke as they are familiar with all its dangers."[120] The adult smoker who started as a youth was a lost cause.

Surveys of child and youth smoking highlighted reasons from students for quitting and the methods they employed. Mendel'son's survey of smoking youth found that only one quit for every nine who smoked. For most, the impetus was illness.[121] In 1902, Nikol'skii published his survey from data obtained at the St. Petersburg Mining Institute. He found only eight students who had quit, citing reasons such as "noticed weakness and the danger of poor effects on the nerves," "to save health and cut unnecessary costs," "health worsened from smoking," "on doctor's advice," "from creed" (*iz ubezhdeniia*), "fiancée forbade smoking," "found it harmful," and "had enough" (*nadoelo*).[122] Their methods ranged from cold turkey to promises to parents, distractions with books, and influence from peers, with multiple citations of developing "strength of will."[123]

Other experts were more measured in their understanding of the difficulty of smoking cessation. Appolov urged nonsmokers to be good examples for smokers, wives to aid husbands, and mothers to help children. Instead of judgment, they should show understanding: "Drunkards and smokers should be pitied because they are slaves to their desires. These unhappy people know themselves that it is evil. . . . We must help them."[124] Buial'skii acknowledged the variable experience, so that for one smoker quitting was "very difficult and boring and another put down the pipe easily and without any cravings [*prinuzhdeniia*]."[125]

The maudlin, and mistitled, "fable-caricature" *Kak oni brosili kurit'* (How they quit smoking) explored not the story of a group of smokers quitting, but instead the story of seven smokers, four of them women, who continued to smoke despite knowledge of its dangers to mind and heart. The characters had concrete discussions of smoking's distasteful odor, its effect on the pregnancy of one of the women, and even the death of another's husband through a tortured process of tongue cancer that involved his tongue being gradually chopped up by surgeons and his eventual starvation. Perhaps in less fable-like and more realistic fashion, every one of the characters continued to smoke.[126] As the main character, the attorney Lobzhinov, lamented, "I don't have the strength of will to quit. I don't have the character. There it is. But I want to smoke. . . . I don't know myself and no one knows who I am. I'm not myself and you're not you . . . and I can't take it any longer. I want to smoke!" When the others all had shamefacedly admitted that none of them had quit either, the entire group enjoyed a smoke together.[127]

Contemporaries suggested numerous substitutes for those experiencing cravings. Krzeminskii, a specialist in nervous illnesses at the University of St. Vladimir, recommended mouthwashes or mints but maintained that quitting without any props was preferable.[128] Grinevskii mentioned the method of Dr. Raspail, which was camphor papirosy or "tar papirosy"— wood sticks smeared with purified tar, which "when sucked on smell[ed] of tarred air." Raspail hypothesized that these sticks produced an experience that "weaken[ed] the urge [*pozyv*] for tobacco." Grinevskii, however, thought the method of little use and instead told smokers to "show yourself that you have strength of will, self-control, and character."[129] For those used to a smoke with a meal, the volume by Krymskii suggested "weak tea, fruit drops, or porridge with sugar," assuring reader that after two or three times, denial would come more easily.[130] Therapies revolved around either simple substitutes for sucking or variations of strengthening the will. Behavioral concepts dominated, despite the emphasis on the chemical poison of nicotine, show-ing that none thought that anything drew the smoker in besides the action.

Pamphlets for antismoking methods, such as Komisarenko's *Pagubnoe privychka* (The ruinous habit), published in nine editions at least, prom-ised help with a system of "real healthfulness and quick action on smokers." Komisarenko did not dismiss craving as insignificant but instead sympa-thized with the "unbearable sorrow" of abstention from nicotine, which often led to returning to the habit. He argued that quitting without some type of aid was impossible: "Every smoker, wishing to quit smoking, needed without fail some method, which accustomed him out of smoking and first destroyed the urge to tobacco and then made it completely impossible." The system consisted of two parts, a mouthpiece and apparatus, which de-livered two or three droplets of his Antinikotin serum through a reservoir. Available through the mail and at pharmacies throughout the capital, the method was buttressed with several pages of testimonials from some of the more than 3,500 satisfied customers, several of whom quit in as few as three days. One husband crowed about how the apparatus had allowed his wife, who had smoked for twenty-five years, to quit. Other satisfied customers mentioned came from the military and judiciary, along with "clerks, clergy, artists, landowners, peasants, tradesman and workers. In a word from the generals to the poorest workers."[131]

Tregubov, another cessation entrepreneur, dismissed apparatuses and medicines as useless in his 1912 pamphlet. He advised the would-be non-smoker to keep tobacco on hand but not smoke it. "Focus on yourself," he wrote, and after the first week it would become easier and easier to forget about smoking. To help he advised avoiding "strong stimulation, sleepless nights and especially all spirits (vodka, wine, and beer) as all this greatly strengthens the desire to smoke."[132] For those powerfully under the thrall of tobacco, he recommended a solution of 2–3% iodine mixed with warm milk three times a day, lily of the valley or valerian caplets, a vegetarian diet, or meditation in front of the mirror regarding the dangers of tobacco (though never before bed).[133] The reference to lily of the valley tablets likely came from the research of the clinician Botkin into the pharmacological uses of the plant, especially for heart conditions.[134] Tregubov further promoted ex-ercise, open air, a "break from regular patterns for five to six days," and most importantly not falling back into old ways, as a person "must be as strong in breaking a habit as in keeping it."[135] Tregubov's method, heavily reliant on behavioral changes, also included chemical components that seemed to follow both current science in Russia and theories from homeopathy.

Not surprisingly, given the pairing of tobacco and alcohol as evils of a common root, therapies offered for alcohol abuse were repurposed to tobacco. Especially prominent in this were the therapies emphasizing the will from neurologists and psychologists working to make a name for themselves in alcoholism treatment. Psychologists had purview over alcohol addiction therapy in late-nineteenth-century Russia, echoing the European fascination with the French theorists of nervous disorders like the neurologist and theorist of hysteria Jean-Martin Charcot (1825–93). Other French theorists worked more directly with addiction. For instance, Theodule Ribot (1839–1916), the editor of *Revue de philosophie positive* and author of the well-received *Les maladies de la volonté* (The diseases of the will) attributed addiction to an "excess of impulse," which could not be resisted, and he diagnosed much of this problem as hereditary degeneracy.[136] American theorists similarly saw drunkenness as a disease that could be passed from parent to child.[137]

American temperance advocates pushed for complete abstention from alcohol as the only cure and the strengthening of will as the course of action.[138] The emphasis on a disciplined will in the American context took on a cast of both middle-class anxiety and capitalist desire for regulated, disciplined, rational behaviors that maximized profits and fought societal disorder.[139] Tobacco treatments often followed a similar course so that treatment for tobacco or alcohol abuse focused not on suppressing desire but rather on strengthening the will. How to strengthen the will, however, remained a slippery therapeutic concept, as the "will" was identified in no consistent way. At times it was more biological, at other points strictly moral. In the late Victorian European context, the two freely intermingled.[140] In terms of smoking treatments, the result was an emphasis on cures that copied treatments for other nervous disorders like neurasthenia, where strengthening the will helped to thwart the markers of the disease.

In Russia, professionals influenced by Ribot contemplated the role of the weakened will in criminality, pathology, and modern life.[141] The weakened will similarly became party to substance abuse and neurasthenia. Lack of will was a root of drunkenness according to a 1905 essay in *Trezvaia zhizn'*.[142] It was the origin of smoking's pull as well.[143] Thus the drunkard and the smoker could look forward to the application of regimens of rest and the strengthening of the body in order to allow the will to recover.[144] In both the cure and the disease echoed methods and conclusions informed by religious ideas of morality and the will. In his 1902 *Kak brosit' kurit'* (How to quit smoking), Aleksandr Iakovlevich Blindovskii foregrounded the necessity for "full and decided *consciousness*" alongside an immediate cessation with no stand-ins. This need not take "a Herculean strength of will" as every person who was "psychologically healthy" presented enough strength of will to quit smoking naturally. Smokers had to understand that "only the physical strength of a person has a limit. The moral strength [was] limitless and subject to man not the other way around." In this construction, will and morals became inextricable. As with Tregubov, Blindovskii advocated quitting with tobacco on hand to be certain of the strength of one's will. As nicotine left the system, the smoking habit would gradually dissipate from the body and the smoker would feel "completely differently in terms of health."[145]

Archpriest Arsenii echoed this belief in strength of character, pointing out that the "organism becomes accustomed to smoking, to nicotine, so that with the lessening of smoking a person for some time has a difficult mood feeling an incomprehensible discomfort and unbearable sadness." As the poison left the body, the will became even stronger, implying that while the will existed as a mental construct, the bodily poison of nicotine could degrade it. He recommended, like the more secular authors, the immediate cessation of use without stand-ins; the best method was "moral discipline over oneself, consciousness that smoking tobacco is improper for a good Christian."[146] The monks of Mount Athos's St. Panteleimon Monastery further commented of those who said they had not the strength, "In those words, you hear the answer of a slave to the flesh, who is not able to preserve within himself the light given him by the maker, the free and reasonable will." In abandoning the will, the monks argued that the smoker let go of that which "distinguishes us from beast and allows one to fight such 'habits.'" As others, they argued this need not take any extraordinary courage: "With just gentle pressure on yourself, you will be free of this false need, which so strongly endangers you and those around you and sometimes makes smokers into criminals."[147] As the anonymous author of a 1904 pamphlet summed it up, a smoker simply needed to say in a disciplined manner, "'I don't want to and will not!' Have the strength of a wolf not a rabbit."[148]

Deficiencies of will created physical, moral, and mental issues according to contemporaries, and therapies for the feminized and rabbit-willed came in many forms. Imperial Russian religious establishments "cured" assaults on the will among alcoholics through regimented rituals such as the spiritual therapies of Father S. Permskii. Permskii was the founder of the St. Sergius Temperance Society, a group advocating recovery through labor alongside self-improvement through cultural activities, religious observation, and a regular diet. The Alexander Nevskii Temperance Society concentrated on a group therapy approach, where social meetings and activities helped to reorient the daily life of the user while at the same time offering constant support.[149]

Group meetings, a staple of later Western therapies, figured prominently in early Russian treatments for the weak will. A. A. Guliaev's 1910 *Zabytyi faktor khristianskogo vospitaniia voli* (Forgotten factors of the Christian development of the will) connected the will and religious teaching through the art of counseling: "Development of the strong spirit and powerful, solid moral character comes from exercises of the will, which consist of . . . joining the educational institutions of the church alongside, especially, attending to worship."[150] A. Virenius, a smoker of twenty years, recommended means associated with strengthening of the will for smokers. After quitting, he wrote, "I again found pleasure in cold water wash and lighter clothing. After two years or so from quitting I instinctively began to be attracted to cold water; I began to swim in the Neva in June."[151] The cold water wash and physical activity appeared often in advice literature regarding strengthening the will and cultivating the quality of "steeliness" of character and body necessary for success.[152] The cold water treatment, along with walks in the brisk air, was the primary means of quitting smoking in the 1890 work by Keibel.[153] This emphasis on bodily tempering and control figured in hygienic recommendations in many countries in the period, as the lack of faith in physicians created a ready audience for health literature and messages of self-control and self-help.[154]

A key method of fighting smoking emerged from neurasthenia treatments: hypnosis. The technique brought tobacco problems under the purview of psychologists and tapped into popular obsessions with the will as a key to treating alcoholism, neurasthenia, and degeneracy.[155] Hypnosis captured the popular imagination and featured in plots of penny novels and chapbooks.[156] A 1901 essay in *Klinicheskii zhurnal* (Clinical journal) advocated hypnosis as a therapy "for nervous disorders, and pathological habits," largely discussing smoking but including cocaine and tobacco as also susceptible to the cure.[157] In the 1905 pamphlet *Lechenie gipnozom morfinistov, alkogolikov i kuril'shchikov* (Healing through hypnosis for morphine addicts, alcoholics, and smokers), M. I. Bereznitskii promoted hypnosis, practiced in the French and German tradition from the foundations laid by Franz Mesmer (1734–1815), as an efficacious treatment for smokers. He claimed to be able to help the motivated patient in as little as one session.[158]

In 1906, Dr. S. D. Vladychko similarly promoted hypnosis as a means for quitting smoking in his publication, *Vlianie tabachnogo dyma na nervnuiu sistemu i organizm' voobshche* (The effect of tobacco smoke on the nervous system and the organism in general), as did others.[159]

Despite the connections made between alcohol and tobacco in terms of dangers and therapies, Russian temperance advocates did not flock to the cessationist cause. In the midst of a perceived crisis of rising alcoholism in the late nineteenth century, the documented increase in tobacco consumption did not elicit the same societal-wide condemnation.[160] Antismoking activists reached nowhere near the success of antialcohol advocates, who achieved prohibition for Russia from 1914–25.[161] This was not from a dearth of examples or international support. Russians could look to the American Anti-Cigarette League, which boasted a membership of 300,000 in 1901 and started international branches in many countries, though none in Russia.[162] Many authors mentioned with approval the antitobacco societies of the United States, France, and Britain as well as antismoking laws instituted in the United States and Germany.[163] The British Anti-Tobacco Society was founded in 1853.[164] An offshoot of the Women's Christian Temperance Union of the United States, the World Women's Christian Temperance Union, included antitobacco messaging that spread throughout Europe, Asia, South America, and the Middle East.[165] One Russian woman attended the 1903 group meeting in Geneva, and the group's 1910 activity report recorded the organization of a branch in Riga and their first antialcohol exhibit in Moscow at the Polytechnic museum. There was no evidence, however, that antitobacco work accompanied these antialcohol efforts as it did in other countries.[166]

As with other substances implicated in the rising debate on addiction, harm, and social responsibility, many issues played a role in the decision of how to deal with tobacco, with political, economic, social, and cultural groups all in contention for their own interests.[167] Russian temperance societies did not follow international patterns to develop from temperance into antitobacco work. Instead, Russian groups often supported tobacco as a preferable alternative to alcohol.[168] The 1904 report for the government-sponsored Guardianship of Popular Sobriety (Popechitel'stvo narodnoi trezvosti) showed that their tearooms and cafeterias sold tobacco and tobacco products.[169] Citizen groups during the Russo-Japanese War, such as the Ufa chapter of the Guardianship of Popular Sobriety, provided tobacco in canteens, buffets, and teahouses to combat the temptation to mobilized soldiers of drink, considered a greater threat to order and discipline.[170] Publications from temperance societies remained largely mute on the tobacco problem, and the issue did not enter into most meetings.[171] Tobacco workers became instead the targets of temperance movements. The first tearoom of a group targeting drinking among women and children in St. Petersburg was established in a tobacco factory.[172]

Attempts to create an antitobacco group in Russia foundered. Grinevskii lamented in November of 1887 that even though the Petersburg papers reported that several "thoughtful" people wanted to start a society against tobacco, no further action ensued.[173] In 1902, another author commented, "In Russia up to today there is still nothing done for the fight with smoking. A society that would fight with smoking does not yet exist. We do not have popular brochures on the dangers of smoking if you do not include those self-published and freely distributed."[174] Bek's estimation of the amount of antitobacco materials in circulation was low, but his assessment of the status of antismoking groups in Russia was not unfair. Compared to foreign counterparts, who pursued legislative action and even obtained restrictions in some measured ways in the early twentieth century, Russian antitobacco work looked rather meager, scattered, and aimless.

Youth smoking animated Western antitobacco activists, feeding into debates about urban problems, degeneracy, and citizenship. In Britain, the Children's Act of 1908 forbade the sale of tobacco to youngsters under sixteen years of age, for reasons both physical and moral and strongly connected to fears of degeneracy.[175] The first anticigarette laws in the United States appeared at the state level in the 1890s in response to a perceived problem of the "cigarette-smoking boy," a rebellious urban urchin who smoked blatantly and lived precociously. In 1893, the state of Washington took the step of making cigarette sales illegal, although the law was declared an illegal infringement on interstate commerce. By 1890 cigarette sales to minors were outlawed in twenty-one states and territories.[176] In the same period, anti–child smoking movements appeared in Germany, Japan, and Portugal, showing the international scope of concern.[177]

Other interests besides morality and individual health influenced lawmakers to take up this question. For example, claims made in Britain that a third of recruits to the Boer War were rejected due to "smoker's heart" fed a desire to stamp out youthful smoking, as did a general belief in the vulnerability of children to tobacco.[178] A Russian pamphlet, *O preduprezhdenii kureniia tabaku v detskom vozraste* (On the prevention of tobacco smoking at a young age) issued in multiple editions, testified to the popularity of the topic in Russia, even if legislation was not quick in coming.[179] As early as 1888, reformers proposed not selling loose *papirosy* and limiting sites for sales as a way to stop children's smoking, but action did not follow.[180] According to a 1912 article in *Pravda,* Senator Vuich and others established an antitobacco league focused on producing "a journal and various styles of cheap brochures propagandizing abstention from tobacco and organiz[ing] a 'club for nonsmoking youth,'" but there are no further references to this endeavor.[181] In the tumultuous years leading up to the war and in the face of increasing disquiet domestically, the effort might have fallen by the wayside or been muscled out by other news.

Religious groups expressed reticence regarding how to best pursue smoking cessation. W. T. Stead, a foreigner who observed a village meeting at Tolstoy's estate, recounted the thorny discussion that followed a motion to forbid smoking in the town over worries of fires. The prosmoking faction in the village, an interesting development considering the enclave's notoriety for its devotion to Tolstoyan asceticism, argued the antismoking rule would escalate problems because smoking boys would simply light up in more hidden, and therefore more dangerous, areas and increase the chance of fires. Tolstoy himself spoke up against compulsion and "succeeded in getting the commune to substitute a voluntary pledge for the proposed law, signed by each of the antismoking agitators, by which they undertook to pay a ruble or to do three days' work if they broke their pledge."[182] Antialcohol work often used sobriety pledges and may have served as an example here.

With rare exception, antismoking activists cautioned that prohibition had proven ineffective and counterproductive for Russia.[183] Priklonskii concluded that by observing the implementation of state measures against tobacco around the world, it was evident that the more severe the restrictions, the more smoking developed.[184] Khmelevskii summed up the history of antitobacco work in Europe: "Persecution for tobacco and forbidding its use had a profound effect on rooting the passion for the plant in Europe; it increased the number of those wishing to try the forbidden weed. The number of users increased daily. To chase the habit was impossible. Those who in the beginning opposed it became addicted to it themselves and therefore, as if in agreement, all of Europe at one time abandoned antitobacco bans."[185] Authors across the period echoed his sentiment that repressive measures were useless.[186] Priklonskii pointed to Russia's specific antitobacco measures and pronounced these as having been "not to any good result."[187] In his *K psikhologii kureniia* (On the psychology of smoking), I. A. Birsthein argued that with youth, repressive measures could actually backfire because young boys embraced the idea of smoking as a "masculine protest."[188] In place of repressive measures, authors advocated further publication of brochures, public health advocacy, and the foundation of societies to spread the message of antismoking.[189]

Russian authors attributed the lack of an antitobacco movement to contention regarding the danger of tobacco and the long tradition of tobacco's medicinal use, but other countries had similar medical histories with tobacco.[190] The scientific communities in other nations were not united against tobacco and yet visible, viable, and effective antitobacco groups had emerged in the United States, Britain, Canada, Australia, France, Japan, and Germany. One difference was that Russian physicians and psychiatrists came out in different forums against government repression, deeming it the source of society-wide psychosis.[191] Additional clues as to why tobacco resistance failed in Russia, despite the widespread nature of the problem, emerge from the Russian temperance movement and the way in which alcohol resistance in Russia was politicized. From the 1840s on, discussions of state profits through the tax system on alcohol led to the equivalence of condemnation of drinking with criticism of the state.[192] In times of upheaval, state liquor stores became the target for crowd attacks. In 1905, 1913, and 1914, crowds engaged in liquor boycotts and ransacked taverns.[193] Temperance groups aligned with liberal sympathies rather than nationalist or conservative agendas became a place for upper-class reformers to engage in antistate agitation but through the veil of moral crusade and paternalistic class actions.[194] Sectarians like Tolstoy or Ioann of Kronstadt, who joined in temperance crusades against the state, caused some clergy of the established church to battle even church-sponsored temperance as possibly tainted by radical politics.[195]

Antialcohol groups often targeted a larger social agenda about lower-class disorder. For instance, the *Pervoe Moskovskoe obshchestvo trezvosti* (First Moscow Temperance Society) and the *Popechitel'stva o narodnoi trezvosti* (Guardianships of Popular Sobriety) resolutely focused on working-class disruption and danger, never mentioning drinking among the middle or upper classes.[196] Undoubtedly tobacco use did not present nearly the problem to public order in the immediate sense that excessive drinking did, nor was it even in league with the widespread problems of urban poverty. Perhaps smoking, seen as a largely upper- and middle-class urban pursuit or a habit that lower-class urbanites could initiate in pursuit of status, did not similarly excite the paternalistic sentiments of reformers. Advertisers were quick to point to smoking as a preferable alternative to other behaviors like drinking or gaming.[197] Australian temperance organizations similarly did not pressure for antitobacco work, and the government seemed uninterested, as the social and public problems of tobacco were not akin to those of alcohol.[198]

The equivocation from specialists regarding the dangers of tobacco, the addictive qualities of it, and how to combat it opened up the entire crusade to some derision. The thundering, often wild claims made by antitobacco activists in Britain had left the leadership and movement susceptible to ridicule.[199] The same would hold true for Russian antismoking advocates who found their concepts mocked by authors and tobacco advocates and manipulated by manufacturers and advertisers. If smoking cessationists had Tolstoy, those who would scorn them had the tragicomic voice of Chekhov. Chekhov, an inveterate if rueful smoker, became so associated with the habit as to have his own apocryphal quotation regarding smoking: "A man who does not smoke or drink, inevitably raises the question, is he a bastard?"[200] Chekhov held a complicated attitude toward tobacco. He had early been an acolyte of Tolstoy and even followed his abstemious ways to a point before rebelling publicly. Chekhov's medical training as well as his flirtation with asceticism gave him an intimate understanding of the antialcohol and antitobacco forces in late-nineteenth-century Russia. He considered the case against tobacco in two works, one ridiculous and one thoughtful, but in both his case lacked vehemence and even brought into question the methods of fighting tobacco and the effects of smoking on health.

Chekhov's most bathetic take on the habit was a one-act, one-man vaudeville written and rewritten between 1886 and 1902, when the final version appeared.[201] The setting was a public health lecture, a popular entertainment of the time that antismoking advocates as well as antialcohol groups readily pursued, along with sing-alongs, plays, tearooms, and museum exhibitions.[202] In it, the hapless Markel Ivanovich Niukhin presented a picture of a henpecked husband of weakened will, a public health speaker with no knowledge of his subject, and a hypocritical, moral scold who did not practice what he preached. Like many of Chekhov's characters, Niukhin evoked a familiar type in the surface story, but beneath the stereotype, dialogue and stage direction revealed psychological turmoil. In a rambling and ridiculous speech, Niukhin confessed, "I'm not a professor of course, and university degrees have passed me by." Admitting that he smoked himself and that he was only speaking because his wife forced him to, his speech devolved quickly into a rambling monologue on bedbugs, twitching eyes, and his wife's boarding school, which he was supposed to promote in his speech. Instead of drumming up business, he painted a portrait of her tyrannical ways, revealing his frailty before her and the terrible, hopeless, unhappiness that bound his life. In the hapless words of this sad, weak man, the only information on tobacco to cross the stage was that "tobacco is, essentially, a plant."[203] Niukhin was as ineffectual as a speaker as he was as head of household.

The silliness of the figure, along with the obviously teasing name of Niukhin, the "snuffer," as taken from the verb for snuff-taking in Russian (*niukhat'*), destroyed any seriousness in the treatment of the base problem. Previous drafts of the story incorporated more information on tobacco's chemistry but further undercut the effect by making the snuff-taking an entire comic scene unto itself, as Niukhin devolved into a sneezing fit after taking snuff that his daughters had doctored with some other noxious material. Their previous effort, he groused, involved face powder.[204] Emasculated by his wife, he was further brought low by his children and their gender-bending pranks. Even his tobacco habit was pathetic, snuff having passed out of fashion almost a century before.

The hypocrisy of the tobacco user preaching abstinence revealed itself in another story from Chekhov, the 1887 "At Home," in which the circuit court prosecutor Evgenii Petrovich Bykovskii confronted his seven-year-old son who had been caught smoking. The story opened as the governess informed Bykovskii of his son's habits and noted that while Bykovskii might not see it as important, she did. Only when the father found out that his son had stolen the tobacco from his own drawer did he decide to speak to the boy, and even then he expressed reticence that mingled distaste for authoritarian schoolmasters with a general disquiet in the severity of the restrictions.

Bykovskii seemed less than upset by the prospect of his son's smoking, even smiling at the image in his mind's eye of the child with a papirosa:

> At the same time, the earnest, anxious face of the governess awakened in him memories of days long past and half forgotten, when smoking at school and in the nursery aroused in masters and parents a strange, almost incomprehensible horror. It really was horror. Children were unmercifully flogged, and expelled from school, and their lives were blighted, although not one of the teachers nor fathers knew exactly what constituted the harm and offence of smoking. Even very intelligent people did not hesitate to combat the vice they did not understand. Bikofski [*sic.*] called to mind the principal of his school, a highly educated, good-natured old man, who was so shocked when he caught a scholar with a cigarette that he would turn pale and immediately summon a special meeting of the school board and sentence the offender to expulsion. No doubt that is one of the laws of society—the less an evil is understood the more bitterly and harshly is it attacked.[205]

Troubled by the thought of the students expelled, the course of their lives ruined, Bykovskii could not justify in his mind the severity of the punishment, which "did a great deal more harm than the crime itself." The confrontation with his son progressed in unexpected directions, to discussions of private property, death, and punishment, but the prosecutor doggedly brought it back around, in a passage presented as a conversation he had with himself:

> "In my day, these questions were settled with singular simplicity," he reflected. "If a youngster was caught smoking he was thrashed. This would, indeed, make a poor-spirited, cowardly boy give up smoking, but a clever and plucky one would carry his tobacco in his boot after the whipping and smoke in an out-house. When he was caught in the outhouse and whipped again he would go down and smoke by the river, and so on until the lad was grown up. My mother used to give me money and candy to keep me from smoking. These expedients now seem to us weak and immoral. Taking up a logical stand-point, the educator of today tries to instill the first principles of right into a child by helping him to understand them and not by rousing his fear or his desire to distinguish himself and obtain a reward."[206]

In the end, Bykovskii resorted to a made-up tale of a kingdom brought to destruction by the early death of a smoking son to convince the lad of the danger in his ways. While the child seemed properly impressed, Bykovskii lamented the use of trickery, concluding that it was a shame that truth and morality were often cloaked in falsification. The story finished with tobacco as a literary device—a catalyst for a revelation by Bykovskii of the unsuit-ability of his professional prosecutorial skills to parenting and, ultimately, of the disconnect between pedagogy, morality, and truth.

In the vaudeville and the short story, Chekhov, a man with medical authority and knowledge, dismissed as trivial or ridiculous the case against tobacco for health, and in the short story he even came out against the coer-cion practiced on boys not to smoke as counterproductive and a cure more harmful than the disease. In both cases, educators capable of cruel rulings based on little evidence became thinly veiled stand-ins for authorities who ruled without compassion, knowledge, or clear outcomes. For Chekhov, any disquiet over tobacco's harms to the body that may have come from his medical training was supplanted by disgust with authoritarian figures in the home, the school, and the state.

Other medical professionals derided the claims of antitobacco advocates as ridiculous or over the top. A review published in the 1912 *Obshchest-vennyi vrach* (Public health doctor) addressed a series of antitobacco and antialcohol posters for schools from a Dr. I. E. Markov of Samara. A com-mission of reviewers concluded that not only were the posters in a lan-guage that "was not popular and would not be understood by the larger population" but also the "majority of the contentions in the posters could not be considered settled and several were outright exaggerations or not in agreement with established objective scientific facts." The commission pronounced Markov's efforts as unlikely to produce good results and decided not to distribute the posters at all.[207] Although none of the posters appeared for examination, the contention among experts regarding what was an effective method for health education and the distaste of many physicians for popular materials that dumbed down or overstated medical information to the public likely appeared in other venues as well. British medical figures similarly resisted some antitobacco advocates for being loose with the science or too fanciful or wild.[208] The more fringe elements of antitobacco campaigns caused push back.[209]

Connoisseurs and manufacturers took advantage of the opening created by a lack of scientific consensus and the reticence of medical authorities and exploited it to put forward the positive attributes of the habit and challenge restrictions on tobacco. Whereas antitobacco authors hung their case on tobacco's contributions to neurasthenia, advertisers instead promoted tobacco as a calming, invigorating, even healthful product to combat the stresses of modern urban life. In some cases, they questioned the claims made against tobacco, challenging the concept that tobacco was sinful, dangerous, agitating, or harmful in a way that mocked the case made by antismoking advocates and belittled the idea of smoking's dangers.

In many advertisements, the travails of modern urban life, and the promised solace of a smoke took center stage. An advertisement for the brand *Iar* promoted its ability to calm the nerves, soothe the back, and lessen fatigue for the beleaguered desk clerk.[210] Using nervousness as a selling point did not distinguish tobacco. Many products promised to cure the ailments of the modern age and alleviate anxieties about the pace of industrialization. A wave of restorative remedies, clinical consultations, advice manuals, and therapeutic gadgets guaranteed relief in advertisements in journals and magazines.[211] What was different with tobacco was the lively counterargument going on about the dangers of the product in terms of manufacture, morals, and health.[212] Advertisers directly addressed the worries for body, mind, and soul trumpeted by antismoking advocates and instead promised, like *Dukat*, that smoking would make life "cheerful" and "easy," or, like *Ottoman*, that it would bring success in terms of "love, money, and honor," not the nervous disposition or declining mental abilities warned of by antismokers.[213]

The sinful nature of smoking received ridicule from other quarters. The tobacco factory Feodosiia of Southern Crimea featured not a dandy asking the viewer, "What to smoke?," but rather Lucifer himself (figure 5.1). The

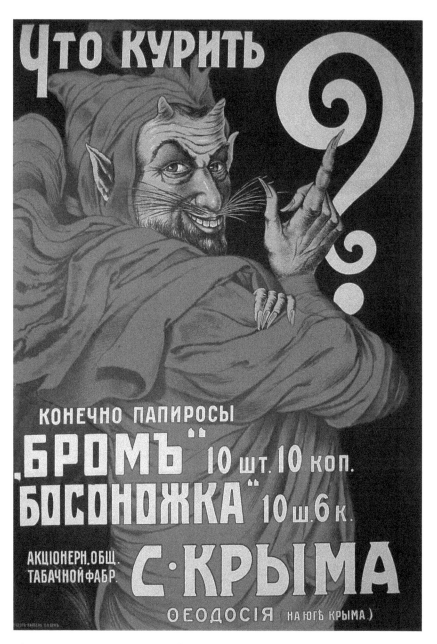

Figure 5.1 *Brom* poster. Prerevolutionary. Collection of Russian State Library, Moscow.

devil, ever the connoisseur, had no questions in his mind: "Of course the papirosy *Brom* and *Bosonozhka.*" The satisfaction Satan takes in "bromine" and "sandals" is obvious not just in his testimonial, but also in his happy demeanor and sturdy form. Bromine, an element whose name derived from the Greek for the sulfuric "stench" of the underworld, celebrated some of the more objectionable elements of smoking, much like Satan had embraced the supposedly damning aspects of the habit. The teasing pose and flirtatious smile could have been a temptation for both men and women, and the prices of the brands—ten for either six or ten kopecks—put them in the midrange. By challenging the religious stalwarts, the advertisement also implied that the user became part of a more secular, modern world. Rather than painting smoking as sinful and harmful, the advertisement instead pushed for a vision of tobacco as secular and playful. Satan was an imp, not a demon.

Women also received the message that tobacco smoking did not bring eternal damnation. Advertisements for the *Eva* brand of papirosy went back to the beginnings of time to deride the idea of tobacco's sinful nature. The use of Eve held implications not just of any sin, but the original one, countering yet another argument of antitobacco authors—that smoking caused sexual debility as part of its triggering of general neurasthenic decline. They urged smokers to realize that instead of being a problem, "it is a sin not to smoke!"[214] Other advertisements went further to boast of enhanced licentious talents that came with the use of their product, for instance utilizing the trope of the cigar or papirosa as stand-in for the phallus or showing one man surrounded by multiple females, implying stamina and attraction.[215] Sensuality had figured in other posters, but the odalisque of the harem promised sensual delight rather than any effects on the physical health of the user.

Advertisers challenged the depiction of smoking as morally dangerous or sexually draining but even more blatantly attacked the vision of tobacco as harmful. In Bogdanov's 1904 advertisement for *Kapriz* (figure 1.2), the poem by Uncle Mikey proposed that "if" tobacco were harmful, then the filtered *Kapriz* answered this making smoking "harmless and affordable"—so much so that "the old and young, and even the children, and even the ill prefer '*Kapriz.*'"

A 1912 advertisement, again by cheerful, nicotinized Uncle Mikey, rolled together the depiction of antismokers as prudes and derision for the perception of tobacco as unhealthful and even the implication that it was sinful in one poem. In it, Uncle Mikey told of enjoying a "good papirosa" as he mocked a bulletin of the French Society against the Use of Tobacco.

Amused, he related with interest the news of an antitobacco song from the group. He confided to the reader that he had rewritten it. In his altered ditty he sang of how *Desert* was "safe," *Eva* "without harm," and *Nora* "without nicotine." He concluded, "You do not have to smoke, but if you smoke Shaposhnikov you can open a path to Eden." Tobacco, like the incense offered up to God, was the key into paradise rather than the reason for man's fall from it.[216]

The most exhaustive depiction of "healthful" smoking came in the form of the 1887 advertisement for the brand *Talisman* of St. Petersburg. The richly detailed poster countered the claims of health authorities by instead showing tobacco as having an almost magical, definitely healthful effect on smokers regardless of gender or class (figure 5.2). The maladies displayed in the crowd on the left range from blindness and baldness to the invalid on the chair in the foreground, suffering from toothache and stomach pain. Behind the poor fellow in the chair stood a trio under the yoke of a more nineteenth-century series of ailments. The two women were cursed with the peculiar sexual ailments of the late-Victorian period; the woman on the left swooned in the throes of hysteria, a symptom of female hypersexuality; the woman on the right suffered from lack of sexual contact and subsequently withered into an old maid. In between these two women of uneasy and too easy virtue stooped the pale, trembling, and desiccated male companion in sexual frailty—the neurasthenic. The hunched shoulders, concave chest, limp, flaccid hand, and general frailty implied, in the context of his companions, expansive problems of health and virility.

A large figure dominated the center of the poster, standing on a podium, which still further emphasized his height and authority. Draped in robes and cape with alchemist's symbols scattered across them, this magical figure served as a transition—a symbol of choice—between the lives shown by the two crowds at his sides. His power rested in the box of papirosy, which he distributed freely to the crowd of infirm nonsmokers, a Christ of the machine age dispersing his white-wrapped healing hosts to the crowd in a modern consumer mass. His wand, drawn as a large papirosy, offered a magical power to tobacco, and the wand's peculiar placement connected it to phallic power.

Through him, the crowd at left might perhaps enter the promised land at right, where a group of virile individuals mixed amiably, chatted energetically, and preened happily, all while enveloped in a dense cloud of smoke. The figures sported ruddy complexions, compared to the pallid group of nonsmokers, and represented all social groups. The countryside woman with her kerchiefed head in the background and the crowd of workers and

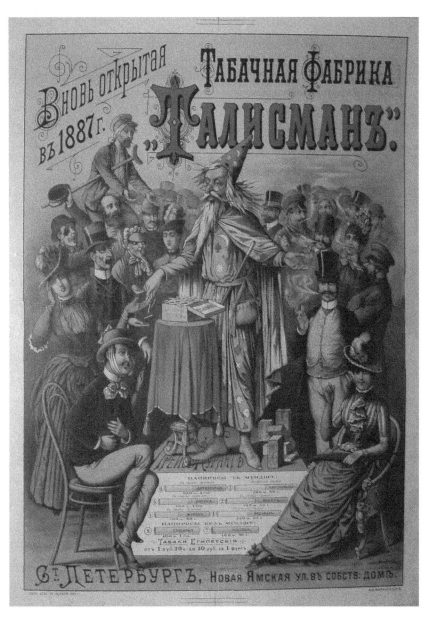

Figure 5.2 *Talisman* poster. 1887. Collection of Russian State Library, Moscow.

a lower-class woman in the middle ground, led to the upper-class figures of the foreground and displayed the egalitarian brotherhood of smokers enjoying a luxury that even the lowliest could taste and with which each could transcend their humble background.

The two most assured figures—the man and woman in the front—stared directly forward, challenging the viewer to interpret them. Their placement mirrored the weak hysteric and feeble neurasthenic of the left-hand side. The man sported the same style of suit, collar, and hat; he differed in pallor, plumpness, and assuredness. The woman had the same face as her invalid counterpart but was now enlivened by health with a lovely "blood and cream" complexion. She conveyed a sexually suggestive assuredness in her posture. Her look and gestures were similar to other smoking women in posters, but here strongly connected to health effects from tobacco. The woman's hand was placed in the foreground spatially covering the genitals of the male in a suggestive cupping, where the papirosa was obscured and visible only close up. This seemed a deliberate sexualization of the image and the mien of the obviously satisfied male smoker with these gestural and spatial overtones underscored the sexual meaning given to tobacco use. *Talisman* cured the ills of the entire crowd, and society as a whole, by bringing all together in health while assuring the next generation. In the world of *Talisman*, the health questions swirling around tobacco were settled.

IF ADDICTION is defined as continued use despite an understanding of tobacco's harmful effects, then late imperial Russian smoking did not meet that standard. No cultural, medical, or social consensus emerged to condemn tobacco soundly. Russian smokers encountered a lively exchange of ideas on tobacco in their churches, theaters, novels, streets, and stores, and this affected their experience of tobacco. The contentious case of tobacco at the turn of the century revealed lively debates among moral reformers, medical theorists, scientific authorities, educated consumers, and motivated manufacturers regarding health, morality, decline, state power, personal satisfaction, religion, and modern life. Not only did they display a familiarity with issues across their respective fields, but by presenting these ideas in either literary parody or advertising copy, they also assumed that the public had more than a passing acquaintance with complex issues across political, social, religious, medical, and cultural boundaries. The lack of a strong medical consensus on tobacco's dangers allowed for this environment of discussion and dissension. Scientific researchers equivocated, and medical authorities suggested moderate or low-inhalation smoking might be safe, if practiced by respectable smokers with suitably expensive tobacco and accessories.

With no agreement regarding smoking's dangers, it was not surprising there was no unanimity regarding its addictive qualities or how to treat dependency. Although religious and moral authorities considered tobacco an intoxicant that enslaved the soul, they recognized no physical compulsion and their moral arguments convinced few. Smoking's dangers and attractions were underplayed and unsurprisingly therapies offered for quitting remained dismissive of the problem. Most simply modified the recommendations for alcoholism's treatments and painted tobacco use as but one more disease of the will, to cure through application of regimen, strengthening of the body, or sessions of hypnosis. Discussions around tobacco use, however, implied a shared understanding of the difficulty for those who wished to quit, even if the difficulty testified to the weakness of the smoker. The therapies proposed did not indicate that psychiatrists, medical doctors, pundits, or priests considered smoking so compelling a problem as to require dramatic intervention.

Scientific and medical authorities did not agree with the antitobacco stances of religious authorities and more strident antitobacco advocates, and even some moralists remained skeptical. Temperance advocates in Russia did not readily condemn tobacco as they did alcohol. Not just a consequence of Russia's past acceptance of tobacco as a medicament, this reflected disquiet among liberal reformers and professionals with state power, greater acceptance of smoking, lack of scientific consensus, and a more successful vision of tobacco as invigorating. Smoking might have been a new form of slavery, but few considered oppressive prohibition as a lesser evil. The tolerance for moderate tobacco use, even among those who did not like tobacco, stood in stark contrast to therapeutic approaches to alcohol dependency where complete abstinence was given as the preferred, and only viable, therapy. In American temperance literature, for instance, moderate drinkers were scorned as the worst of users.[217]

Rather than a source for neurasthenia or a danger to the soul, tobacco was portrayed by advocates as a cure for nervousness, boredom, and sexual weakness. Advocates, and even some with seemingly ambivalent attitudes toward use, painted a vision of tobacco's opponents as misguided on policy at least and prudes and hypocrites at worst. Nothing was sacred in the battle as even Tolstoy was the butt of the joke when a brand of papirosy appearing "in honor" of the stridently antitobacco author came out in 1911.[218] Manufacturers readily embraced the depiction from some moralists that tobacco use was sinful in images and copy that playfully mocked the stridency of the opposition and turned it into a marketing tool. In the marketplace of ideas, outside the chemical draws and cultural cues of dependency, smokers could readily find support for continued use.

EPILOGUE

Revolution and Cessation

Russian leaf and style of smoke differed noticeably from that of Western Europe and the United States, creating a physically singular, possibly more addictive, papirosa. The unique style of smoke was further distinguished by social, cultural, and political meanings embedded in late imperial Russian developments. The mode of production distinguished Russian papirosy as a consequence of the perspective of Russian manufacturers on the costs of hand labor versus machine labor as well as the opportunities for development brought by rapid industrialization. The social costs of this choice as well as the revolutionary concepts and progressive rhetoric that surrounded them made Russian smoking different not just for Russian bodies but also for Russian society. The sourcing of leaf from within its own borders but originating in areas of contested imperial power invested Russian smoking with powerful patriotic significance that could be physically experienced in smell and taste. The politics of empire met those of class in the concepts of connoisseurship, social distinction, gender divisions, and liberal attainment that flowed alongside the smoke.

Not only political, social, and physical foundations for distinctive Russian smoking could be found in the late imperial period. The encounter of Russians with tobacco began with distaste from authorities of both church and state, and the force of antitobacco efforts remained wed to commentary about the effects of consumption on morality and citizenship for years. Yet the rise of the medical and psychiatric professions in Russia and their interests in social change framed the tobacco problem in the language of neurasthenia, national decline, and degeneracy. Even as religious and social commentators pushed an image of smoking as a danger to soul, body, and state, scientific authorities wavered on the shores of moderation while marketers and other cultural figures ridiculed abstemious cautions as the domain of prim scolds or hypocritical paternalists. Wary of authoritarian tendencies in their state, Russians did not embrace governmental solutions to smoking, and manufacturers waded into this morass of indecision with sharp appeals that mocked or upended the case against tobacco.

The exceptional contours of Russia's tobacco story continued after 1914 as the tsar cracked down on alcohol use with a prohibition that would stand into the 1920s, but as before, measures against tobacco did not materialize alongside those for alcohol.[1] Instead, tobacco became part of soldiers' rations and experienced a general rise in production. In addition to the tobacco ration for soldiers, tobacco collection campaigns sponsored by the government and private citizens seeded the front lines with papirosy, creating new users and further cementing an image of tobacco as the valorous companion of the man in uniform. A postcard appeal for a collection drive urged the public to help soldiers weather the tedium of the trench with the help of tobacco (figure E.1). The postcard showed two men, relaxed and contemplative, one with pipe and one with papirosa in the shelter of a dugout trench. A care package at bottom held the tobacco, the smoke of which the seated soldier let out in a puff that spelled out "Thank you."

Russia's frontline soldiers did not smoke alone. The worries for tobacco's effects on national potency had lost out to the long-held belief in its connections to bold men in uniform not just in Russia but also in most of the combatant nations of the war.[2] Many philanthropic groups worked to satisfy the tobacco needs of the fighting man, allowing for patriotic spirit to be demonstrated one papirosa at a time. A book of artists' autographs came out in 1915 Moscow, which was to be sold and then have the profits used for the purchase of tobacco for the men.[3] The volume seemed an odd choice for fundraising but the crossover of popular entertainment, consumer culture, and tobacco donations was an easy leap. Care had to be taken, however, regarding issues of class and taste. One foreigner noted that the Russian soldiers did not always take well to the donated smokes, "for the troops disliked finely made cigarettes, preferring the very strong, cheap Russian papirosy made from vile-smelling makhorka."[4] The tastes cultivated before the war and the associations of class, solidarity, and manliness of the late tsarist years were not dispelled by the whiff of gunpowder.

Tobacco served the wartime needs of the state not just by comforting men in uniform. At the beginning of the war, the tsar prohibited alcohol sales to stabilize the domestic social situation, but it was a hard blow to the economic situation of the state. Alcohol excise taxes provided substantial

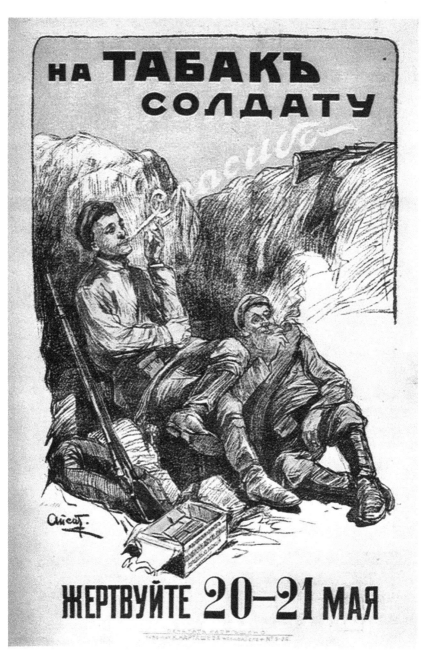

Figure E.1 "Spasibo." Tobacco for soldiers postcard. Artist A. P. Apsit, published by Moscow Committee for Supply of Tobacco to Soldiers on the Front Lines. Prerevolutionary. Author's collection.

revenues now desperately needed as the Russian state went to war. Officials scrambled to find sources for revenue and tobacco provided one stream, and they raised excise taxes on tobacco and especially makhorka products substantially. Factories in the capital made out well in the system, but those in other areas, like Iaroslavl, took the changes as a real blow. The tax problems hampered the industry as did raw material shortages and transport difficulties as railways became overburdened with wartime traffic. International markets also suffered as rich tobacco areas in the Balkans became battlegrounds and tobacco production was targeted.[5] The drafting of qualified workers furthered the feminization of the industry and also impacted quality and production as new workers attempted to come up to speed and replace experienced workers in an environment of difficulty and scarcity.[6]

A steep decline in output in papirosy began in 1917.[7] Problems supplying papers, the drafting of skilled workers, and difficulties at factories led to a move from finished papirosy to rough, makhorka tobacco, as seen in table 6.1. The production of crumbled tobacco took five times less worker time than that of papirosy.[8]

Tobacco shortages made their way from the home front to the battle front. So bad was it that a 1917 story in *Pravda* reported on tactics of the enemy involving the perceived scarcity of tobacco among Russian troops. In the month before the revolution, soldiers in Bubnov supposedly yelled out to their Russian adversaries that they had thrown tobacco and papirosy into the trenches and that they should all jump out and look for them. The Russian troops did not fall for the trick, but the desperate tobacco situation was obviously bad enough to be seen even across no man's land.[9]

Only the inability of Russia to maintain production of nearly all manufactured goods led to any disruption in the march of tobacco into further usage. Faced with prohibitions on alcohol, food shortages, and stressful situations, many Russians on the home front relished a bit of luxurious tobacco even as free papirosy to soldiers recruited new users on the front lines. The tobacco industry weathered problems better than most. Raw material stores

Table E.1 Tobacco worked from 1913 to 1919

	1913	*1914*	*1915*	*1919*
Tobacco (in pounds)	6,811,704	5,942,448	5,520,348	2,819,700
Papirosy (in thousands)	13,859,864	15,339,109	17,228,522	5,161,097
Makhorka	3,386,499	3,609,807	3,426,510	963,000

S. Narkir'er, *Proizvodstvo tabachnykh fabric RSFSR v 1919 godu (v tsifrakh)* (Moscow: Vyschii sovet narodnogo khoziastva, 1921), 23.

allowed the industry to continue production as other groups struggled, but manufacture still suffered in comparison to peacetime numbers. By 1919, tobacco output was at 46.1 percent of prerevolutionary-era levels.[10] The public, and military, smoked whatever they could get.[11] Papirosy, which had already reached nearly half of tobacco production, surpassed that threshold sometime during the period of war, revolution, and civil war, so that by the 1920s they exceeded 80 percent of worked tobacco.[12] Papirosy smoking was now a habit embedded in Russian bodies, psyches, and society.

The outbreak of World War I briefly quelled the labor discontent that had characterized the industry beginning in the 1890s, but by 1915, things soon returned to their previous seething status. Despite the vicious crackdowns of the late nineteenth century and the post-1905 period, the women of tobacco still marched and organized. In August 1915, the workers of Asmolov again brought demands to management and this time won a 15 percent raise. With such victories to buoy them, they continued to agitate into 1916 and 1917.[13] In February 1917, workers of Laferm and other tobacco concerns went on strike.[14] Women workers had become a larger and larger percentage of the workforce as their men had gone to war, and the marches of this women's day quickly turned into something

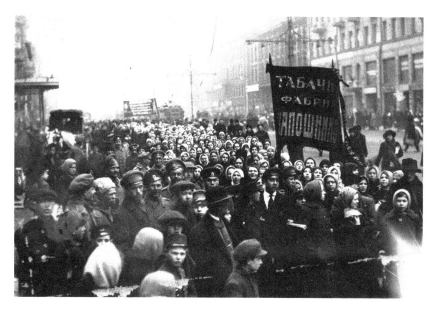

Figure E.2   Shaposhnikov factory women, March 19, 1917. "Notes of a Boring Person—St. Petersburg Demonstrations of 1917," https://fotki.yandex.ru/next/users/humus777/album/442440/view/1109403. Accessed June 26, 2017.

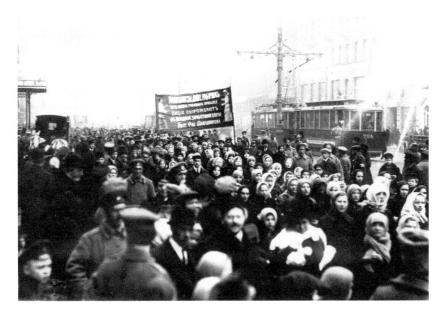

Figure E.3   Shaposhnikov factory women, March 19, 1917. "Notes of a Boring Person—St. Petersburg Demonstrations of 1917," https://fotki.yandex.ru/next/users/humus777/album/442440/view/1109401. Accessed June 26, 2017.

far more. Not just any action, the celebration of International Women's Day in St. Petersburg in 1917 sparked the general strike that would bring down the tsarist regime.[15] As women marched from factory to factory demanding bread and pulling others onto the street, the government proved unable to maintain control, and the autocracy crumbled. Further agitation in March pushed the provisional government to grant women the vote. The women of Shaposhnikov, with banners and in large numbers, were there (figures E.2 and E.3).[16]

The revolution did not end tobacco worker activity. On June 8, 1917, 14,000 female tobacco workers agitated for better wages and social programs, and a *Pravda* article observed that the women seemed poised for even larger activities.[17] Clearly, the Bolsheviks were ready for more. In October of 1917 they overturned the provisional government and took over the state and economy. Shaposhnikova, the tobacco queen, did not live to see the turmoil of 1917 and what it would do to the empire she had ruled. She passed away in February of that tumultuous year, missing the chaos of the provisional government and the upheaval of the Bolshevik takeover in October. Nor would she see the nationalization of her factory, as it was renamed first after Lev Trotsky and then, after his star fell, after Clara Tsetkin. She did not witness the transfer of Gabai into the firm Iava or of Asmolov into the stalwart Nasha Marka (also known as the Don State Tobacco Factory). Perhaps this was all to the best for the tobacco queen, because the Bolsheviks had no patience for royalty. As factories changed hands, owners fell from grace. Following the revolutions of 1917, the owners of the Dunaev factory of Iaroslavl, now labeled "exploiters," journeyed to prison camps or became workers themselves. A few even served in the hotel their family had once purchased with their tobacco fortune.[18]

Hierarchies were upended, the names of the factories and brands changed, the supply of paper and leaf waxed and waned, but papirosy continued to be produced in largely the same way as they had been during the tsarist period—with unique materials from Russian growers using a largely female workforce. Like their queen, the women workers of tobacco ended up on the wrong side of history. Few were Bolsheviks and some even came out for the opposition. Tobacco workers from Laferm agitated alongside the soldiers of Kronstadt in the 1921 rebellion against the Soviet government and for freedoms of speech, the press, and association.[19] A memo to Lenin and Stalin detailed the spread of anarchist materials at Laferm even as the state attempted to frighten the rioters back into obedience.[20] While the soldiers and tobacco workers forced a softening of economic policy, they did not end up as winners, and as the Bolsheviks quashed the rebellion the female tobacco workers were pushed into the stereotyped roles of all women workers—backwards, unskilled, and unworthy of interest.[21]

The Bolshevik Revolution ushered into power a new state with its own conflicted relationship to tobacco. In 1918, Lenin and his fellows established the People's Commissariat for Public Health, with its head Dr. N. A. Semashko.[22] Lenin and Semashko were both ardent antismokers. Lenin so hated the habit that he forced smokers at meetings to stand near the fireplace and send their exhalations up the flue.[23] The triumph of public health as a major policy point closed one chapter on tobacco's relationship to state and citizen and brought a new era for antitobacco advocacy. In 1920, at Lenin's urgings, Semashko attempted to push through a ban on further agricultural expansion into tobacco with hopes of rationing it for adults and pushing a restriction on purchase of tobacco by children.[24]

He failed. Instead, tobacco's immediate economic importance trumped long-term public health, and ties to valorous military, and now revolutionary, figures became even more pronounced and celebrated. Tobacco scented the revolution. John Reed recalled the hall of the Petrograd Soviet after the seizure of power: "There was no heat in the hall but the stifling heat of unwashed human bodies. A foul blue cloud of cigarette smoke rose from the mass and hung in the thick air."[25] Just as easily, tobacco's politics changed. The frontiers celebrated in nineteenth-century imperial imagery now became Soviet frontiers. The political frontlines of communism were heralded in new brand names—*Komsomolskii* (Komsomol), *Trudovye* (labor), *Smychka* (worker peasant alliance). Technological achievements, the frontier of the science-obsessed Soviet regime, also merited commemoration with papirosy brands—*Aeroport* (airport) *Belomorkanal* (White Sea Canal), and *Sputnik* (satellite). And other horizons beckoned. Instead of pushing to the south and east, the north and, later, space—*Sever* (north), *Kosmos* (cosmos)—called out to smokers. [26]

Even as Semashko failed in pursuing a full state policy against tobacco, antitobacco messages became intrinsic to Soviet descriptions of a healthful life. The impact of having the leader of the Commissariat of Health openly rail against tobacco cannot be underestimated. Still coded in the language of neurasthenia, the poison nicotine retained center stage in descriptions of tobacco's dangers. The recommendations for young pioneers included cautions not to smoke or drink, and advice to women, in the guise of health recommendations for future mothers, outlined the many dangers of tobacco through the institutions and propaganda of the Department for the Protection of Mothers and Infants.[27] These appeals, at least, did seem to have some effect. No more advertisements with cheeky children sneaking a smoke made it into the public sphere, and although images of masculine, patriotic smoking remained, representations of respectable female smoking declined to almost nothing.

Despite these victories, the Soviet state would be very slow to respond to the global revolution in attitudes toward tobacco brought on by new research into the connections of smoking and cancer in the 1950s and 1960s. While elsewhere the tobacco industry led the resistance to cessation efforts, the Soviet Union did not have a similarly independent, profit-motivated group. Instead, a tumult of social, cultural, medical, and individual reticence hampered the antitobacco movement. Springing in part from science that was filtered through political visions, pushed into Pavlovian knots, and periodically purged; in part from physicians that were poorly trained, barely paid, and generally disrespected; in part from the old and hoary slogans of poison and neurasthenic decline that continued to frame public health appeals against tobacco; and perhaps also from leaders who smoked with vigor and enthusiasm, the political and social will to confront tobacco was wanting. It would not be until 1978 that the Soviets would finally put forward a policy on smoking and the dangers of tobacco use on a unified, national scale, over ten years after the United States' similar report from their surgeon general in 1964 and two decades after British and American researchers had outlined with sobering numbers the many health dangers of tobacco.[28]

The lag in policy echoed a political, public, medical, and social disinterest in confronting tobacco even as demographers and experts noted the alarming decline in popular health in the Soviet Union.[29] At least some of this reticence to act, as well as the difficulties that would come in trying to eradicate smoking after 1978, emerged out of the foundations for tobacco outlined in this book. Papirosy established themselves as the primary form of tobacco consumption earlier in Russia than did cigarettes in any other Western nation. Even before they became the norm of consumption, the image of tobacco to Russian empire, manhood, and power had become part of representations of the state, masculinity, and the military. Cultural figures, marketers, and users themselves embedded smoking in representations of class, hospitality, social interaction, and urban life. The distinctive Russian papirosy had so well established itself so early and with such depth in the bodies and habits of Russians and in the political, economic, social, and cultural life of the nation that to fight it would require a strength of will by state and individuals that would take some decade to form, even as the body count continued to rise.

Notes

INTRODUCTION

1. In memoirs, first-time smokers report a harsh feel and unpleasant taste. As smokers become accustomed to the habit, they begin to discern tastes that are more enjoyable, yet these can be individual. The experience I describe here is a personal one, but I benefited greatly in the construction of this introduction from the guidance and insight of the University of Pittsburgh's Kenneth A. Perkins, PhD, who served as a consultant for this book.

2. The cigarette of the past almost certainly did not burn with as smooth a draw as the smoke of today, and likely popped, crackled, and went out far more often.

3. M. V. Butashevich-Perashevskii recalled the moment he *slyshal* (heard) tobacco smoke in Peter and Paul fortress in the 1840s, as quoted in Igor Bogdanov, *Dym otechestva, ili kratkaia istoriia tabakokureniia* (Moscow: Novoe literaturnoe obozrenie, 2007), 161.

4. The unpleasant first cigarette is one of the "visceral forms of sales resistance" common to many drugs. David T. Courtwright, *Forces of Habit: Drugs and the Making of the Modern World* (Cambridge, MA: Harvard University Press, 2002), 104.

5. The cardboard tube was called the *gil'za*, the tobacco portion the *kurka*. Wherever possible, I use "papirosy" for Russian smokes and "cigarette" for Western smokes. Westerners often used the term "cigarette" to refer to what was likely a Russian papirosa. In those cases, I have kept the original. Adolf Fedorovich Grinevskii, *Bros'te kurit'! O vrede kureniia tabaku dlia zdorov'ia*, 2 ed. (Moscow: I. Efimov, 1905), 12–13; *Kratkii ocherk tabakokureniia v Rossii, v minuvshev 19-m stoletii: Za period vremeni s 1810 po 1906 god* (Kiev: Petr Barskii, 1906), 7; S. V. Lebedev, N. O. Osipov, N. I. Prokhorov, and V. G. Shaposhnikov, "Tobacco," in *Entsiklopedicheskii slovar XXXII*, ed. F. A. Brokgauz and I. A. Efron (St. Petersburg: I. A. Efron, 1901), 421.

6. Robert N. Proctor, *Golden Holocaust: Origins of the Cigarette Catastrophe and the Case for Abolition* (Berkeley: University of California Press, 2011), 28–30.

7. Courtwright, *Forces,* 17–18, 114.

8. Kathleen Sebelius, *How Tobacco Smoke Causes Disease: The Biology and Behavioral Basis for Smoking-Attributable Disease; A Report of the Surgeon General* (hereafter SGR) (Rockville, MD: U.S. Department of Health and Human Services, 2010), 111; Jordan Goodman, *Tobacco in History: The Cultures of Dependence* (London: Routledge, 1993), 5–6.

9. Nicotine is less effective in non-tobacco products, according to some research. Sebelius, *SGR*, 110.

10. Jordan Goodman, "Webs of Drug Dependence: Towards a Political History of Smoking and Health," in *Ashes to Ashes: The History of Smoking and Health*, ed. S. Lock, L. A. Reynolds, and E. M. Tansey (Amsterdam: Rodopi, 1998), 16. Carol Benedict argues that the cigarette is not inherently modern, but instead it is the match that makes it more revolutionary. The more addictive quality of inhaled smoking tobacco does change the relationship of the user to the product; see her *Golden-Silk Smoke: A History of Tobacco in China, 1550–2010* (Berkeley: University of California Press, 2011), 180–81.

11. N. I. Umnova, "Tabachnaia promyshlennost za 15 let (c.1890–1904)," in *Sbornik statei i materialov po tabachnomu delu*, ed. S. A. Egiz (St. Petersburg: V. F. Kirshbaum, 1913), 99–140.

12. Arcadius Kahan, *Russian Economic History: The Nineteenth Century* (Chicago: University of Chicago Press, 1989), 63.

13. E. S. Krymskii, *Vred dlia zdorov'ia ot kureniia i niukhaniia tabaku i sredstva perestat' kurit'* (Zvenigorodka: E. S. Krymskii, 1889), 4; Egiz, *Sbornik statei*, iii.

14. Lev Borisovich Kafengauz, *Evoliutsiia promyshlennogo proizvodstva Rossii (posledniaia tret' XIX v.–30-e gody XX v.)* (Moscow: Epifaniia, 1994), 156, 198, 265.

15. Goodman, *Tobacco*, 94. China seems to have come close behind Russia in the market turn to cigarettes. Benedict, *Golden-Silk Smoke*, 133–39.

16. I. Tregubov, *Normal'nyi sposob brosit' kurit'* (Batum: D. L. Kapelia, 1912), 3; Ivan Ivanovich Priklonskii (Dr.), *Upotreblenie tabaka i ego vrednoe na organizm cheloveka vliianie* (Moscow: K. Tikhomirov, 1909), 5; "Russian Paper Trade: The Manufacture of Paper Cigarette Tubes," *World's Paper Trade Review*, March 29, 1907: 8.

17. Students of Grammatchikov and Ossendovskii, "K voprosu o vliianii kureniia na organizm cheloveka," *Vrach* 1 (1887): 4–8.

18. Proctor, *Golden*, 33–34.

19. Courtwright, *Forces,* 97–98.

20. Benedict, *Golden-Silk*, 29–30. See also Joseph C. Winter, "Introduction to the North American Tobacco Species," and Alexander von Gernet, "North American Indigenous *Nicotiana* Use and Tobacco Shamanism: The Early Documentary Record, 1520–1660," in *Tobacco Use by Native North Americans: Sacred Smoke and Silent Killer,* ed. Joseph C. Winter (Norman: University of Oklahoma Press, 2000), 3–4, 65.

21. Sebelius, *SGR*, 31, 32.

22. Neal L. Benowitz, "Nicotine Addiction," *New England Journal of Medicine* 362 (2010) 2295–2303.

23. K. Fagerstrom and T. Eissenberg, "Dependence on Tobacco and Nicotine Products: A Case for Product-Specific Assessment," *Nicotine and Tobacco Research* 14 (2012): 1382–90.

24. Sebelius, *SGR*, 118.

25. Allan M. Brandt, *The Cigarette Century: The Rise, Fall, and Deadly Persistence of the Product That Defined America* (New York: Basic Books, 2007), 358.

26. Barbara Hahn, *Making Tobacco Bright: Creating an American Commodity, 1617–1937* (Baltimore, MD: Johns Hopkins University Press, 2011), 5–6.

27. Courtwright, *Forces,* 56–57; Benedict, *Golden-Silk,* 29–30; Egiz, *Sbornik statei*, iv. Chernigov, Poltava, Voronezh, Tambov, and Samara grew makhorka. The best was *rubanka*—strong and easily stored. The most sowed was the middling "silver" sort. V. G. Kotel'nikov, *Vozdelyvane prostago tabaka-makhorki*, 2nd ed. (St. Petersburg: Izd. A. F. Devriena, 1899), iii; for comparative flavor see Lynn T. Kozlowski, Jack E. Henningfield, and Janet Brigham, *Cigarettes, Nicotine, and Health: A Biobehavioral Approach* (Thousand Oaks, CA: Sage, 2001), 15.

28. The Russian sorts were Bakun, Shnurovkii, or Russian-Samara. Kotel'nikov, *Vozdelyvanie*, 9–11.

29. D-r. Rokau, *Interesnaia i liubopytnaia istoriia kurivshikh', niuchavshikh' i zhevashikh' tabak': S legendarnymi pravdivym skazaniem o ego pagubnom' vlianii na zdorov'e cheloveka* (Moscow: A. V. Kudriavtseva, 1885/6), 3; Iu. P. Bokarev, "Tobacco Production in Russia," in

Tobacco in Russian History and Culture: From the Seventeenth Century to the Present, ed. Matthew P. Romaniello and Tricia Starks (New York: Routledge, 2009), 148–157, esp. 149; Goodman, *Tobacco,* 4.

30. Proctor, *Golden,* 364.

31. K. Dmitriev, *Kak vozdelyvat' tabak i podgotovliat' ego v prodazhu* (Moscow: I. S. Gabai, 1894), 30–31; Mary C. Neuberger, *Balkan Smoke: Tobacco and the Making of Modern Bulgaria* (Ithaca, NY: Cornell University Press, 2013), 209; Proctor, *Golden,* 364.

32. Proctor, *Golden,* 380. In some reports early Russians urinated on tobacco as part of the curing process. This may have added ammonia, which "frees" nicotine to create greater psychoactive effects. For Russia see Matthew P. Romaniello, "Customs and Consumption: Russian Tobacco Habits in the Seventeenth and Eighteenth Century," in *The Global Lives of Things: Materiality, Material Culture and Commodities in the First Global Age,* ed. Anne Gerritsen and Giorgio Riello (London: Routledge, 2015), 183–97. On urination on tobacco in other cultures see Proctor, *Golden,* 396.

33. Courtwright, *Forces,* 56.

34. Sources indicate Russians inhaled fully despite the nicotine content. Hahn argues that standards for cultivation and controls were still in flux in the 1800s. Memoirs implied that at least the broad distinction of Russian and Western tobacco existed. *Making Tobacco.* 2–7.

35. Only two scholars have engaged Russian tobacco history—one is Bogdanov in his delightful popular history *Dym*; the other is A. V. Malinin, whose two works, *O chem umolchal MINZDRAV* (Moscow: Russkii tabak, 2003) and *Tabachnaia istoriia Rossii* (Moscow: Russkii Tabak, 2006), are both published by the press "Russian tobacco," funded by industry groups. A short historical introduction appeared in L. N. Federenko, *Kurenie v Rossii* (Rossiiskaia akademiia obrazovaniia iuznoe otdelenie. Slaviansk-na-kubain: Slavianskii filial Armavirskogo gosudarstvennogo pedagogicheskogo instituta, 2002). The singular scholarly work on tobacco use in Eastern Europe is Neuberger's *Balkan Smoke.*

36. World Health Organization, *WHO Report on the Global Tobacco Epidemic, 2013* (Geneva, Switzerland: World Health Organization, 2013); World Health Organization, *European Tobacco Control Status Report 2013* (Geneva, Switzerland: World Health Organization, 2013).

37. Sebelius, *SGR,* 181; J. E. Rose, "Multiple Brain Pathways and Receptors Underlying Tobacco Addiction," *Biochemical Pharmacology* 74 (2007): 1263–70.

38. This change was not made, but the discussion indicates the difficulty of assessing only one cause to dependency. See K. Fagerstrom "Determinants of Tobacco Use and Renaming the FTND to the Fagerstrom Test for Cigarette Dependence," *Nicotine Tobacco Research* 14 (2012): 75–78. A full explanation of the test can be found in Sebelius, *SGR,* 106–7.

39. Priscilla Parkhurst Ferguson, "The Senses of Taste," and Mark S. R. Jenner, "Follow Your Nose? Smell, Smelling, and Their Histories," *American Historical Review* 116 (2011): 371, 337.

40. Carolyn Korsmeyer, *Making Sense of Taste: Food and Philosophy* (Ithaca, NY: Cornell University Press, 1999).

41. Diane Ackerman, *A Natural History of the Senses* (New York: Random House, 1990), 30.

42. This was an argument made by Marshall McLuhan and Walter Ong, but roundly critiqued in more recent works like that of Mark M. Smith in *Sensing the Past: Seeing, Hearing, Smelling, Tasting, and Touching in History* (Berkeley: University of California Press, 2007) and "Making Sense of Social History," *Journal of Social History* 37, no. 1 (2003): 165–86; and in his "Producing Sense, Consuming Sense, Making Sense: Perils and Prospects for Sensory History." *Journal of Social History.* 40:4 (2007): 841–58; "The Senses in History." *The American History Review.* 116:2 (2011): 307–400; "The Senses in American History: A Round Table." *The Journal of American History.* 95 (2008): 378 451.

43. A large literature addresses these issues. See, for example, Alain Corbin, *The Foul and the Fragrant: Odor and the French Social Imagination* (Cambridge, MA: Harvard University Press, 1986); David S. Barnes, *The Great Stink of Paris and the Nineteenth-Century Struggle against*

Filth and Germs. (Baltimore, MD: Johns Hopkins Press, 2006); Hans J. Rindisbacher, *The Smell of Books: A Cultural-Historical Study of Olfactory Perception in Literature* (Ann Arbor: University of Michigan Press, 1992); Constance Classen, David Howes, and Anthony Synnott, *Aroma: The Cultural History of Smell* (London: Routledge, 1994); David Howes, ed. *Empire of the Senses: The Sensual Culture Reader* (2004; repr., London: Bloomsbury, 2014); Alexander M. Martin, "Sewage and the City: Filth, Smell, and Representations of Urban Life in Moscow, 1770–1880," *Russian Review* 67 (2008): 243–74.

44. Martin, "Sewage and the City," 243–74; and his "Introduction: The Sensory in Russian and Soviet history," as well as Alison K. Smith's "Fermentation, Taste, and Identity," and Aaron B. Retish's "The Taste of *Kumyshka* and the Debate over Udmurt Culture," in *Russian History through the Senses: From 1700 to the Present,* ed. Matthew P. Romaniello and Tricia Starks (London: Bloomsbury, 2016), 1–19, 45–66, 141–64. See also Alison K. Smith, *Recipes for Russia: Food and Nationhood under the Tsars* (DeKalb: Northern Illinois University Press, 2008).

45. Sebelius, *SGR*, 182.

46. Dong-Chul Seo and Yan Huang, "Systematic Review of Social Network Analysis in Adolescent Cigarette Smoking Behavior," *Journal of School Health* 82 (2012): 21–27; N. A. Christakia, J. H. Fowler, "The Collective Dynamics of Smoking in a Large Social Network," *New England Journal of Medicine.* 358 (2008): 2249–58; S. C. Hitchman et al., "Socioeconomic Status and Smokers' Number of Smoking Friends: Findings from the International Tobacco Control (ITC) Four Country Survey," *Drug and Alcohol Dependence* 143 (2014): 158–66; S. T. Higgins, R. Redner, J. S. Priest, J. Y. Bunn, "Socioeconomic Disadvantage and Other Risk Factors for Using Higher-Nicotine/Tar-Yield (Regular Full-flavor) Cigarettes," *Nicotine and Tobacco Research* 19(12) (2017): 1425–33; R. Hiscock et al., "Socioeconomic Status and Smoking: A Review," *Annals of New York Academy of Science* 1248 (2012): 107–23.

47. Sebelius, *SGR*, 117–19, 131, 10506, 170.

48. See, for example, S. Tormazov, *Zagadka kurenie* (St. Petersburg: M. O. Vol'f', 1907), 306. A larger discussion appears in chapter 5.

49. Mary Douglas, *The World of Goods* (New York: Basic Books, 1979).

50. Jan de Vries, *The Industrious Revolution: Consumer Behavior and the Household Economy, 1650 to the Present* (Cambridge: Cambridge University Press, 2008), 161.

51. For a dog-leg the user rolled the edge of a scrap paper around their finger tip to form a pipe-like bowl, twisted the rest into a pipe stem, and then filled the small bowl with tobacco.

52. Sebelius, *SGR,* 120.

53. Daniel Miller, *Stuff* (Cambridge, Polity, 2010), 23–31.

54. Violin, Ia. A., *Tabak i ego vred dlia zdorov'ia* (Kazan: Shtaba zapasnoi armii, 1920), 4.

55. Proctor, *Golden*, 6.

56. Sebelius, *SGR,* 105–6, 117–99.

57. Grinevskii, *Bros'te*, 14.

58. See, for example, Iain Gately, *Tobacco: The Story of How Tobacco Seduced the World.* (New York: Grove Press, 2001); Hahn, *Making Tobacco*; Richard Kluger, *Ashes to Ashes: America's Hundred-Year Cigarette War, the Public Health, and the Unabashed Triumph of Philip Morris.* (New York: Alfred A. Knopf, 1996); Neuberger, *Balkan Smoke*; Proctor, *Golden.*

59. See, for example, A. K. Demin, ed. *Kurenie ili zdorov'e v Rossii* (Moscow: Fond Zdorov'e i okruzhaiushchaia sreda, 1996); A. K. Demin, et al. *Rossiia: Delo tabak, rassledovanie massovogo ubiistva* (Moscow: RAOZ, 2012); Cassandra Tate, *Cigarette Wars: The Triumph of "The Little White Slaver"* (New York: Oxford University Press, 1999); Pamela E. Pennock, *Advertising Sin and Sickness: The Politics of Alcohol and Tobacco Marketing, 1950–1990* (DeKalb: Northern Illinois University Press, 2007); Robert N Proctor, *The Nazi War on Cancer* (Princeton, NJ: Princeton University Press,1999).

60. See, for example, Sander L. Gilman and Xhou Zun, eds. *Smoke: A Cultural History of Smoking Around the World* (London: Reaktion books, 2004); Goodman, *Tobacco*; Matthew

Hilton, *Smoking in British Popular Culture, 1800–2000* (Manchester: Manchester University Press, 2000); Richard Klein, *Cigarettes Are Sublime* (Durham, NC: Duke University Press, 1993); Jarrett Rudy, *The Freedom to Smoke: Tobacco Consumption and Identity.* (Montreal: McGill-Queen's University Press, 2005); Steven B. Bunker, *Creating Mexican Consumer Culture in the Age of Porfirio Diaz* (Albuquerque: University of New Mexico Press, 2012). Andrei Valer'evich Shapovalov, *Ocherki istorii i kul'tury potrebleniia tabak v Sibiri: XVII–pervaia polovina XX vv.* (Novosibirsk: Progress-servis, 2002).

61. Ben Eklof, Josh Bushnell, and Larissa Zakharova, eds., *Russia's Great Reforms, 1855–1881* (Bloomington: Indiana University Press, 1994).

62. Janet M. Hartley, *Siberia: A History of the People* (New Haven, CT: Yale University Press, 2014), 163–83; Alec Nove, *An Economic History of the U.S.S.R.* (London: The Penguin Press, 1969), 13–14.

63. Alison K. Smith, *For the Common Good and Their Own Well-Being: Social Estates in Imperial Russia* (Oxford: Oxford University Press, 2014), 123–48; Joseph Bradley, *Muzhik and Muscovite: Urbanization in Late Imperial Russia* (Berkeley: University of California Press, 1985), 4; Harley D. Balzer, ed., *Russia's Missing Middle Class: The Professions in Russian History* (Armonk, NY: M. E. Sharpe, 1996), 89–116; see also Thomas C. Owen, "Impediments to a Bourgeois Consciousness in Russia, 1880–1905: The Estate Structure, Ethnic Diversity, and Economic Regionalism"; Samuel D. Kassow, James L. West, and Edith W. Clowes, "Introduction: The Problem of the Middle in Late Imperial Russian Society," and Sidney Monas, "The Twilit Middle Class of Nineteenth-Century Russia," all in *Between Tsar and People: Educated Society and the Quest for Public Identity in Late Imperial Russia,* eds. Edith W. Clowes, Samuel D. Kassow, and James L. West (Princeton, NJ: Princeton University Press, 1991), 3–14, 28–37, and 75–89; Mark D. Steinberg, *Petersburg Fin de Siècle* (New Haven, CT: Yale University Press, 2011), 1–9.

64. Mark D. Steinberg, *Proletarian Imagination: Self, Modernity, and the Sacred in Russia, 1910–1925* (Ithaca, NY: Cornell University Press, 2002), 2–9

65. See the opportunities for identity creation in the urban environment highlighted by Lynda Need in "Mapping the Self: Gender, Space and Modernity in Mid-Victorian London," in *Rewriting the Self: Histories from the Renaissance to the Present,* ed. Roy Porter (London: Routledge, 1997), 184–85.

66. Laura Engelstein, *The Keys to Happiness: Sex and the Search for Modernity in Fin-de-Siècle Russia* (Ithaca, NY: Cornell University Press, 1992), 1–13; Louise McReynolds, *Russia at Play: Leisure Activities at the End of the Tsarist Era* (Ithaca, NY: Cornell University Press, 2003), 3–6; Christine Ruane, *The Empire's New Clothes: A History of the Russian Fashion Industry, 1700–1917* (New Haven, CT: Yale University Press, 2009), 1–3; Anna Fishzon, *Fandom, Authenticity, and Opera: Mad Acts and Letter Scenes in Fin-de-Siècle Russia* (New York: Palgrave Macmillan, 2013), 15; Sally West, *I Shop in Moscow: Advertising and the Creation of Consumer Culture in Late Tsarist Russia* (Dekalb: Northern Illinois University Press, 2011), 5.

67. Barbara Alpern Engel, *Breaking the Ties that Bound: The Politics of Marital Strife in Late Imperial Russia* (Ithaca, NY: Cornell University Press, 2011), 2–4.

68. Engelstein, *Keys,* 1–13; Julie V. Brown, "Revolution and Psychosis: The Mixing of Science and Politics in Russian Psychiatric medicine, 1905–13," *Russian Review* 46 (1987): 283–302; Nancy Mandelker Frieden, *Russian Physicians in an Era of Reform and Revolution, 1856–1905* (Princeton, NJ: Princeton University Press, 1981); John F. Hutchinson, *Politics and Public Health in Revolutionary Russia, 1890–1918* (Baltimore, MD: Johns Hopkins University Press, 1990); Richard Stites, *The Women's Liberation Movement in Russia: Feminism, Nihilism, and Bolshevism, 1860–1930* (Princeton, NJ: Princeton University Press, 1978); Barbara Alpern Engel, *Mothers and Daughters: Women of the Intelligentsia in Nineteenth-Century Russia* (Cambridge: Cambridge University Press, 1983), 3.

69. Simon Pawley, "Revolution in Health: Nervous Weakness and Visions of Health in Revolutionary Russia, c. 1900–31," *Historical Research* 90 (2017): 191–209; Daniel Beer, *Renovating*

Russia: The Human Sciences and the Fate of Liberal Modernity, 1880–1930 (Ithaca, NY: Cornell University Press, 2008), 11–13, 31–32; Robert A. Nye, *Crime, Madness, and Politics in Modern France: The Medical Concept of National Decline* (Princeton, NJ: Princeton University Press, 1984).

70. Ferguson, "Senses of Taste," 373.

71. Goodman, *Tobacco*, 101–4; Robin Walker, *Under Fire: A History of Tobacco Smoking in Australia* (Carlton, Victoria: Melbourne University Press, 1984), 1–8; Benedict, *Golden-Silk*, 131–48; Howard Cox, *The Global Cigarette: Origins and Evolution of British American Tobacco, 1880–1945* (New York: Oxford University Press, 2000), 19–45; John C. Burnham, *Bad Habits: Drinking, Smoking, Taking Drugs, Gambling, Sexual Misbehavior, and Swearing in American History* (New York: New York University Press, 1993), 86–111; Roberta G. Ferrence, *Deadly Fashion: The Rise and Fall of Cigarette Smoking in North America* (New York: Garland Publishing, 1989); Gerard S. Petrone, *Tobacco Advertising: The Great Seduction* (Atglen, PA: Schiffer Publishing, 1996), 65–69; Nannie M. Tilley, *The R. J. Reynolds Tobacco Company* (Chapel Hill: University of North Carolina Press, 1985), 29–94. For the inverse story of the fall, see Frank V. Tursi, Susan E. White, and Steve McQuilken, *Lost Empire: The Fall of R. J. Reynolds Tobacco Company* (Rochester, WA: Gorham Printing, 2000).

72. Availability is crucial to uptake of drugs according to Courtwright, *Forces*, 189.

73. For comparison see the stories told in Courtwright, *Forces*; Gately, *Tobacco*; Gilman and Xun, *Smoke*; Goodman, *Tobacco*; V. G. Kiernan, *Tobacco: A History* (London: Hutchinson Radius, 1991).

74. Benedict, *Golden-Silk*. 199–239.

1. CULTIVATED

1. Klein identifies the fictitious soldier as a Turkish Zouave, but the Turks did not establish a Zouave regiment until the 1880s. This would have to be a French Zouave. See *Cigarettes*, 135. Proctor wrote of an Egyptian soldier who, in the 1832 Siege of Acre, in the war between the Egyptians and Ottomans, improvised paper rolled tobacco after a broken pipe. Either way the Zouave retained the popular imagination. *Golden*, 28.

2. Burnham, *Bad Habits*, 89.

3. Fernand Braudel, *Civilization and Capitalism: 15th–18th Century.* Vol. 1. *The Structures of Everyday Life: The Limits of the Possible* (Berkeley: University of California Press, 1992), 263.

4. *Kratkii cherk tabakokureniia v Rossii*, 6–7.

5. Bogdanov, *Dym*, 52.

6. Konstantine Klioutchkine, "'I Smoke, Therefore I Think': Tobacco as Liberation in Russian Nineteenth-Century Literature and Culture," in *Tobacco in Russian History and Culture: From the Seventeenth Century to the Present,* ed. Matthew P. Romaniello and Tricia Starks (New York: Routledge, 2009), 93.

7. Aleksandr Snopkov, Pavel Snopkov, and Aleksandr Shkliaruk, *Reklama v plakate: Russkii torgovo-promyshlennyi plakat za 100 let/Advertising Art in Russia.* (Moscow: Kontakt Kul'tura, 2007), plate 17, p. 19

8. Courtwright, *Forces,* 15–16.

9. Kiernan, *Tobacco*, 42, 138–40.

10. Ravenholt, "Tobacco's Global Death March" 219.

11. Kiernan, *Tobacco,* 42.

12. As quoted in ibid., 140.

13. "Referaty," *Pedagogicheskii sbornik, izdavaemyi pri glavnom upgravlenii voenn-uchebnykh zavedenii* Knizhka 368 (September 1897): 505.

14. Klioutchkine, "I Smoke, Therefore I Think," 90.

15. F. B. Biriukova, "Kurenie kak fenomen povsednevnoi zhizni Rossii v kontse XVIII-seredeine XIX v," in *Istoriia Rossiiskoi povsednevnosti: Materialy dvadtsat' shestoi vserossiiskoi*

zaochnoi nauchnoi konferentsii, ed. S. D. Morozova and V. B. Zhiromska (St. Petersburg: Nestor, 2013), 56.

16. Willard Sunderland, "Shop Signs, Monuments, Souvenirs: Views of the Empire in Everyday Life," in *Picturing Russia: Explorations in Visual Culture,* ed. Valerie A. Kivelson and Joan Neuberger (New Haven, CT: Yale University Press, 2008), 104–8; Jeffrey Brooks, *When Russia Learned to Read: Literacy and Popular Literature, 1861–1917* (Evanston, IL: Northwestern University Press, 2003), xix.

17. Jeffrey Auerbach argued that, for Britain, "imperialism was as much a cultural project as a military endeavor. . . . Imperialism is constructed as much in the mind as it is a physical reality." "Art, Advertising, and the Legacy of Empire," *Journal of Popular Culture* 35, no. 4 (Spring 2002), 20.

18. Brooks, *When Russia Learned to Read,* 223.

19. See similar arguments made in Bunker, *Creating,* 14.

20. Stephen M. Norris outlined this debate in the introduction to his work on visual culture, *A War of Images: Russian Popular Prints, Wartime Culture, and National Identity, 1812–1945.* (DeKalb: Northern Illinois University Press, 2006), 7–8.

21. S. V. Lebedev, N. O. Osipov, N. I. Prokhorov, and V. G. Shaposhnikov, "Tobacco," in *Entsiklopedicheskii slovar XXXII*, ed. F. A. Brokgauz and I. A. Efron (St. Petersburg: I. A. Efron, 1901), 421.

22. Iu. P. Bokarev, "Tobacco Production in Russia: The Transition to Communism," in *Tobacco in Russian History and Culture: From the Seventeenth Century to the Present*, ed. Matthew P. Romaniello and Tricia Starks (New York: Routledge, 2009), 148.

23. O. J. Frederiksen, "Virginia Tobacco in Russia under Peter the Great," *Slavonic and East European Review. American Series.* 2 (March 1943): 40–56.

24. *O razvedenii i fabrikatsii tabaka* (Moscow: Aleksandr Semen, 1852), 125–53.

25. S. A. Egiz, "Programma opisaniia morfologicheskikh priznakov form *nicotiana rustia* L. I. *niocitana tabacum* l," in *Sbornik statei i materialov po tabachnomu delu*, ed. S. A. Egiz (St. Petersburg: V. F Kirshbaum, 1913), 60–161.

26. Kotel'nikov, *Vozdelyvanie,* 9–11.

27. V. N. Liubimenko, *Tabak* (Petrograd: M. S. Sabashnikovy, 1922), 11.

28. *Stranichka iz istorii promyshlennosti iugo-vostochnoi Rossii: Tabachnaia fabrika F. K. Shtaf v Saratove* (Saratov: F. M. Kimmel', 1896), 15–16.

29. See the exhaustive list in Mikhail Vasil'evich Kechedzhi-Shapovalov, *Tabakovodstvo v Rossi* (St. Petersburg: Ulei, 1912), 1–2.

30. "Tabachnaia promyshlenost' v Rossii: Statiia vtoraia i posledniaia," *Otechestvennyia zapiski: Ucheno-literaturnyi zhurnal'* 28 (1845), 23–28.

31. John King Fairbank, Katherine Frost Bruner, and Elizabeth MacLeod Matheson, eds., *The I. G. in Peking: Letters of Robert Hart, Chinese Maritime Customs, 1868–1907.* vol. 1 (Cambridge, MA: The Belknap Press of Harvard University Press, 1975), 574.

32. Henry Sutherland Edwards, *The Russians at Home: Unpolitical Sketches,* 2nd ed. (London: Wm. H. Allen and Co, 1861), 409.

33. John Bain, *Cigarettes in Fact and Fancy* (Boston: H. M. Caldwell Co, 1906), 24.

34. W. A. Brennan, *Tobacco Leaves: Being a Book of Facts for Smokers* (Menasha, WI: Index Office, Inc. 1915), 63, 136.

35. Lebedev, et al., "Tobacco," 421.

36. Malinin, *Tabachnaia istoriia Rossii*, 201.

37. "Russian Paper Trade: The Manufacture of Paper Cigarette Tubes," *The World's Paper Trade Review*, March 29, 1907, 8.

38. Lebedev, et al., "Tobacco," 421; Brennan, *Tobacco Leaves*, 136

39. *O razvedenii i fabrikatsii*, 68.

40. Ibid., 126–51; for a more thorough discussion of the flavoring of Russian tobacco, see Tricia Starks, "The Taste, Smell, and Semiotics of Cigarettes," in *Russian History through the*

Senses: From 1700 to the Present, ed. Matthew P. Romaniello and Tricia Starks (London: Blooms-bury Academic, 2016), 97–115.

41. Bogdanov, *Dym,* 148.

42. Ibid., 49–51.

43. Alexander M. Martin, *Enlightened Metropolis: Constructing Imperial Moscow, 1762–1855* (Oxford: Oxford University Press, 2013), 68–69.

44. Bogdanov, *Dym,* 115.

45. Malinin, *Tabachnaia istoriia Rossii,* 79.

46. Evgenii Popov, *Nachnite bor'bu so strast'iu k tabaku.* 3rd ed. (Perm: Gubernskoe prav-lenie, 1887), 15; Bek (Prof.), *Kurenie: V obshchedostupnom izlozhenii.* Bezplatnoe prilozhenie k zhurnalu "Narodnoe zdravie" (St. Petersburg: S-Peterburgskaia elektropechatnia, 1902), 25; V. I. Korno and M. G. Kitainer, *Balkanskaia Zvezda: Stranitsy istorii* (Iaroslavl: Niuans, 2000), 51–54; Bogdanov, *Dym,* 97.

47. Bruce W. Menning, *Bayonets before Bullets: The Imperial Russian Army, 1861–1914* (Bloomington: Indiana University Press, 2000), 51–86; *Kratkii ocherk tabakokureniia v Rossii,* 7–8.

48. F. V. Greene, *Sketches of Army Life in Russia* (New York: Charles Scribner's Sons, 1880), 8.

49. Ibid., 5–6.

50. The National Archives, CO 389, Board of Trade: Entry Books, 15, ff. 185–89, "Whitehall to the Lords Commission on the state of Trade between Russia and England," August 10, 1697. Citation courtesy Matthew P. Romaniello.

51. Kiernan, *Tobacco,* 173–82.

52. Marc Vigié and Muriel Vigié, *L'herbe à Nicot: Amateurs de tabac, fermiers généraux et contrebandiers sous l'Ancien Régime* (Paris: Fayard, 1989).

53. Peter Bartrip, "Pushing the Weed: The Editorializing and Advertising of Tobacco in the *Lancet* and the *British Medical Journal,* 1880–1958," in *Ashes to Ashes The History of Smoking and Health,* ed. S. Lock, L. A. Reynolds, and E. M. Tansey (Amsterdam: Rodopi, 1998), 107.

54. Martin, *Enlightened Metropolis,* 163–65.

55. Richard Sobel, *They Satisfy: The Cigarette in American Life* (Garden City, NY: Anchor Press/Doubleday, 1978), 10.

56. Korno and Kitainer, *Balkanskaia Zvezda,* 54.

57. I. V. Bratiushenko, "Ofitserskie ekonomicheskie obshchestva v gody Russko Iaponskoi I pervoi mirovoi voin," *Voprosy Istorii* (00428779) 2004, no. 7: 104–15.

58. K. Markovich, *Otchet: Po sboru papiros, tabaku i kuritel'nykh prinadlezhnostei, proizve-dennomu v g. Rostove n/D. i po nekotorym stantsiiam Vladinavnazskoi zheleznoi dorogi* (Rostov na Don: Pechantia S. P. Iakovleva, 1904), 6.

59. Aleksandr Khokhrev, "Tabak v stile Shaposhnikova," *Territoriia biznesa: Zhurnal delo-vykh liudei* 9, no. 34 (September 2009): 85.

60. By 1914 there were thirty-one advertising firms in Moscow and thirty-six in St. Pe-tersburg. The relative novelty of the industry allowed women to find opportunities. Women owned five of the thirteen firms in Moscow. West, *I Shop in Moscow,* 12; Sally West, "Con-structing Consumer Culture: Advertising in Imperial Russia to 1914" (PhD diss., University of Illinois–Urbana-Champaign, 1995), 36; Sally West, "The Material Promised Land: Advertis-ing's Modern Agenda in Late Imperial Russia," *Russian Review* 57 (July 1998): 345. See also on the long dureé comparison of tobacco advertising and cessation propaganda, O. I. Budanova, "Problema tabakokureniia v otechestvennom plakate: Ot reklamy tabaka do antitabachnoi pro-pagandy," in *Rumiantsevskie chteniia 2015,* comp. E. A. Ivanova (Moscow: Pashkov dome, 2015), 3–38.

61. West, "The Material Promised Land," 345–63.

62. Ekaterina Klimova, "Russkii reklamnyi plakat: Stanovlenie zhanra," in *Reklamnyi Plakat v Rossii, 1900–1920-e,* comp. Ekaterina Klimova and Irina Zolotinkina, ed. Anastasiia Rudakova (St. Petersburg: Palace Editions, 2010), 7.

63. Klimova, "Russkii reklamnyi plakat," 7; Nina Baburina and Svetlana Artamonova, ed. *Russkii reklamnyi plakat* (Moscow: Kontakt-kul'tura, 2001). 5.

64. Klaus Vashik and Nina Baburina, *Real'nost' utopii: Isskusstvo Russkogo plakata XX veka* (Moscow: Progress-Traditsiia, 2003), 42.

65. Irina Zolotinkina, "Smitrii Balanov i biuro reklam Leningradskogo Otkomkhoza," in *Reklamnyi Plakat v Rossii, 1900–1920-e*, comp. Ekaterina Klimova and Irina Zolotinkina, ed. Anastasiia Rudakova (St. Petersburg: Palace Editions, 2010), 15; Sally West, "The Material Promised Land: Advertising's Modern Agenda in Late Imperial Russia," *Russian Review* 57 (July 1998): 348.

66. Brooks, *When Russia Learned to Read*, 109–18.

67. Jeff Sahadeo, *Russian Colonial Society in Tashkent, 1865–1923* (Bloomington: Indiana University Press, 2007), 155.

68. West, "The Material Promised Land," 345; Elena Chernevich, ed., *Russkii graficheskii dizain, 1880–1917* (Moscow: Vneshsigma, 1997), 101–2; West, *I Shop in Moscow*, 57; West, "Constructing Consumer Culture," 30.

69. I. N. Paltusova, *Torgovaia reklama i upakovka v Rossii, XIX–XX vv.* (Moscow: GIM, 1993), 6.

70. Vashik and Baburina, *Real'nost' utopii*, 31.

71. Roland Marchand, *Advertising the American Dream: Making Way for Modernity, 1920–1940* (Berkeley: University of California Press, 1985).

72. West, *I Shop in Moscow*, 77–90.

73. Ibid., 51.

74. West, "Constructing Consumer Culture," 11.

75. Brandt, *Cigarette Century*, 32.

76. *Peterburskaia gazeta* data collected by West, *I Shop in Moscow*, 14; West, "Constructing Consumer Culture," 308.

77. Sample pack from Chernevich, *Russkii graficheskii dizain*, 101.

78. Violin, *Tabak*, 4.

79. Olga Maiorova, *From the Shadow of Empire: Defining the Russian Nation through Cultural Mythology, 1855–1870* (Madison: University of Wisconsin Press, 2010), 190.

80. Judith Deutsch Kornblatt, *The Cossack Hero in Russian Literature: A Study in Cultural Mythology* (Madison: The University of Wisconsin Press, 1992), 17, 61; Maiorova, *From the Shadow*, 72, 190; Norris, *A War of Images*, 81.

81. Korno and Kitainer call him a "krest'ianin." The renaming is not explained. Another history posits it was renamed for an old brand. Even so, the symbolism and timing assure a new contextual meaning. Korno and Kitainer, *Balkanskaia Zvezda*, 29–37, 58–62; West, *I Shop in Moscow*, 106.

82. Kornblatt, *The Cossack*, 4–5, 16–17; Maiorova, *From the Shadow*, 42, 119, 190. Norris argues that the images of the Russo-Turkish War as a holy war trickled down to the peasantry, and these advertising images would imply that, indeed, the concept infused society. *A War of Images*, 80–106, 83–87, especially the discussion of Russia's fight with France over Palestine.

83. Bogdanov, *Dym*, 72.

84. West, *I Shop in Moscow*, 192.

85. Kornblatt, *The Cossack*; Norris, *A War of Images*, 81.

86. Bogdanov, *Dym*, 183.

87. Titles reported included *Diadia Mikhei za granitsei; Diadia Mikhei v derevne; Diadia Mikhei v Peterburge: Fel'eton-reklamy Diadi Mikhei; Puteshevstvie za tabakami na Vostok, 1903–1904*, as reported in L. M. Turchinskii, comp, *Russkie poety XX veka: Materialy dlia bibliografii* (Moscow: Znak, 2007), 105.

88. Sally West, "Constructing Consumer Culture," 42; West, *I Shop in Moscow*, 117–18; Bogdanov, *Dym*, 183.

89. "A Trip to the East for Tobacco with Uncle Mikey," *Put' pravdy*, May 18, 1914, 4.

90. Bogdanov, *Dym*, 185.

91. A high quality reproduction of the Suvarov pack was not available. Konstantine Klioutchkine, "'I Smoke, Therefore I Think,'" 86.

92. Bogdanov, *Dym*, 73.

93. Norris, *A War of Images*, 88–89, 92–98.

94. Baburina and Artamonova, *Russkii reklamnyi plakat*, plate 32.

95. Norris, *A War of Images*, 121, 149.

96. Dobryi molodets, *Moskovskii listok*, March 13, 1913: 1. West employs the terminology of "borrowed interest" to understand this process. *I Shop in Moscow*, 180.

97. Sahadeo, *Russian Colonial Society*, 21, 146, 152.

98. Vashik and Baburina, *Real'nost' utopii*, 35.

99. Klimova, "Russkii reklamnyi plakat," 10.

100. West, *I Shop in Moscow*, 179.

101. According to Norris, the French were depicted as *basurman* in 1812, but by the Crimean war the "savage infidel" had become a Muslim Turk in popular prints. *A War of Images*, 62–63.

102. West, *I Shop in Moscow*, 174–75

103. A hunting trip on his eastern excursion grounded. "Puteshestvie na vostoke," *Put' pravdy*, May 18, 1914, 4.

104. Hilton, *Smoking*, 97–99.

105. West, *I Shop in Moscow*, 117.

106. Ibid., 205–8

107. Rudy, *Freedom*, 120–21.

108. Albanskii advertisement, *Restorannoe delo* 10 (1912): 1.

109. Dolores Mitchell, "Images of Exotic Women in Turn-of-the-Century Tobacco Art," *Feminist Studies* 18, no. 2 (1992): 340.

110. Adeeb Khalid, "Russian History and the Debate over Orientalism," *Kritika: Explorations in Russian and Eurasian History* 1, no 4 (2000): 691–700; Peter Scott, "Prisoners of the Caucasus: Ideologies of Imperialism in Lermontov's 'Bela,'" *PMLA* 107, no. 2 (March 1992): 246–60, especially 247–48.

111. A. Appolov, comp. *Perestanem kurit'! Shto takoe tabak i kakoi vred ot nego byvaet* No. 148 (Moscow: I. D. Sytin, 1904), 3; Ivan Davidson Kalmar, "The *Houkah* in the Harem: On Smoking and Orientalist Art," in *Smoke: A Global History of Smoking*, ed. Sander Gilman and Zhou Xun (London: Reaktion Books, 2004), 218–20.

112. Mitchell, "Images of Exotic Women," 331.

113. Korsmeyer, *Making Sense of Taste*, 169, 170.

114. Jeffrey Auerbach, "Art, Advertising, and the Legacy of Empire," *Journal of Popular Culture* 35, no. 4 (Spring 2002), 20.

115. Kalmar, "The *Houkah* in the Harem," 220.

116. West, *I Shop in Moscow*, 63–74; *Podrobnyi ukazatl' po otdelam vserossiiskoi promyshlennoi i khudozhestvennoi vystavki 1896 g. v Nizhnev-novgorode: Otdel IX Proizvodstva fabrichno-remeslennyia* (Moscow: Russkago t-va pechatnago i izdatel'skago dela', 1896).

117. Elizabeth D. Harvey, "The Portal of Touch," *American Historical Review* 116, no. 2 (2011): 397.

118. Auerbach, "Art, Advertising, and the Legacy of Empire," 12.

119. Ibid., 12–15.

120. Kalmar, "The *Houkah* in the Harem," 220; Auerbach, "Art, Advertising, and the Legacy of Empire," 12.

121. West, *I Shop in Moscow*, 62–94

122. Uncle Mikey, "Tobacco in Russia: An Historical-Poetic Investigation," *Restorannoe Delo* 2 (1912): 2.

123. Vashik and Baburina, *Real'nost' utopii*, 33. Missing is the overtly racist imagery in other popular prints. See Norris, *A War of Images*, 107–33

124. Auerbach, "Art, Advertising, and the Legacy of Empire," 20.
125. Norris explores the image of the soldier in Russian national identity in the nineteenth century in his *War of Images*. Kornblatt traced the Cossack through nineteenth-century Russian literature in *The Cossack*. Maiorova noted this tendency in Russian fiction of the later period in *From the Shadow*, 41–48.
126. Norris, *A War of Images*, 7–8.
127. West, *I Shop in Moscow*, 7.
128. Mitchell, "Images of Exotic Women," 334–40.

2. PRODUCED

1. *Ocherk 25-letnei deiatel'nosti tabachnoi fabriki A. N Shaposhnikova v S.-Peterburge, 2 Ianvaria 1873–1898.* (St. Petersburg: Eduarda Goppe, 1897), 7–13.
2. Bogdanov, *Dym*, 182–89; A. A. Arakelov, "Monopolizatsiia tabachnoi promyshlennosti Rossii," *Voprosy istorii* 9 (1981), 17–27; Aleksandr Khokhrev, "Tabak v stile shaposhnikova," *Territoriia biznesa: Zhurnal delovykh liudei* 9, no. 34 (September 2009): 82–85; *Ocherk 25-letnei deiatel'nosti*, 19; Marina Romanova, "Tabachnyi kapitan," *Pravda*, December 3, 2001, http://www.pravda.ru/society/03-12-2001/836632-0/; N. Maslov, "Iz proshlogo nashei tabachnoi promyshlennosti," *Vestnik tabachnoi promyshlennosti* 1–2 (1925): 17–27; Malinin, *Tabachnaia istoriia*, 243–53.
3. Gabai was also run by a widow; Malinin, *Tabachnaia istoriia*, 232. Few women were so enmeshed in the industry elsewhere—only Mrs. Frederick Coudert-Brennig, who ran advertisements in 1910s New York for "Brennig's Own" high priced hand-rolled Turkish cigarettes. Petrone, *Tobacco*, 219.
4. Neuberger, *Balkan Smoke*, 3.
5. Boris B. Gorshkov, *Russia's Factory Children: State, Society, and Law, 1800–1917*. (Pittsburgh: University of Pittsburgh Press, 2009), 1.
6. Matthew P. Romaniello, "Muscovy's Extraordinary Ban on Tobacco," in *Tobacco in Russian History and Culture from the Seventeenth Century to the Present*, ed. Matthew P. Romaniello and Tricia Starks (New York: Routledge, 2009), 9–25; Jacob M. Price, "The Tobacco Adventure to Russia: Enterprise, Politics, and Diplomacy in the Quest for a Northern Market for English Colonial Tobacco, 1676–1722," *Transactions of the American Philosophical Society* 51 (1961): 62–63.
7. The year 1714 or 1715 is given in "Tabachnaia promyshlenost' v Rossii: Statiia pervaia," *Otechestvennyia zapiski: Ucheno-literaturnyi zhurnal'* 28 (1845), 12. Korno and Kitainer give the date as 1716. *Balkanskaia Zvezda*, 20. Matthew P. Romaniello argued that the German, British and Dutch production techniques were very similar; "'Tobacco! Tobacco!' Exporting New Habits to Siberia and Russian America," *Sibirica* (Summer 2017): 1–26.
8. S. V. Lebedev, N. O. Osipov, N. I. Prokhorov, and V. G. Shaposhnikov, "Tobacco," in *Entsiklopedicheskii slovar XXXII*, ed. F. A. Brokgauz and I. A. Efron (St. Petersburg: I. A. Efron, 1901), 429.
9. Dmitriev, *Kak vozdelyvat'*, 6.
10. I. M. Dogel, *Tabak, kak prikhot' i neschastie cheloveka: Rech', chitannaia na godichnom akt Kazanskago universiteta, 1884.* 3rd ed. (Kazan: Imperatorskii universitet, 1886), 17; "Tabachnaia promyshlenost' v Rossii: Statiia vtoraia i posledniaia," *Otechestvennyia zapiski: Ucheno-literaturnyi zhurnal'* 28 (1845), 23; M. Chulkhov, *Istoriia zakonodatel'stva: Tabachnoi promyshlennosti v Rossii do Ekateriny II* (Kazan: Ivan Dubrovin, 1855); A. Krylov, *Tabak: Prakticheskoe rukovodstvo k vozdelyvaniiu tabaka* (Moscow: N. Ris', 1869).
11. "Tabachnaia promyshlenost' v Rossii," 14; V. E. Ignatiev, "Kurenie," in *Entsiklopedicheskii slovar*, ed. By F. A. Brokgauz and I. A. Efron v. XVII (St. Petersburg: I. A. Efron, 1896), 81.
12. Bogdanov, *Dym*, 66.
13. Price, "The Tobacco Adventure to Russia," 95.

14. "Tabachnaia promyshlenost' v Rossii," 18–19. Malinin included the date 1819 for when the Imperial Moscow Society for Agriculture began importing American tobacco seed, but this 1845 essay presented an earlier start. *Tabachnaia istoriia Rossii*, 81.

15. Kotel'nikov, *Vozdelyvanie*, 4–7.

16. M. V. Dzhervis, *Russkaia tabachnaia fabrika v XVIII I XIX vekakh* (Leningrad: Akademii nauk SSSR, 1933), 6.

17. Malinin, *Tabachnaia istoriia Rossii*, 80–82.

18. Dzhervis, *Russkaia tabachnaia fabrika*, 33.

19. Dogel, *Tabak,* 42.

20. I. Stal'skii, comp., *Donskaia gosudarstvennaia tabachnaia fabrika: Ocherk po materialam starykh kadrovikov DGTF A. K. Vasil'eva, E. I. Riabininoi, O. P. Ogarenko, i V. I. Shcherbakova* (Rostov-na-Don: Gosizdat, 1938), 3–4.

21. Worker memoir from "Dobrynin" in GARF f. R-5667 op. 10 d. 83 l. 2; see also Markovich, *Otchet*, 6.

22. V. I. Lenin, "Razvitie kapitalizma v Rossii," in *Polnoe sobranie sochinenii,* vol. 3 (Moscow: Gosizdat, 1958), 543; English translation: V. I. Lenin, "The Development of Capitalism in Russia," in *Collected Works*, 4th ed. (Moscow: Progress Publishers, 1964), 542–43.

23. Keibel, *Kak nam' sleduet' kurit' shtoby umen'shit' vred tabaka dlia zdorov'ia* (St. Petersburg: V. Bezobraz, 1890), 8.

24. West, *I Shop in Moscow*. Jewish ownership became a strong feature of postrevolutionary tobacco concerns. In 1924, 17.7 percent of tobacco shops were owned by Jewish "Nepmen." Yuri Slezkine, *The Jewish Century* (Princeton, NJ: Princeton University Press, 2004), 218; see also *Kratkii ocherk deiatel'nosti tabachnoi fabrik "Brat'ev Kogen'"* (Kiev: I. I. Chokolov, 1897).

25. Khokhrev, "Tabak v stile shaposhnikova," 82–85.

26. Korno and Kitainer, *Balkanskaia Zvezda*, 29–32.

27. Bogdanov, *Dym*, 96.

28. Korno and Kitainer, *Balkanskaia Zvezda*, 37; Liubimenko, *Tabak*, 12, 15.

29. V. V., *Kurite skol'ko khotite: Istoriia upotrebleniia tabaka, psikhologicheskiia osnovy etoi privychki, bezvrednost' eia i vashneishiia gigienicheskiia pravila kureniia.* (St. Petersburg: Gosudarstvennaia tipografiia, 1890), 16.

30. Lebedev et al., "Tobacco," 428–36.

31. Iu. P. Bokarev, "Tobacco in Russia," unpublished manuscript, last modified May 20, 2008.

32. Malinin noted that because a government official oversaw the *banderol* process, factories did not work at night or on holidays. This indicated central control, not localized control, of tax farming. *Tabachnaia istoriia Rossii,* 104.

33. Dzhervis, *Russkaia tabachnaia fabrika*, 12.

34. V. N. Liubimenko, *Tabachnaia promyshlennost' v Rossii* (Petrograd: Komis. Po izuch. Estest. Proizvoditel'nykh sil Rossii, 1916), 5.

35. Osipov, "Tobacco in Russia," 429; see also K. I. Karafa-Korbut, *Ustavy ob aktsiznykh sborakh*. Tom iii (St. Petersburg: I. I Zubkova, 1914), 1–175.

36. Krymskii, *Vred*, 4.

37. Lebedev, et al., "Tobacco," 431–35. See also Evgenii Ragozin, *Istoriia tabaka i sistemy naloga na nego v Evrope i Amerike* (St. Petersburg: A. Benke, 1871).

38. Bogdanov, *Dym*, 13.

39. Even the Russo-Turkish war did not cause a great set back, and growth generally continued. Dzhervis, *Russkaia tabachnaia fabrika,* 14–19.

40. *Kratkii ocherk tabakokureniia v Rossii*, 8; Lebedev et al., "Tobacco," 431.

41. Krymskii, *Vred,* 17.

42. In the US, in 1864, a tax on cigarettes joined an 1862 tax on cigars. After the war, the tobacco taxes rose in 1865 and 1875. R. T. Ravenholt, "Tobacco's Global Death March," *Population and Development Review,* 16, no. 2 (June 1990): 219.

43. Liubimenko, *Tabachnaia promyshlennost'*, 65.

44. Kate Transchel, *Under the Influence: Working-Class Drinking, Temperance, and Cultural Revolution in Russia, 1895–1932* (Pittsburgh: University of Pittsburgh Press, 2006), 32; For the problems of evaluating the "drunken budget" see Mark Lawrence Schrad, *Vodka Politics: Alcohol, Autocracy, and the Secret History of the Russian State* (Oxford: Oxford University Press, 2014), 112–17.

45. Liubimenko, *Tabak,* 35.

46. Dzhervis, *Russkaia tabachnaia fabrika,* 16.

47. Kafengauz, *Evoliutsiia,* 52.

48. Greene, *Sketches,* 14.

49. V. I. Zasidatel-Krzheminskii, *Tabachnoe otravlenie: V sviazi s ucheniem ob angionevrozakh i bolezn'iu Raynand* (St. Petersburg: Prakticheskaia meditsina, 1911), 3.

50. Iu. P. Bokarev, "Tobacco Production in Russia: The Transition to Communism," in *Tobacco in Russian History and Culture,* ed. Matthew P. Romaniello and Tricia Starks (New York: Routledge, 2009), 149.

51. Tregubov, *Normal'nyi sposob*, 3; Priklonskii, *Upotreblenie*, 5; Greene, *Sketches,* 14.

52. The source for this statistic was not given. Bogdanov, *Dym,* 78.

53. Kafengauz, *Evoliutsiia,* 156, see for example the tax evasion of later decades 295.

54. Allan M. Brandt, "Blow Some My Way: Passive Smoking, Risk and American Culture," in *Ashes to Ashes: The History of Smoking and Health*, ed. S. Lock, L. A. Reynolds and E. M. Tansey (Amsterdam: Rodopi, 1998), 164.

55. "Russian Paper Trade: The Manufacture of Paper Cigarette Tubes," *The World's Paper Trade Review* 29 March 1907: 8.

56. Ignatiev, "Kurenie," 72–75.

57. 1.2 funt per day. N. I. Vorshinina, "K statistike kuriashchikh tabak," *Vrach* 30 (1891): 58.

58. Lebedev et al., "Tobacco," 433.

59. Kafengauz, *Evoliutsiia,* 156.

60. Liubemenko produced slightly varied numbers for the total 1910 tobacco production. This might have been a result of the difference of the book publication points (1916 and 1922) or an error. The difference was of about seven thousand pounds. Liubimenko, *Tabachnaia promyshlennost'*, 64

61. Liubemenko, *Tabak,* 27.

62. Lebedev et al., "Tobacco," 421–22.

63. Rose L. Glickman, *Russian Factory Women: Workplace and Society, 1880–1914* (Berkeley: University of California Press, 1984), 42.

64. Goodman, *Tobacco,* 230–31; Ravenholt, "Tobacco's Global Death March" 219; Proctor, *Golden,* 39–40.

65. Bunker, *Creating,* 18.

66. Goodman, *Tobacco,* 102, 230–31.

67. Umanova, "Tabachnaia promyshlennost'," in *Sbornik statei i materialov po tabachnomu delu,* ed. S. A. Egiz (St. Petersburg: V. F. Kirshbaum, 1913), 129.

68. Lebedev et al., "Tobacco," 422.

69. Umanova, "Tabachnaia promyshlennost'," 130–31.

70. Neuburger, *Balkan Smoke,* 68–69.

71. Patricia A. Cooper, *Once a Cigar Maker: Men, Women, and Work Culture in American Cigar Factories, 1900–1919* (Urbana: University of Illinois Press, 1987), 218–46.

72. This is in line with Chinese production for other goods, but tobacco came to China with Duke's mechanization. Kenneth Pomeranz, *The Great Divergence: China, Europe, and the Making of the Modern World Economy* (Princeton, NJ: Princeton University Press, 2000); Benedict, *Golden-Silk,* 131–33. Hand rolling still ruled China's rural market.

73. Dzhervis, *Russkaia tabachnaia fabrika,* 18.

74. Kafengauz, *Evoliutsiia*, 108; Bonnell, "Introduction," *The Russian Worker*, 1–2.

75. Victoria E. Bonnell, "Introduction," in *The Russian Worker: Life and Labor under the Tsarist Regime*, ed. Bonnell (Berkeley: University of California Press, 1983), 1–2.

76. Victoria E. Bonnell, *Roots of Rebellion: Workers' Politics and Organizations in St. Petersburg and Moscow, 1900–1914* (Berkeley: University of California Press, 1983), 216.

77. Dzhervis, *Russkaia tabachnaia fabrika*, 17.

78. Malinin, *Tabachnaia istoriia Rossii*, 100.

79. *Podrobnyi ukazatel'*, 39.

80. Stal'skii, *Donskaia*, 5.

81. Dzhervis, *Russkaia tabachnaia fabrika*, 18–19.

82. Stal'skii, *Donskaia*, 5.

83. Khokhrev, "Tabak v stile shaposhnikova," 110.

84. Malinin, *Tabachnaia istoriia Rossii*, 111.

85. Rudy, *Freedom*, 120; Hilton, *Smoking*, 26.

86. Katyk gilzy, *Moskovskii Listok*, January 2, 1896, 4; Malinin, *Tabachnaia istoriia Rossii*, 109; West, *I Shop in Moscow*, 108–9.

87. N. Umnov, "Fabrichnaia pererabotka i oborduovanie tabachnykh fabric v 1890–1909 godakh," *Vestnik tabachnoi promyshlennosit* 3 (1925): 18–29; V. G. Novikova and N. N. Shchemelev, *Nasha marka: Ocherki istorii Donskoi gosudarstvennoi tabachnoi fabriki* (Rostov: Rostovskoi knizhnoe izd., 1968), 57.

88. *Ustav tovarishchestva fabrik tabachnikh izdelii pod firmoiu "Laferm": Vysochaishe utverzhdennyi vo 2-i den' Ianvaria 1870 goda*. (St. Petersburg: Brat'i Shumakher, 1883); *Ustav tovarishchestva tabachnoi fabriki "Dukat" v Moskve* (Moscow: Russkoe tovarishchestvo, 1910); *Ustav tovarishchestva tabachnoi fabriki "Brat'ia Shapshal"* (St. Petersburg: Rumanov, 1905).

89. Arakelov, "Monopolizatsiia," 17–27; Natalia Gurushina, "Free-Standing Companies in Tsarist Russia," in *Three Free-Standing Company in the World Economy, 1830–1996*, ed. Mira Wilkins and Harm Schröter (Oxford: Oxford University Press, 1998), 190. Reports in newspapers tracked the progress of the merger, Leontiii Chev-skii and S. S. Danilov, "Novyi sindikat," *Pravda*, May 4, 1912, 1; "Tabachnyi sindikat," *Pravda*, July 1, 1912, 3; "K slukham o 'raspade v tabachnom sindikate," *Pravda*, July 1, 1912, 14; "Tabachnyi sindikat," *Pravda*, August 15, 1912, 14.

90. Gurushina, "Free-Standing Companies in Tsarist Russia," 191.

91. "Pokhod na kuril'shchikov" *Pravda*, May 3, 1912, 11; Bogdanov, *Dym*, 189.

92. Arakelov, "Monopolizatsiia," 26–27.

93. *Zhurnal: Sostoiavshagosia 24 Fevralia–8 Marta 1914 g. pri Glavnom Upravlenii neokladnykh sborov i kazennoi prodazhi pitei soveshchaniia po voprosu o vliianii tabachnago ustava na tabakovodstvo i fabrikatsiiu tabaka* (St. Petersburg: Ministerstva Finansov, 1914), 381

94. Arakelov, "Monopolizatsiia," 26.

95. Papirosy production rose by 7.6 times. Arakelov, "Monopolizatsiia," 18.

96. Korno and Kitainer, *Balkanskaia Zvezda*, 3.

97. Umnova, "Tabachnaia promyshlennost," 140.

98. Edwards, *The Russians*, 408–9.

99. Brennan, *Tobacco Leaves*, 32–33.

100. Bain, *Cigarettes*, 63–66.

101. Benedict, *Golden-Silk*, 135.

102. Petrone, *Tobacco*, 112

103. Barbara Alpern Engel, *Between the Fields and the City: Women, Work and Family in Russia, 1861–1914* (Cambridge: Cambridge University Press, 1996), 203.

104. Bogdanov, *Dym*, 151.

105. Malinin, *Tabachnaia istoriia Rossii*, 104.

106. Novikova and Shchemelev, *Nasha marka*, 10.

107. Bogdanov, *Dym*, 126.

108. S. V. Kifuriak and O. I. Kokoulin, *Tabachnaia fabrika "Iava"* (Moscow: Pishchevaia pro-myshlennost, 1978), 16; A. A. Nosova, "38 let raboty na fabrike," *Tabak* 1 (1953): 16–17; D. P. Pavlov, "52 goda v riadakh tabachnikov," *Tabak* 1 (1953): 19–21.

109. A. D. Ipatov, comp. *Bylye gody: Vospominaniia starykh rabochikh tabachnykh fabrik g. Saratova* (Saratov: Saratovskoe oblastnoe izdatelstvo, 1937), 10; for a more laudatory account, see *Stranichka iz istorii promyshlennosti iugo-vostochoi Rossii: Tabachnaia fabrika F. K. Shtaf d Saratove* (Saratov: F. M. Kimmel', 1896).

110. Novikova and Shchemelev, *Nasha marka*, 10.

111. Worker memoir as a lightly fictionalized story in GARF f. R-5667 op 10 d 83 l. 7.

112. Ipatov, *Bylye gody*, 19.

113. Ibid., 20.

114. Ibid., 26.

115. V. V. Sviatlovskii, *Materialy dlia otsenki zdorov'ia rabochikh na sveklosakharnykh zavo-dakh i na tabachnykh fabrikakh: Izdanie zhurnala "Zemskii Vrach"* (Chernigov: Gubernskaia pravleniia, 1889), 22.

116. Novikova and Shchemelev, *Nasha marka*, 16.

117. Kolyshko, a journalist for *Ocherki sovremennoi Rossii*, as quoted in Korno and Kitainer, *Balkanskaia Zvezda*, 72.

118. Ipatov, *Bylye gody*, 17.

119. Bonnell, *The Russian Worker*, 190.

120. Stal'skii, *Donskaia*, 9.

121. Ipatov, *Bylye gody*, 20.

122. Maria Konstantinovna Valitskaia, *Izsledovanie zdorov'ia rabochikh' na tabachnykh' fab-rikakh': Nabliudeniia proizvedeny na 12 tabachnykh' fabrikakh' iuga Rossii 3-mia risunkami i 1-i diagrammoi* (St. Petersburg: Tovarishchestvo Parovoi Skoropechatni Iavlonskii i Tserott', 1889), 12.

123. Stal'skii, *Donskaia*, 10

124. Korno and Kitainer, *Balkanskaia zvezda*, 102.

125. Ipatov, *Bylye gody*, 21.

126. Ibid., 15

127. Bonnell, "Introduction," *The Russian Worker*, 17–18.

128. Lebedev et al., "Tobacco," 434.

129. Ibid.

130. N. M. Druzhinin, *Okhrana zhenskogo i detskogo truda v fabrichnoi promyshlennosti Ros-sia: Diplomnoe sochinenie* (Moscow: ZAO, 2005), 43–44.

131. Bradley, *Muzhik and Muscovite*, 185–88.

132. Ipatov, *Bylye gody*, 13.

133. Sobel, *They Satisfy*, 31; Leonard Rogoff, "Jewish Proletarians in the New South: The Durham Cigarette Rollers," *American Jewish History* 1/4 (1994): 141–157.

134. Novikova and Shchemelev, *Nasha marka*, 11.

135. Glickman, *Russian Factory*, 97.

136. L N. Tolstoi, *Polnoe sobranie sochinenii,* vol. 25 (Moscow: Gosizdat, 1937), 302–7. In English see Lev N. Tolstoy, *What Shall We Do Then? On the Moscow Census. Collected Articles*, trans. Leo Weiner (Boston: Dana Estes and Company, 1904), 187–88.

137. Tolstoi, *Polnoe sobranie sochinenii*, 305.

138. Ibid.

139. Bradley, *Muzhik and Muscovite*, 220–21, 276–77.

140. Translation from S. An-sky, *The New Way* (1907), as quoted in Valerii Dymshits, "'Broth-ers and Sisters in Toil and Struggle': Jewish Workers and Artisans on the Eve of Revolution," in *Photographing the Jewish Nation: Pictures from S. An-sky's Ethnographic Expeditions*, ed. Eugene M. Avrutin et al. (Lebanon, NH: Brandeis University Press, 2009), 80.

141. Samuel Gompers, *Seventy Years of Life and Labor: An Autobiography*, ed. Nick Salvatore (Ithaca, NY: Cornell University Press, 1984), 17.

142. Engel, *Between the Fields*.

143. Valitskaia, *Izsledovanie zdorov'ia rabochikh'*, 13.

144. Ipatov, *Bylye gody*, 9.

145. Ibid.

146. Stal'skii, *Donskaia*, 6.

147. Ipatov, *Bylye gody*, 13.

148. A. I. Voinich, "Porshloe i nastoiashchee," *Tabak* 1 (1953): 18.

149. Sheila Fitzpatrick and Yuri Slezkine, eds., *In the Shadow of Revolution: Life Stories of Russian Women from 1917 to the Second World War* (Princeton, NJ: Princeton University Press, 2000), 244.

150. Novikova and Shchemelev, *Nasha marka*, 13–15; Ipatov, *Bylye gody*, 12, 15, 18; S. Kifuriak and Kokoulin, *Tabachnaia fabrika "Iava*," 30–31; Stal'skii, *Donskaia*, 6; Gorshkov, *Russia's Factory Children*, 60.

151. Novikova and Shchemelev, *Nasha marka*, 13–15.

152. Nosova, "38 let raboty na fabrike," 16. See similarly Voinich, "Porshloe i nastoiashchee," 18.

153. Gorshkov, *Russia's Factory Children*, 72.

154. Bonnell, "Introduction," *The Russian Worker*, 9.

155. Stal'skii, *Donskaia*, 8.

156. Ipatov, *Bylye gody*, 24.

157. Gorshkov, *Russia's Factory Children*, 167.

158. Ibid., 47–48.

159. Glickman, *Russian Factory*, 12–13, 85–86.

160. "Tabachnaia fabrika 'Ottoman,'" *Pravda*, July 21, 1912, 14. See also "Tabachnaia fabrika Brat'ev Shapshal," *Pravda*, June 15, 1912, 12.

161. "Zhenskii trud S.-Peterburg: Tabachnaia fabrika Bogdanova," *Rabotnitsa* 1 (1914): 9–10.

162. Malinin, *Tabachnaia istoriia Rossii*, 102.

163. Novikova and Shchemelev, *Nasha marka*, 14.

164. Ipatov, *Bylye gody*, 15.

165. Ibid., 27.

166. Iulius Bartolomeo, *Demon v vodke i v tabake ili tabak i vino, to i drugoe, kaka medlennyi iad, razrushaiushchii zdorov'e, sily, i sokrashchaiushchii zhizn' chelveka* (Moscow: I. E. Shiuman, 1871), 68.

167. Mount Athos St. Panteleimon Monastery, *Bros'te kurit'! O vrede kureniia tabake dlia zdorov'ia*, 6th ed. (Moscow: I. Efimov, 1905), 12.

168. F. A. Udintsev, *O vrede kureniia (Nauchno-populiarnyi ocherk)* (Kiev: Imperatroskii universitet sv. Vladimira, 1913), 9.

169. Sviatlovskii, *Materialy*, 18–19.

170. Ibid., 19–20.

171. Ibid., 25–30.

172. Rokau, *Interesnaia i liubopytnaia istoriia*, 80–81.

173. "K voprosu o vliianii kureniia na organism cheloveka," *Vrach* 1 (January 1887): 4–8. For more on the dangers of the factory see Ev. Belov, "25 let rabotu po tabakovodstvu," *Tabak* 2 (1939): 26–27.

174. *O razvedenii i fabrikatsii tabaka*, 308.

175. Ibid., 307.

176. Valitskaia, *Izsledovanie zdorov'ia rabochikh'*, 3; See for example the citation in S. P. Botkin, *Vrednye posledstviia ot kureniia tabaku* (Moscow: P. V. Bel'tsova, 1914), quotations page 5, 27, see also 7, 26.

177. Valitskaia, *Izsledovanie zdorov'ia rabochikh'*, 28–29.

178. Ibid., 30–34.

179. Her findings are further reported in Sviatlovskii, *Materialy,* 20–21; Valitskaia, *Izsledovanie zdorov'ia rabochikh',* 20.

180. Valitskaia, *Izsledovanie zdorov'ia rabochikh',* 23–26.

181. Engel, *Between the Fields,* 159.

182. Stal'skii, *Donskaia,* 12.

183. Hirsz Abramowich, *Profiles of a Lost World: Memoirs of East European Jewish Life before World War II* (Detroit: Wayne State University Press, 1999), 132. See also Rochelle Goldberg Ruthchild, *Equality and Revolution: Women's Rights in the Russian Empire, 1905–1917* (Pittsburgh: University of Pittsburgh Press, 2010), 175.

184. Valitskaia, *Izsledovanie zdorov'ia rabochikh',* 11.

185. Sviatlovskii, *Materialy,* 22.

186. Novikoff, "The Temperance Movement in Russia," *The nineteenth century* 12 (1882): 439–59.

187. Krymskii, *Vred,* 22.

188. Sander S. Gilman, "Smoking Jews on the Frontier," in *Jewish Frontiers: Essays on Bodies, Histories, and Identities* (New York: Palgrave Macmillan, 2004), 95–109, see figures on 97.

189. Gilman, "Smoking Jews," 98.

190. "Russian Paper Trade: The Manufacture of Paper Cigarette Tubes," *The World's Paper Trade Review,* March 29, 1907: 8.

191. "1871 g. Noiabria 19.—Predstavlenie Vilenskogo gubernatora E. P. Steblina-Kamenskogo ministru vnutrennikh del A. E. Timashevu o stachke rabochikh tabachnoi fabriki duruncha I Shismana v Vil'ne s trebovaniem povysheniia zarabotnoi platy," in *Rabochee dvizhenie v Rossii v XIX veke: Sbornik dokumentov i materialov,* ed. A. M. Pankratova, tom. 2, 1861–1884, chast. 1, 1861–1874 (Moscow: Gosizdat, 1950), 275–76.

192. "Vypiska iz gazety *Uait* from 1913 on Sheremetevskii tobacco factory in Grodno," GARF f. R-6889 op. 1 d. 294 l.1–2.

193. Ipatov, *Bylye gody,* 53.

194. Glickman, *Russian Factory,* 124–25.

195. Stal'skii, *Donskaia,* 9.

196. Glickman, *Russian Factory,* 127.

197. Ipatov, *Bylye gody,* 52.

198. Stal'skii, *Donskaia,* 9.

199. Ipatov, *Bylye gody,* 31–32.

200. Bonnell, "Introduction," *The Russian Worker,* 22–23.

201. Kifuriak and Kokoulin, *Tabachnaia fabrika "Iava,"* 31.

202. Ipatov, *Bylye gody,* 32–33

203. Bonnell, "Introduction," *The Russian Worker,* 23–24.

204. For activist complaints, see "Tabachnaia fabrika brat'ev Shapshal," *Pravda,* June 15, 1912, 12. For worker testimony, see Stal'skii, *Donskaia,* 11.

205. Bonnell, "Introduction," *The Russian Worker,* 23.

206. Korno and Kitainer, *Balkanskaia Zvezda,* 73.

207. Bonnell, "Introduction," *The Russian Worker,* 20–21.

208. Stal'skii, *Donskaia,* 7.

209. Sviatlovskii, *Materialy,* 22.

210. Nosova, "38 let raboty na fabrie," 16.

211. Valitskaia, *Izsledovanie zdorov'ia rabochikh',* 12.

212. Sviatlovskii, *Materialy,* 22.

213. A. I. Il'inskii, comp., *Tri iada: Tabak, alkogol' (vodka), i sifilis (O vliianii ikh na byt' i zdorov'e cheloveka i ego potomstva i o tom—kak predokhranit sebia ot prichiniamago imi vreda)* 2nd ed. (Moscow: Kh. Barkhudarian, 1898), 4.

214. A. I. Il'inskii, comp., *Polezno, ili vredno kurit', niukhat' i zhevat' tabak.* (Moscow: I. D. Sytin, 1888), 43.

215. Druzhinin, *Okhrana,* 60.

216. Ibid., 53.

217. Evgenii Popov, *Deti! Nikogda ne nachinaite kurit' tabak.* 2nd ed. (Perm: P. F. Kamenskii, 1884), 6.

218. Appolov, *Perestanem kurit'!*, 40. See also D. P. Nikol'skii, *O tabake i vrede ego kureniia* (St. Petersburg: Ministerstva vnutrennikh del, 1894), 9–10.

219. "K voprosu o vliianii kureniia na organism cheloveka," *Vrach* 1, no. 1 (January 1887): 6.

220. Vladimir M-ov', *Neskol'ko slov o tabake i ego upotreblenii (Otdel'nyi ottisk iz zhurnala Staroobriadets no. 5 za 1906 g)* (Nizhnyi Novgorod: I. M. Mashkistov, 1906), 4.

221. Students of Grammatchikov and Ossendovskii, "K voprosu o vliianii kureniiia na organizm cheloveka," *Vrach* 1 (1887): 6.

222. Il'inskii, *Polezno*, 43–44.

223. Druzhinin, *Okhrana*, 65–69.

224. Beliakov, *Tabak*, 44.

225. Appolov, *Perestanem kurit'!*, 41.

226. Proctor, *Golden,* 36–38; Walker, *Under Fire*, 57.

227. *Kratkii ocherk tabakokureniia v Rossii*, 10.

228. John Martin Crawford, ed., *The Industries of Russia: Manufactures and Trade with a General Industrial Map* (St. Petersburg: Department of Trade and Manufacture of the Imperial Ministry of Finance, 1893), 241.

229. Gorshkov, *Russia's Factory Children*, 75–76.

230. Bogdanov, *Dym*, 46.

231. Crawford, *Industries*, 239; Bogdanov, *Dym*, 46.

232. Crawford, *Industries*, 241.

233. Feodorva Fedotovich Ivankin and Leonid Dmitrii Romanovich, *Tabak i spichki v Rossii, 1875–1920 gg.* (Moscow: Staraia basmannaia, 2009), 4.

234. Bogdanov, *Dym*, 140.

235. Proctor, *Golden,* 27.

236. Bonnell, "Introduction," *The Russian Worker*, 3–7; Druzhinin, *Okhrana*, 84.

237. Gorshkov, *Russia's Factory Children,* 123–37, 146–57.

238. Ibid., 111.

239. Patrick Beaver, *The Match Makers: The Story of Bryant and May* (London: Henry Melland Limited, 1985); John Emsley, *The Shocking History of Phosphorus: A Biography of the Devil's Element* (Basingstoke: Macmillan Publishing, 2000).

240. *Ocherk 25-letnei deiatel'nosti*, 8.

241. Ibid., 7–8.

242. Bogdanov, *Dym,* 182.

243. Korno and Kitainer, *Balkanskaia Zvezda*, 74–90.

244. Sviatlovskii, *Materialy*, 23–24.

245. Malinin, *Tabachnaia istoriia*, 214.

246. Stal'skii, *Donskaia,* 30.

247. Keibel, *Kak nam' sleduet'*, 16,

248. *Ocherk 25-letnei deiatel'nosti*, 1–13.

249. Sally West, "The Material Promised Land: Advertising's Modern Agenda in Late Imperial Russia," *Russian Review* 57 (July 1998): 351; Martin, *Enlightened Metropolis*, 149; Fishzon, *Fandom*, 19–46.

250. "In Syria," *Restorannoe Delo* 5 (1912): 1.

251. Novikova and Shchemelev, *Nasha marka*, 10.

252. Druzhinin, *Okhrana*.

253. Reginald E. Zelnick, *Labor and Society in Tsarist Russia: The Factory Workers of St. Petersburg, 1855–1870* (Stanford: Stanford University Press, 1971), 63.

254. See the essays Michael F. Hamm, "Continuity and Change in Late Imperial Kiev," Frederick W. Skinner, "Odessa and the Problem of Urban Modernization," and Audrey

Altstadt-Mirhadi, "Baku: Transformation of a Muslim Town," in *The City in Late Imperial Russia,* ed. Michael F. Hamm (Bloomington: Indiana University Press, 1986), 103, 119, 232–33, and 282–318.

255. Glickman, *Russian Factory,* 162–65; Laura Engelstein, *Moscow, 1905: Working-Class Organization and Political Conflict* (Stanford: Stanford University Press, 1982), 15; Gorshkov, *Russia's Factory Children,* quotation, 10; description, 166–73.

256. The piece appeared in *Zemliz i volia.* The first was an 1871 tobacco strike of five workers in Vilnius. See "1871 g. Noiabria," in *Rabochee dvizhenie v Rossii v XIX veke: Sbornik dokumentov i materialov,* ed. A. M. Pankratova, tom. 2 (Moscow: Gosizdat, 1950), 275.

257. *Zemlia i volia* (1879), no. 3, cited in V. Iakovlev, ed., *Revoliutsionnaia zhurnalistika 70-kh godov* (Paris, 1905), pp. 296–98, as cited in Glickman, *Russian Factory,* 162.

258. "1884 g. Maia 5.—Raport Moskosvkogo ober-politseimeistera A. A. Kozlova Moskovskomu general-gubernatoru V. A. Dolgorukovu o stachke rabochikh na tabachnoi fabrike M I. Bostandzhoglo v Moskve v sviazi s umen'sheniem rastsenok" [sekretno] in *Rabochee dvizhenie v Rossii v XIX veke: Sbornik dokumentov i materialov,* ed. A. M. Pankratova, tom. 2, 1861–1884, chast. 2, 1875–1884 (Moscow: Gosizdat, 1950), 553–54.

259. Novikova and Shchemelev, *Nasha marka,* 21–24.

260. Alexander Polunov, *Russia in the Nineteenth Century: Autocracy, Reform, and Social Change, 1814–1914* (London: M. E. Sharpe, 2005), 125–38, 181–200.

261. I. M. Pushkareva et al., eds. *Rabochee dvizhenie v Rossii: 1895–Fevral' 1917 g.,* Khronika vyp. 1 1895 (Moscow: Pervaia obraztsovaia tipografiia, 1992), 91, 102.

262. Anna Hillyar and Jane McDermid, *Revolutionary Women in Russia, 1870–1917: A Study in Collective Biography* (Manchester: Manchester University Press, 2000), 71–72.

263. Pushkareva, *Rabochee dvizhenie v Rossii: 1895–Fevral' 1917 g.,* 93.

264. Laferm was located on Vasilevsky Island between the mining institute and the university and across the Neva from Palace Square. See Allan M. Vladimir, *On the Dilemmas of Russian Marxism, 1895–1903: The Second Congress of the Russian Social Democratic Labour Party: A Short History of the Social Democratic Movement in Russia* (CUP Archive, 1969), x.

265. Jane McDermid and Anna Hillyar, *Midwives of the Revolution; Female Bolsheviks and Women Workers in 1917* (Athens: Ohio University Press, 1999), 69.

266. Pushkareva, *Rabochee dvizhenie v Rossii: 1895–Fevral' 1917 g.,* 99–100.

267. Glickman, *Russian Factory,* 163. Defenestration of a packing machine is described in A. M. Kirsanov, "Pervaia Leningradskaia tabachnaia fabrik v proshlom i nastoiashchem," *Tabak* 1(1953): 13–15.

268. The letter from "A Worker" in *Zhizn' Tabachnika* (1907), no. 1: 4 was referenced in Glickman, *Russian Factory,* 203.

269. V. I. Lenin, "Lenin's May Day Leaflet," April 1896, https://www.marxists.org/archive/lenin/works/1896/apr/19.htm.

270. She later took to the Menshevik faction. McDermid and Hillyar, *Midwives of the Revolution,* 69.

271. Glickman, *Russian Factory,* 182–83; Leopold H. Haimson, "Russian Workers' Political and Social Identities: The Role of Social Representations in the Interaction between Members of the Labor Movement and the Social Democratic Intelligentsia," in *Workers and Intelligentsia in Late Imperial Russia: Realities, Representations, Reflections,* ed. Reginald E. Zelnik (Berkeley: University of California Press, 1999), 152–53.

272. Kifuriak and Kokoulin, *Tabachnaia fabrika "Iava,"* 31.

273. Novikova and Shchemelev, *Nasha marka,* 29–30.

274. Stal'skii, *Donskaia,* 13.

275. Glickman, *Russian Factory,* 164.

276. Article for Uait journal for 1913 in GARF f. R-6889 op. 1 d. 294 l.1–2.

277. Novikova and Shchemelev, *Nasha marka,* 33.

278. Ibid., 34.

279. Bonnell, *Roots of Rebellion*, 81–84, 128–29.

280. The story, V. Temnykh's "V prokhodnoi. Ocherk iz fabrichnoi zhizni," from *Russkoe Bogatstvo* (1903), no. 3: 78, is quoted at length in Glickman, *Russian Factory*, 184–86.

281. V. Karelina, "Rabotnitsy v Gaponovskikh obshchestvakh," in *Rabotnitsa v 1905 g. v S.-Peterburge: Sbornik statie i vospominanii*, ed. P. F. Kudelli (Lenignrad: Priboi, 1926), 14–26.

282. Can Nacar, "Labor Activism and the State in the Ottoman Tobacco Industry," *International Journal of Middle East Studies* 46 (2014): 533–51.

283. Ipatov, *Bylye gody*, 38.

284. Engelstein, *Moscow*, 83–84.

285. Ibid., 173, 233; Bonnell, *Roots of Rebellion*, 129, 137, 162, 206, 216

286. Rabochii, "Tovarishcham fabr. Bobrova," *Zhizn tabachnika* 1 (1907): 5; Bonnell, *Roots of Rebellion*, 216.

287. Bonnell, *Roots of Rebellion*, 216–17.

288. Karelina, "Rabotnitsy," 64–67.

289. The other delegates included Boldyreva (textiles), Anna Barkova, Tatiana Razueva, and Valentina Bagrova. Glickman, *Russian Factory*, 194–95. See Kudelli, *Rabotnitsa v 1905*, 75–78, 85–86.

290. A. M. Barkova (iz oprosa), in *Rabotnitsa v 1905*, ed. Kudelli, 75–78.

291. Bonnell, *Roots of Rebellion*, 338.

292. Stal'skii, *Donskaia*, 7.

293. Sahadeo, *Russian Colonial Society in Tashkent*, 126.

294. Barkova, as quoted in Kudelli, *Rabotnitsa v 1905*, 62.

295. *Asmolovskie devushki prosiat' piataka; Asmolov rasserdils'ia—poslal kazaka"* Novikova and Shchemelev, *Nasha marka*, 39–53.

296. Hillyar and McDermid, *Revolutionary Women*, 123.

297. Ipatov, *Bylye gody*, 37.

298. Ibid., 46.

299. In the US, attacks on tobacco tended to be on the product rather than the producers as the source of "evil"; Burnham, *Bad Habits*, 94–95.

300. Korno and Kitainer, *Balkanskaia Zvezda*, 100.

301. Ipatov, *Bylye gody*, 37.

302. Ibid., 40–41.

303. Ibid., 39.

304. Glickman, *Russian Factory*, 197.

305. Donald A. Filtzer, *A Dream Deferred: New Studies in Russian and Soviet Labour History* (Bern: Peter Lang, 2008), 33. See also *Ustav bol'nichnoi kassy pri tabachnoi fabrike Ottoman, t-va Laferm', nakhodiashcheisia v S. Peterburge, Kolokol'naia ul, No. 8* (St. Petersburg: Br. V. I. Linnik, 1913).

306. "Tabachnaia fabrika Shaposhnikova," *Pravda*, June 10, 1912, 12.

307. "Na fabrikakh i zavodakh: kontora tabachnoi f-ki A. N. Shapohshnikov i Ko," *Pravda*, August 7, 1912, 11.

308. "Tovarishchestvo Laferm," *Pravda*, June 9, 1912, 11.

309. Rochelle Goldberg Ruthchild, "Women's Suffrage and Revolution in the Russian Empire, 1905–1917," *Aspasia* 1 (2007): 13.

310. "V tabachnom proizvodstve. Tabachn. Fabr. T-va br. Shapshal," *Pravda*, April 12, 1913, 5; "V tabachnom proizvodstve: Tabachnaia fab. T-va br. Shapshal," *Pravda*, March 21, 1913, 8; March 24, 1913, 11; March 30, 1913, 12, and March 31, 1913, 12.

311. "Tozhe 'Prestuplenie,'" *Severnaia Pravda*, August 8, 1913, 317.

312. "V tabachnom proizvodstve: Tabachnaia fab. Laferm," *Pravda*, June 27, 1913, 3; "Spravka obshchestva zavodchikov a fabrikantov o zabastovkakh na Peterburgskikh fabrikakh i zavodakh v Iiule 1913 g," in *Rabochee dvizhenie v Petrograde v 1912–1917: Dokumenty i materialy*, ed. Iu. I. Korablev (Leningrad: Lenizdat, 1958), 127.

313. Laferm workers earlier organized funds for families of ill or out-of-work coworkers. "Tabachnaia fabr. 'Laferm," *Pravda*, August 15, 1912, 11; Glickman, *Russian Factory,* 212.

314. Polkovnik Popov, "Doklad nachal'nika Peterburgskogo okhrannogo otdeleniia ministru vnutrennikh del o zabastovke rabochikh Narvskoi zastavy v sviazi s otravleniiami na Rossiisko-Amerikanskoi rezinovoi manufacture 'Treugol'nik' i ob otravleniikakh tabachnykh fabrikakh 'Laferm' A. N. Shaposhnikova i Ko," in *Rabochee dvizhenie v Petrograde*, ed. Korablev, 167–68; Glickman, *Russian Factory,* 213; *Zhurnal: Sostoiavshagosia 24 Fevralia–8 Marta 1914,* 381.

315. Glickman, *Russian Factory,* 212.

316. Bonnell, *Roots of Rebellion,* 257–58; 313; 338.

317. "Professional'noe dvizhenie v Peterburge," *Rabochii put,* October 26, 1917, 9.

318. Barbara Evans Clements, *Bolshevik Women* (Cambridge: Cambridge University Press, 1997), 168.

319. P. Kvadelli, "Rabotnitsy v 1905 godu," in *Rabotnitsa*, ed. Kudelli, *Rabotnitsa v 1905,* 8.

320. Ruthchild, *Equality and Revolution,* 6–8.

3. TASTED

1. In Russia, see D. N. Zhatkin and A. P. Dolgov, "Peri v Russkoi poezii," *Russkaia rech'* 3 (2007), 3–8; in Europe, see Robert Schumann's *Paradise and the Peri* (1843), Gilbert and Sullivan's *Iolanthe: The Peer and the Peri* (1882), or Paul Dukas's *La Péri* (1912).

2. Benedict, *Golden-Silk*, 5.

3. Steinberg, *Petersburg,* 47–56.

4. Lynda Nead, *Victorian Babylon: People, Streets and Images in Nineteenth-Century London* (New Haven, CT: Yale University Press, 2000), 57–84.

5. Fishzon, *Fandom,* 79–111, 113–47.

6. Benedict, *Golden-Silk,* 8.

7. Transchel, *Under the Influence,* 39.

8. Nove, *Economic History,* 17–26

9. Maiorova, *From the Shadow,* 3–8.

10. McReynolds, *Russia at Play,* 5–8; Fishzon, *Fandom,* 15; West, *I Shop in Moscow,* 5.

11. Zolotyia advertisement, *Put' pravdy,* April 22, 1914, 8.

12. Ibid.

13. Bradley, *Muzhik and Muscovite,* 220–21, 276–77.

14. "Furor," *Moskovskii listok,* February 6, 1896, 4.

15. West, *I Shop in Moscow,* 126.

16. Safo advertisement, *Restorannoe delo* 1 (1912): back cover.

17. West, *I Shop in Moscow,* 112–19.

18. Smith, "Fermentation," 45–66.

19. Ackerman, *A Natural History,* 138–43.

20. Korsmeyer, *Making Sense of Taste,* 1–2; Smith, *Sensing the Past,* 75–91.

21. Rudy, *Freedom,* 109.

22. Martin, *Enlightened Metropolis,* 156, 220–97.

23. Cathy A. Frierson, *All Russia is Burning! A Cultural History of Fire and Arson in Late Imperial Russia* (Seattle: University of Washington Press, 2002), 36.

24. "Tabachnaia promyshlenost' v Rossii: Statiia pervaia," *Otechestvennyia zapiski: Ucheno-literaturnyi zhurnal'* vol. XXVIII (1845), 1–20.

25. "Tabachnaia promyshlenost' v Rossii," 17, quotation page 28.

26. Bain, *Cigarettes,* 176–77.

27. "Tabachnaia promyshlenost' v Rossii," 28.

28. Liubimenko, *Tabachnaia promyshlennost',* 46.

29. V. E. Ignatiev, "Kurenie," in *Entsiklopedicheskii slovar,* ed. By F. A. Brokgauz and I. A. Efron v. XVII (St. Petersburg: I. A. Efron, 1896), 73. The process continues today. Sebelius, *SGR,* 44–45.

30. Nikol'skii, *O tabake.*

31. Iu. P. Bokarev, "Tobacco in Russia," unpublished manuscript, last modified May 20, 2008.

32. Allan M. Brandt, "Blow Some My Way: Passive Smoking, Risk and American Culture," in *Ashes to Ashes: The History of Smoking and Health*, ed. S. Lock, L. A. Reynolds, ad E. M. Tansey (Amsterdam: Rodopi, 1998), 164.

33. Classen, Howes, and Synnott, *Aroma*, 78–84;

34. Smith, *Sensing the Past*, 59–74. Claire Shaw, "Deafness and the Politics of Hearing," in *Russian History through the Senses from 1700 to the Present*, ed. Matthew P. Romaniello and Tricia Starks (London: Bloomsbury, 2016), 193–217.

35. Rindisbacher, *The Smell of Books*, 120, 125, 141–42.

36. Catriona Kelly, *Refining Russia: Advice Literature, Polite Culture, and Gender from Catherine to Yeltsin* (Oxford: Oxford University Press, 2001), 156–229; P. I. Novoderevenskii, *Iskusstvo krasivo odevat'sia: Prakticheskiia ukapaniia dlia muzhchin, kak odevat'sia deshevo i iziashchno, ne podvergaia sebia ekspluatatsii portnykh.* (Narva: R. Peder, 1903).

37. Hilton, *Selling to the Masses: Retailing in Russia, 1880–1930* (Pittsburgh: University of Pittsburgh Press, 2011), 9.

38. Corbin, *The Foul,* 149–50

39. McReynolds, *Russia at Play,* 55.

40. Mary Douglas argues for the ritual and symbolic nature of dirt, here expanded to smoke. *Purity and Danger: An Analysis of Concepts of Pollution and Taboo* (Reprint, London: Routledge, 2002), passim.

41. A. Komilfil'do, *Khoroshii ton* (1911), as referenced in McReynolds, *Russia at Play*, 55.

42. Benedict, *Golden-Silk,* 73–81.

43. Bogdanov, *Dym*, 55–57

44. S. V. Lebedev, N. O. Osipov, N. I. Prokhorov, and V. G. Shaposhnikov, "Tobacco," in *Entsiklopedicheskii slovar XXXII*, ed. F. A. Brokgauz and I. A. Efron (St. Petersburg: I. A. Efron, 1901), 418.

45. Katyk gilzy, *Moskovskii Listok*, January 2, 1896, 4.

46. A. Sobornov, "Sanitarnyia melochi," *Zdorov'e* 51 (1883): 3–4.

47. Ignatiev, "Kurenie," 72–75.

48. Rudy, *Freedom*, 131.

49. Dogel, *Tabak,* 21.

50. Krymskii, *Vred*, 22.

51. Nikol'skii, *O tabake*, 5.

52. Ibid.

53. Liubimenko, *Tabachnaia promyshlennost'*, 40.

54. Ignatiev, "Kurenie," 72.

55. Konstantine Klioutchkine, "'I Smoke, Therefore I Think,'" in *Tobacco in Russian History and Culture*, 83, 87.

56. Quoted in Bogdanov, *Dym*, 161.

57. The 1912 account of a strike of 200 workers noted that they achieved the "laughable" concession of being able "to wash hands for five minutes and to smoke on stairs and near ventilation." See "Likvidatsiia zabostovki na fabrike Erikson," *Pravda*, June 21, 1912, 10.

58. Anatoli Evgen'evich Ivanov, "Studencheskaia 'samopomoshch' v vyshei shkole Rossiiskoi imperii, Konets XIX–nachalo XX veka," *Otechestvennaia Istoriia* 4 (September 2002): 35–50.

59. Alexander Bestuzhev-Marlisnkii, *The Test* (1838–39), as quoted and translated by Klioutchkine, "'I Smoke, Therefore I Think,'" 88.

60. S. Tormazov, *Zagadka kureniia* (St. Petersburg: M. O. Vol'f, 1907), 7.

61. Tormazov, *Zagadka,* 7.

62. *Gadalka* (fortune teller) papirosy from Kharkov featured a golliwog in one of their posters.

63. Paltusova, *Torgovaia reklama,* 3.

64. See the analysis of John MacKay, *True Songs of Freedom: Uncle Tom's Cabin in Russian Culture and Society* (Madison: University of Wisconsin Press, 2013).

65. S. A. Beliakov, *Tabak i vliianie kureniia ego na zdorov'e cheloveka* (Samara: Zemskaia tipografiia, 1904), 21.

66. Klioutchkine, "'I Smoke, Therefore I Think,'" 91, 94; Briukova, "Kurenie," 58–59.

67. Edward H. Judge, *Plehve: Repression and Reform in Imperial Russia, 1902–1904* (Syracuse, NY: Syracuse University Press, 1983), 7; Bain, *Cigarettes,* 139.

68. Bogdanov, *Dym,* 68–69

69. Olga Matich, "Gender Trouble in the Amazonian Kingdom: Turn-of-the-Century Representations of Women in Russia," in *Amazons of the Avant-Garde: Alexandra Exter, Natalia Goncharova, Liubov Popova, Olga Rozanova, Varvara Stepanova, and Nadezhda Udaltsova,* ed. John E. Bowlt and Matthew Drutt (New York: Guggenheim Museum Publications, 2000), 78–81.

70. West, *I Shop in Moscow,* 182.

71. P. N. Berdov, "Iz materialov Pushkinskogo iubileia, 1899 g.," in *Pushkin: Vremennik Pushkinskoi komissii* (Moscow: Izd-vo AN SSSR, 1937), [Vyp.] 3, pp. 401–14. On the centennial in advertising generally, see West, *I Shop in Moscow* 213–14.

72. West, *I Shop in Moscow* 214–15; N. M. Karas, *Uvlekatel'nyi mir Moskovskoi reklamy XIX-nachala XX veka* (Moscow: Muzei istorii goroda Moskvy, 1996), 70, plate 3.

73. Advertisement for Shaposhnikov factory, *Restorannoe delo* 3 (1912): 3

74. Diadia Mikhei (S. A. Korotkii), "Tabachnoe zelie na Ruski: Istoriko-poeticheskoe izsledovanie," *Restorannoe Delo* 2 (1912): 2.

75. Zhadzhi-oglu gilzy poster, 1909, Vashik and Baburina, *Real'nost' utopii,* 35, plate 35.

76. A large scan of the painting is available for examination, along with commentary, at the Tretyakov Gallery website, http://www.tretyakovgallerymagazine.com/articles/2-2015-47/human-comedy-and-drama-life-art-pavel-fedotov (accessed November 28, 2017).

77. Hilton, *Smoking,* 33–35.

78. Aleksandr Khokhrev, "Tabak v stile shaposhnikova," *Territoriia biznesa: Zhurnal delovykh liudei* 9, no. 34 (September 2009): 83.

79. Klimova, "Russkii reklamnyi plakat"; Vashik and Baburina, *Real'nost' utopii,* 39.

80. Chernevich, *Russkii graficheskii dizain,* 39.

81. Hilton, *Smoking,* 53.

82. See also Vashik and Baburina, *Real'nost' utopii,* 34, plate 33.

83. Klioutchkine, "'I Smoke, Therefore I Think,'" 89–90. Dan Healey, *Homosexual Desire in Revolutionary Russia: The Regulation of Sexual and Gender Dissent* (Chicago: University of Chicago Press, 2001), 37.

84. Ibid., 95.

85. Bogdanov, *Dym,* 67.

86. Klioutchkine, "'I Smoke, Therefore I Think,'" 95.

87. S. Troinitskii, *Farforovyia tabakerki imperatorskago ermitazha* (Petrograd: Starye gody, 1915), 5–7.

88. Douglas Smith, "Conspicuous Consumption at the Court of Catherine the Great: Count Zakhar Chernyshev's Snuffbox," in *Picturing Russia,* 67–70.

89. Troinitskii, *Farforovyia tabakerki,* 5–7.

90. The first chapter featured a lithograph of a smoking man lounging on a couch with a three- to five-foot-long pipe, while behind him another three pipes, as well as bottles and a table, stand ready. See Bussiron, *O vliianii tabaku kuritel'nogo, niukhal'nogo i tsigar, na zdorov'e nravstvennost' i um' cheloveka* (St. Petersburg: K. Zhernakov, 1845), 1.

91. Greene, *Sketches*, 5–6.

92. Bonnell, *Russian Worker*, 106.

93. Chernevich, *Russkii graficheskii dizain*, 101–2; Paltusova, *Torgovaia reklama*, 6.

94. Bogdanov, *Dym*, 114.

95. L. Bardovskaia, *Sekret dvortsovoi tabakerki* (St. Petersburg: Tsarskoe selo, 2002), 18; Veniamin Kozharinov, *Russkaia parfiumeriia: Illiustrirovannaia istoriia* (Moscow: Neisvestnaia Rossiia Chastnaia Kollektsiia, 2005), 16–17.

96. Kozharinov, *Russkaia parfiumeriia*, 16.

97. Petr Iv. Poliakov, *Ne kuri, ne niukhai i ne zhui tabaku (Pis'mo uchenogo i opytnogo vracha)* (Graivoron: I. S. Banin, 1891), 16.

98. Vl. O. Trakhtenberg, *Kak oni brosili kurit'* (St. Petersburg: Trud, 1904), 2.

99. Rudy, *Freedom*, 32

100. Ibid., 78.

101. Philippe Perrot, *Fashioning the Bourgeoisie: A History of Clothing in the Nineteenth Century*, trans. Richard Bienvenu (Princeton, NJ: Princeton University Press, 1994), 107; Rudy, *Freedom*, 32.

102. Bogdanov argued that this may have given a ritual space to smoking, elevating it from a simple act of leisure. Since smoking in most accounts is associated with work and intellectual activity, and in the West the smell is singled out as the reason for segregation, scent seems a more likely causal factor. *Dym*, 43.

103. Rudy, *Freedom*, 32.

104. *Kratkii ocherk tabakokureniia v Rossii*, 14.

105. Greene, *Sketches*, 225.

106. West, *I Shop in Moscow*, 156; for *Kabinetnaia* see figure 4.12.

107. Popov, *Nachnite bor'bu*, 25.

108. Bogdanov, *Dym*, 78.

109. Popov, *Nachnite bor'bu*, 3.

110. Courtwright, *Forces of Habit*, 101–2.

111. Greene, *Sketches*, 89–90.

112. Henri Troyat, *Daily Life in Russia under the Last Tsar*, trans. Malcolm Barnes (Stanford: Stanford University Press, 1961), dinner 27, prison 59, merchants' club 46, soldiers 113, students 161.

113. *Kratkii ocherk tabakokureniia v Rossii*, 14; "Tabachnaia promyshlenost' v Rossii: Statiia pervaia," *Otechestvennyia zapiski: Ucheno-literaturnyi zhurnal'* 28 (1845): 18.

114. Rudy, *Freedom*, 38–43.

115. Tregubov, *Normal'nyi sposob*, 9.

116. "Na fabrikakh i zavodakh," *Pravda*, June 9, 1912, 12.

117. "Govoriat, veroiatno . . ." *Pravda*, June 25, 1912, 14.

118. "O Shtrafakh," *Pravda*, March 11, 1913, 2.

119. Alexander M. Martin, "Sewage and the City: Filth, Smell, and Representations of Urban Life in Moscow, 1770–1880," *Russian Review* 67 (2008): 243–74.

120. Bogdanov, *Dym*, 57, 95.

121. Lebedev et al., "Tobacco," 429.

122. Martin, *Enlightened Metropolis*, 55–59.

123. Transchel, *Under the Influence*, 24; Martin, *Enlightened Metropolis*, 114.

124. The original may have used the term papirosy. The translation here is from Bonnell, *The Russian Worker*, 63.

125. D. Nikol'skii, *O kurenii tabaka sredi uchashchikhsia* no. 42 (St. Petersburg: Russkago vracha, 1902), 12.

126. Ignatiev, "Kurenie," 75.

127. Bogdanov, *Dym*, 57.

128. Popov, *Nachnite bor'bu*, 3.

129. Brandt, "Blow Some My Way," 164.

130. Kozharinov, *Russkaia parfiumeriia*, 4.

131. West, *I Shop in Moscow*, 154–55.

132. Bek, *Kurenie*, 22.

133. *Sladkiia* and *Krema* from the Shaposhnikov factory, and *Desert* from Kolobov and Bobrov.

134. Steinberg, *Proletarian Imagination*, 93.

135. Corbin, *The Foul*, 149.

136. Arsenii, *Bros'te kurit' tabak'* (Moscow: A. I. Cnegireva, 1907), 4.

137. Martin, "Sewage and the City," 243–74.

138. Popov, *Nachnite bor'bu*, 3–4; Bogdanov, *Dym*, 25.

139. Bonnell, *The Russian Worker*, 61.

140. N. P. Preis, *Tabak i vino—vragi chelovechestva*, 5th ed. (Kharkhov: Pechatnoe delo, 1902), iii.

141. I. V. Ponomarev, *Stikhi o kurenii tabaka: Na pol'zu blizhnemu* (Kamyshin: Lebedeva i Fadeev, 1904), 3–9.

142. On melancholy and boredom see Steinberg, *Petersburg*, 238–45.

143. Patricia Meyer Spacks, *Boredom: The Literary History of a State of Mind* (Chicago: University of Chicago Press, 1995), 3–23.

144. Hilton, *Smoking*, 106

145. McReynolds, *Russia at Play*, 95–96, 201–2.

146. Bonnell, *The Russian Worker*, 11–14; West, *I Shop in Moscow*, 103, 104, 123–25; Sally West, "Constructing Consumer Culture: Advertising in Imperial Russia to 1914" (PhD diss., University of Illinois–Urbana-Champaign, 1995), 241.

147. Bonnell, *The Russian Worker*, 10.

148. Rudy, *Freedom*, 20–21.

149. Louise McReynolds, "Visualizing Masculinity: The Male Sex That Was Not One In Fin-de-Siècle Russia," in *Picturing Russia: Explorations in Visual Culture*, ed. Valerie A. Kivelson and Joan Neuberger (New Haven, CT: Yale University Press, 2008), 133–38; Catriona Kelly, "'The Lads Indulged Themselves, They Used to Smoke. . .' Tobacco and Children's Culture in Twentieth-Century Russia," in *Tobacco in Russian History and Culture: From the Seventeenth Century to the Present*, ed. Matthew P. Romaniello and Tricia Starks (New York: Routledge, 2009), 158–82.

150. O. Dedelin, *Kak uchit'sia ot' kureniia* (trans. from the German) (Moscow: Izdaniia, 1909), 5.

151. I. A. Birshtein, *K psikhologii kureniia* (Moscow: Moskovskii voennyi okrug, 1913), 1.

152. *Damskii mir*, March 3, 1909, 33.

153. See the runs of these advertisements in *Niva* in 1907 and 1910; and *Rodina* in 1910.

154. West, *I Shop in Moscow*, 109.

155. Glickman, *Russian Factory*, 131.

156. For fuller discussion of the case for women's smoking see Tricia Starks, "A Community in the Clouds: Advertising Tobacco, Gender, and Liberation in Pre-Revolutionary Russia," *Journal of Women's History* 25, no. 1 (Spring 2013): 62–84.

157. S. N. Kaznakov, *Paketovyia tabekerki imperatorskogo farforovogo zaboda* (Sirius: St. Petersburg, 1913), 35–36.

158. Klioutchkine, "'I Smoke, Therefore I Think,'" 96–97; V. I. Dalia, *Tolkovyi slovar' zhivago velikoruskago iazyka*, vol. II (Moscow: Lazarevskii institute vostochnykh iazykov, 1863), 20.

159. A. N. Savinov, "Petr Efimovich Zabolotskii, 1803–1866," in *Russkoe iskusstvo: Ocherki o zhizni i tvorchestve khudozhnikov, Pervaia polovina deviatnadtsatogo veka*, ed. A. I. Leonov (Moscow: Gosizdat Isskustvo, 1954), 677–80.

160. Bunker, *Creating*, 30.

161. Petrone, *Tobacco,* 215.

162. Bendeict, *Golden Silk Smoke,* 199–236.

163. Patricia Herlihy, *Odessa: A History, 1794–1914* (Cambridge, MA: Harvard University Press, 1986), 130; Bogdanov, *Dym,* 67.

164. Engel, *Mothers,* 64, 80, 114.

165. Klioutchkine, "'I Smoke, Therefore I Think,'" 97–98.

166. Stites, *The Women's Liberation Movement in Russia,* 102.

167. See for example, V. G. Avseenki, "Zloi dukh: Roman," *Russkii vestnik* 152 (April 1881), 630, or D. V. Grigorovich, "Zamshevye liudi (Zapoza) Komediia v 5 destviiakh," *Polnoe sobranie sochineneii D. V. Grigorovicha v 12 tomakh* tom. 11 (St. Petersburg: A. F. Marksa, 1896), 1–5; Engelstein, *Keys,* 1.

168. Laurie Bernstein, *Sonia's Daughters: Prostitutes and Their Regulation in Imperial Russia* (Berkeley: University of California Press, 1995), 35, 43; Steinberg, *Petersburg,* 190, 196.

169. Edwards, *The Russians,* 424.

170. Quoted in Bogdanov, *Dym,* 58. For women's smoking elsewhere see Kiernan, *Tobacco,* 84–85

171. Krymskii, *Vred,* 18.

172. Ibid., 15–16.

173. "Znatnyia kuril'shchitsy," *Modnyi svet'* 32 (1902): 343.

174. Annette M. B. Meaken, *Woman in Transition* (London: Methuen and Co., 1907), 135–36.

175. Kiernan, *Tobacco,* 96.

176. Grinevskii, *Bros'te,* 15.

177. Barbara T. Norton and Jehanne M. Gheith, eds., *An Improper Profession: Women, Gender, and Journalism in Late Imperial Russia* (Durham, NC: Duke University Press, 2001).

178. In regards to women's voting see Ruthchild, *Equality and Revolution,* 1–10; on smoking, see Starks, "A Community in the Clouds," 64

179. Mitchell, "Images of Exotic Women," 327.

180. Juliana Sivulka, *Soap, Sex, and Cigarettes: A Cultural History of American Advertising* (Belmont, CA: Wadsworth Publishing Company, 1998), 86–88; Dolores Mitchell, "Women and Nineteenth-Century Images of Smoking," in *Smoke: A Global History of Smoking,* ed. Sander Gilman and Zhou Xun (London: Reaktion Books, 2004), 300, 302; Petrone, *Tobacco,* 221–22; Hilton, *Smoking,* 150–51.

181. "Docheri Skifskago tsaria," *Put' pravdy,* April 22, 1914, 8.

182. Hilton, *Smoking,* 32.

183. G. T. Lowth, *Around the Kremlin; or, Pictures of Life in Moscow* (London: Hurst and Blackett, 1868), 247–48.

184. Klimova and Zolotinkina, *Reklamnyi plakat v Rossii,* 39, plate 32.

185. Quoted in Bogdanov, *Dym,* 67.

186. West, "Smokescreens," 105–6.

187. Baburina and Artamonova referred to this as the "elegant Amazonian." *Russkii reklamnyi plakat,* 6.

188. Rudy, *Freedom,* 4.

189. Sally West, "The Material Promised Land: Advertising's Modern Agenda in Late Imperial Russia," *Russian Review* 57 (July 1998): 347.

4. CONDEMNED

1. *Mukhomora* (from Tazhik) refers to the psychoactive mushroom fly agaric. *Zatemnenii* has appeared as "blurring" and could be "dimming" or "shadowing," but "clouding" approximates both obscuring and darkening. L. N. Tolstoy, "Dlia chego liudi odurmanivaiutsia," *Polnoe sobranie sochinenii,* tom. 27 (Moscow: Gosizdat, 1937), full essay 269–85, quotations pp. 269 and 271.

2. Ibid., tobacco section, 275–78; quotations pp. 269, 270, and 272.

3. Ibid., 276.

4. Ibid., 275–76.

5. Ibid., 277–79; A. B. Biriukova, "Kurenie kak fenomen povsednevnoi zhizni Rossii v kontse XVIII–seredine XIX v.," in *Istoriia rossiiskoi povsednevnosti: Materialy dvadtsat' shestoi vserossiiskoi zaochnoi nauchnoi konferentsii,* ed. S. D. Morozov and V. B. Zhiromska (St. Petersburg: Nestor, 2013), 51–52.

6. Tolstoi, "Dlia chego," 276.

7. Tolstoy occasionally indulged his lusts, but preached denial. Leo Tolstoy Jr., "Why Tolstoy Gave Up Meat, Tobacco, and Spirits," *Chambers's Journal* (December 1939): 934–35.

8. Ibid.; Ronald D. LeBlanc, "Tolstoy's Way of No Flesh: Abstinence, Vegetarianism, and Christian Physiology," and Darra Goldstein, "Is Hay Only for Horses? Highlights of Russian Vegetarianism at the Turn of the Century," in *Food in Russian History and Culture,* ed. Musya Glants and Joyce Toomre (Bloomington: Indiana University Press, 1997), 81–102, 103–23.

9. Patricia Herlihy, *The Alcoholic Empire: Vodka and Politics in Late Imperial Russia* (Oxford: Oxford University Press, 2002), 111–14.

10. Ibid., 111.

11. Beer, *Renovating Russia,* 7–11; Mount Athos' St. Panteleimon Monastery, *Bros'te kurit!,* 9.

12. Courtwright, *Forces,* 181; Mount Athos, *Bros'te kurit,* 8–9.

13. Beer, *Renovating Russia,* 51-53. Healey, *Homosexual Desire,* 77–92.

14. Herlihy noted a similar rise in anti-alcohol tracts in the three decades before 1914. See *The Alcoholic Empire,* 3. The Russian State Library collection revealed a significant increase in titles after 1900, but this could be a reflection more of items preserved than production.

15. Brooks, *When Russia Learned to Read,* xiii–xvi, 4.

16. Simon Pawley, "Revolution in Health: Nervous Weakness and Visions of Health in Revolutionary Russia, c. 1900–31," *Historical Research* 90 (2017): 195–96. See, for example, *O tabake* (Moscow: I. D. Sytkin i ko., 1890); *O tabake i vrede ego kureniia* (prerevolutionary pocket book with no author, publisher, or date).

17. Brooks, *When Russia Learned to Read,* 337–88.

18. Robert Otto, *Publishing for the People: The Firm Posrednik, 1885–1905.* (New York: Garland Publishing, 1987), 135, 173.

19. Mount Athos St. Panteleimon Monastery, *Kakoi vred prinosit cheloveku tabak?* (Odessa: E. I. Fesenko, 1896); Mount Athos St. Panteleimon Monastery, *O p'ianstve i drugikh bogoprotivnykh privychkakh kurenii tabaka, skvernoslovii, penii mirskikh pesen, igrishchakh, kataniiakh, sueverii i bozhbe. S ukazaniem dvukh dobrodetelei, kotoryia legko dovodiat do istinnago schastiia* (Moscow: I. Efimov, 1901); see also Arseniia Igumena (Nastoiatelia voskresenskago monastyria), *O poroke tabakokureniia* (St. Petersburg: A. S. Suvorina, 1905).

20. Botkin borrowed from A. K. Kasatkin's *O vrede kureniia tabaka* (St. Petersburg, 1910) and E. I. Fesenko's *Bros'te kurit'* (Odessa: P. V. Bel'tsov, 1914) as sources, Botkin, *Vrednye posledstviia,* 2–31.

21. Brooks, *When Russia Learned to Read,* 246–68.

22. P. K. Komisarenko, *Pagubnaia privychka,* 9th ed. (Moscow: A. I. Momontov, 1913).

23. "Plakaty dlia bor'by s kuren'em tabaku i alkogolizmom (glavnym obrazom v shkolakh)," *Obshchestvennyi vrach* (April 1912): 34.

24. M. Valitskaia, *O vrede kureniia tabaku (Doklad, chitannyi v Pedagogicheskom musee Solianago gorodka v S.-Pb-ge). Iz No. 7 i 8 Zemskago vracha za 1890* (Kiev: Chernigovskoe gubernskoe upravleniie, 1890).

25. Beliakov, *Tabak.*

26. "O vrede tabaka," *Krest'ianin"* 33 (1908): 531.

27. *Tabak: Sredstvo izbavit'sia ot mnogikh boleznei* (Kazan: Imperatorskii Universitet, 1888), republished in 1890 as *O Tabake* (Moscow: I. D. Sitkin i co., 1890).

28. For Valitskaia, see Sviatlovskii, *Materialy,* 20–21. For Il'inskii, see Vitol'd Khmelevskii, *O stoikosti i kolichestvennom opredelenii nikotina v trupakh zhivotnykh, otravlennykh' etim' alkoloidom': Dissertatsiia na stepen doktora meditsiny* (St. Petersburg: Russkaia skoropechantia I. S. Pakhimova, 1876), 19. For Filaret, see A. L. Mendel'son, "K voprosu o vliianii kureniia na zdorov'e: Doklad II sektsii Obshchestva okhraneniia narodnago zdraviia," *Zhurnal Russkago obshchestva Okhraneniia narodnago zdraviia: Dopushchen Uchenym Komitetom Ministerstva Narodnago Prosveshcheniia dlia fundamental'nykh bibliotek srednikh uchebnykh zavedenii, muzhskikh i zhenskikh* 9 (September 1897): 583; for Tolstoy see Appolov, *Perestanem kurit'!,* 17.

29. Mendel'son, "K voprosu," 583–99.

30. Tricia Starks, *The Body Soviet: Propaganda, Hygiene, and the Revolutionary State* (Madison: University of Wisconsin Press, 2008), 39–42.

31. Mendel'son, "K voprosu," 588.

32. Mendel'son quoted P. I. Vershinin from *Sanitarnoe Delo,* Feb. 3, 1891. See "K voprosu," 587.

33. Mendel'son, "K voprosu," 586–87.

34. Rudy, *Freedom,* 25–26.

35. Mendel'son, "K voprosu," 589–91, 596

36. Ibid., 592, 596–99.

37. Ibid., 583.

38. For example, S. B., *Torzhestvo tabaku fiziologiia tabaku, trubku, sigar, papiros, pakhitos i tabakerki,* trans. from the French (St. Petersburg: Vnutr. strazhi, 1863); Parant, *O tabake,* trans. from the French (St. Petersburg: Smirnov, n.d.—prerevolutionary); Dedelin, *Kak uchit'sia.*

39. Bussiron, *O vlianii tabaku,* 13; Bartolomeo, *Demon,* 67; M-ov', *Neskol'ko slov,* 3.

40. Popov, *Nachnite bor'bu,* 7; Appolov, *Perestanem kurit'!,* 10; Beliakov, *Tabak* 34; M-ov', *Neskol'ko slov,* 6; Tregubov, *Normal'nyi sposob,* 8; A. Blindovskii, *Kak brosit kurit* (Kiev: A. O. Shterenzon, 1912), 4; Udintsev *O vrede,* 6;

41. Popov, *Deti!* 4; M-ov', *Neskol'ko slov,* 3; Appolov, *Perestanem kurit'!,* 10.

42. Popov, *Deti!* 4; Bussiron, *O vlianii tabaku,* 14; Popov, *Nachnite bor'bu,* 8–9; Priklonskii, *Upotreblenie tabaka,* 24; Vvedenskii (Sviashchennik), *O kurenii tabaku,* Otdela rasprostraneniia dukhovno-nravstv. knig. pri Mosk. Obshchestve Liubit. Dukhovn. Prosveshcheniia, 5th ed. (Moscow: Dormam, 1915), 3.

43. Zasidatel'-Krzheminskii, *Tabachnoe otravlenie,* 7.

44. Poliakov, *Ne kuri,* 3, quotation p. 8.

45. Bek, *Kurenie,* 4–14; Rokau, *Interesnaia,* 1–3.

46. Dogel, *Tabak,* 3–12, 51–53.

47. Rokau, *Interesnaia,* 1–7; Bek, *Kurenie,* 4–18.

48. Udintsev, *O vrede,* 11.

49. "Barbarities to Smokers," *New York Times,* April 5, 1896, 1.

50. Rokau, *Interesnaia,* 14; Jacob M. Price, "The Tobacco Adventure to Russia: Enterprise, Politics, and Diplomacy in the Quest for a Northern Market for English Colonial Tobacco, 1676–1722," *Transactions of the American Philosophical Society* 51 (1961), 17–18; The punishments were witnessed by Adam Olearius, *The Travels of Olearius in Seventeenth-Century Russia,* trans. Samuel H. Baron (Stanford: Stanford University Press, 1967), 29, 145–46.

51. Bek, *Kurenie,* 16; Rokau, *Interesnaia,* 31. Repeated in *Dvadtstipiatiletie tabachnoi fabriki V. I. Asmolova v Rostov na Donu. (Kratkii istoricheskii ocherk fabriki) izdanie v pamiat iubileinago goda* (Moscow: A. Gatnukh, 1882), 8.

52. A. Virenius, *Kurenie tabaka* (St. Petersburg: N. V. Gasvskii, 1907), 8

53. Mount Athos, *Bros'te kurit,* 14.

54. Tregubov, *Normal'nyi sposob,* 8.

55. M-ov', *Neskol'ko slov,* 5; Bartolomeo, *Demon,* 67; Bussiron, *O vlianii tabaku,* 13.

56. Zasidatel'-Krzheminskii, *Tabachnoe otravlenie,* 7.

57. On Mikhail, Popov, *Nachnite bor'bu*, 19; from medical authorities, Botkin, *Vrednye posledstviia*, 28; Nik. Pav. Preis, *Tabak—vrag chelovechestva (Avto-kompiliativnyi sbornik)* (Khar'kov: Pechatnoe delo, 1902), 25; Rokau, *Interesnaia*, 13–14; Priklonskii, *Upotreblenie*, 37. See also Nikol'skii, *O tabake*, 10–11; N. P. Pomerantsev, *O tabake i vrede ego kureniia: Beseda s uchenikami v–viii klassov Shelaputinskoi gimnazii gimnazicheskago vracha* (Moscow: M. M. Tarchigin, 1908), 8; from Old Believers and other religious groups, M-ov', *Neskol'ko slov*, 7; Mount Athos Skete of St. Il'inskii, *Kurenia tabaku, kak odna iz neprostitel'nykh prikhotei cheloveka*. 2nd ed., # 62 (Odessa: D. Pliushchev, 1896), 53; Aleksandr Zybin, comp., *Tabak, kak pagubnaia strast', i ego vrednoe vliianie na dukhovnuiu iI telesnuiu zhizn' cheloveka* (Kungur: M. Letunov, 1907), 10.

58. Ponomarev, *Stikhi*, 17.

59. "Bol'shoi pozhar na Vyborskoi storone," *Pravda*, August 13, 1912, 10; Grinevskii, *Bros'te*, 49; Bogdanov, *Dym*, 55; Frierson, *All Russia is Burning!*, 83.

60. Popov, *Nachnite bor'bu*, 18.

61. His full title read "instructor of hygiene at the Kharkhov City Trade School and Kharkhov City Fourth (4-x) class school and instructor of hygiene for worker's and tradesmen of Kharkhov," Preis, *Tabak—vrag*, 26; Dogel, *Tabak*, 53.

62. Popov, *Nachnite bor'bu*, 15, see also *Tabak*, 5.

63. M-ov', *Neskol'ko slov*, 6.

64. Nikol'skii, *O tabake*, 3; Appolov, *Perestanem kurit'!*, 6–7.

65. Mount Athos, *Kurenia tabaku*, 57–58.

66. Dogel, *Tabak*, 55; Grinevskii, *Bros'te*, 25; Ponomarev, *Stikhi*, 44.

67. Popov, *Nachnite bor'bu*, 15; Ponomarev, *Stikhi*, 12; Priklonskii, *Upotreblenie*, 38; Pomerantsev, *O tabake*, 8.

68. Rokau, *Interesnaia*, 114.

69. Ponomarev, *Stikhi*, 9; Vvedenskii, *O kurenii tabaku*, 12–15.

70. Nikol'skii, *O tabake*, 10; Ponomarev, *Stikhi*, 12–13.

71. Popov, *Nachnite bor'bu*, 16; Ponomarev, *Stikhi*, 13.

72. Benedict, *Golden-Silk*, 8.

73. Tate, *Cigarette Wars*, 54–55.

74. *Tabak*, 2.

75. V. Mikhailovskii, *Tabak i vrednoe vliianie ego na cheloveka*, 5th ed. (St. Petersburg: E. A. Pozdniakov, 1894), 23–25.

76. Arsenii, *Bros'te kurit' tabak'*, 5.

77. Vvedenskii, *O kurenii tabaku*, 23.

78. Popov, *Nachnite bor'bu*, 22–23.

79. Nikol'skii, *O tabake*, quotation p. 4, 2–4; see also Mount Athos, *Kurenia tabaku*, 25–26.

80. Pomerantsev, *O tabake*, 8.

81. Popov, *Nachnite bor'bu*, 4.

82. Grinevskii, *Bros'te*, 26.

83. Krymskii, *Vred*, 29.

84. A. F. Gamalei, *Ob upotreblenii spiritnykh napitkov i kurenii tabaku iz.* zhurnala *Ogni* (n.p.: A. M. Ponomareva, n.d.—voennyi tsensor), 4. An antitobacco tract translated in 1912 indicated a similar fight in Britain. F. Dziuvett, *Beregite vashe zdorov'e: Shto nado delat' shtoby byt' zdorovym, Azbuka gigieny dlia detei v shkole i sem'e (So svedeniiami o vrede alkogolia i tabaka)*, perevod s angliiskago P. Khlebnikova Biblioteka I. Gorbunova-Posadova dlia detei i dlia iunoshestva, no 197 (Moscow: I. N. Kushnerev i ko., 1912), 13; see also mentions of European and British regulation in V. E. Ignatiev, "Kurenie," in *Entsiklopedicheskii slovar*, ed. By F. A. Brokgauz and I. A. Efron v. XVII (St. Petersburg: I. A. Efron, 1896), 73. In the United States see Petrone, *Tobacco*, 234–36. For general regulation of scent in the city, see David Howes and Constance Classen, *Ways of Sensing: Understanding the Senses in Society* (London: Routledge, 2014), 97–114.

85. Edwards, *The Russians*, 408–9.

86. Petrone, Tobacco, 14.

87. Grinevskii, *Bros'te*, 17–18.

88. Ibid., 27. Troyat wrote of the special cars in his memoir from his 1902 trip.

89. Preis, *Tabak—vrag*, 44.

90. Gamalei, *Ob upotreblenii*, 3–4.

91. Corbin, *The Foul*, 149–51.

92. Nicotine discovery, Mount Athos St. Panteleimon Monastery, *P'ianstvo i kurenie tabaku i ikh vrednye posledstviia* 2 ed. (Moscow: I. Efimov, 1904), 37; Danger of poison, Bartolomeo, *Demon*, 3–4; Rokau, *Interesnaia*, 39–40; Il'inskii, *Polezno*; Grinevskii, *Bros'te*, 4–5; Bek, *Kurenie*, 23–25; Botkin, *Vrednye posledstviia*, 5;

93. Sebelius, *SGR*, 29–32; V. I. Mezhov, *Iadovityia svoistva tabaka i gibel'noe vliianie ikh na chelovecheskii organizm* (St. Petersburg: V. Bezobrazov i comp., 1871)

94. Bussiron, *O vlianii tabaku*, 8; Beliakov, *Tabak*, 27–33; Aleksandr Tugendgol'd', *Fiziologicheskiia izseldovaniia o deistvii nikotina* (Moscow: V. Grachev, 1864), dogs: 15–22, frogs: 25–58, rabbits: 58–86; I. Buial'skii, *O vrede ot izlishnego kureniia tabaka*, no. 170, *Sanktpetersburg Vedomostei* (St. Petersburg: Akademii nauk, 1859), 7–8; Khmelevskii, *O stoikosti*, 13 horses; 39–45 dogs;

95. Popov, *Nachnite bor'bu*, 3–4; M-ov', *Neskol'ko slov*, 1–2.

96. Botkin, *Vrednye posledstviia*, 9.

97. Bek, *Kurenie*, 23. Nicotine is important to addiction, but for cancers, the crucial element is the almost seventy carcinogens enter the lungs with every tobacco smoke inhalation. Sebelius, *SGR*, 225. For the discovery of tars, see Proctor, *Golden*, 156. For further attacks, Evlogii Episkop, *Tabak i ego vrednoe vliianie na cheloveka* (Saratov: A. F. Vinkler, 1914).

98. *P'ianstvo i kurenie tabaku i ikh vrednye posledstviia*, 2nd ed (Moscow: I. Efimov, 1904), 38; Il'inskii, *Polezno*, 11.

99. Preis, *Tabak—vrag*, 10–11.

100. Appolov, *Perestanem kurit'!*, 9.

101. Il'inskii, *Polezno*, 12.

102. Susan K. Morrissey, *Suicide and the Body Politic in Imperial Russia* (Cambridge: Cambridge University Press, 2006); Steinberg, *Petersburg*, 157–97.

103. Zybin, *Tabak*, 7. See similarly Krymskii, *Vred*, 10.

104. M-ov', *Neskol'ko slov*, 2–3.

105. L. A. Zolotarev, comp. *O preduprezhdenii kureniia tabaku v detskom vozrast': Populiarno-nauchnyi ocherk dlia roditelei i vospitatelei*, 2nd ed. (Moscow: I. N. Kushnerev, 1914).

106. Zolotarev, *O preduprezhdenii*, 26.

107. Il'inski, *Polezno*, 34.

108. Buial'skii, *O vrede*, 8.

109. Rokau, *Interesnaia*, 39.

110. Zasidatel'-Krzheminskii, *Tabachnoe otravlenie*, tobacco heart: 8; eyes: 10; nervous system: 11, 21–24; sex organs: 12.

111. Ignatiev, "Kurenie," 74.

112. Krymskii, *Vred*, 9.

113. Ibid., 10–11.

114. Mount Athos, *Bros'te kurit*, 7.

115. Beliakov, *Tabak*, 38; Nikol'skii, *O tabake*, 7.

116. Il'inskii, *Tri iada*, 32–33; Il'inski, *Polezno*, 25–26, 60; see also Grinevskii, *Bros'te*, 7; Krymskii, *Vred*, 12; Botkin, *Vrednye posledstviia*, 16.

117. Poliakov, *Ne kuri*, 5.

118. As reported in R. Magnus and D. A. Kamenskii, "Nikotin," in *Real'naia entsiklopediia prakticheskoi meditisny*, ed. M. B. Bliumenau, vol. 13 (St. Petersburg: Prakticheskaia Meditsina, 1909), 160–61.

119. Ignatiev, "Kurenie," 74.

120. Nikol'skii, *O tabake*, 6.

121. Students of Grammatchikov and Ossendovskii, "K voprosu o vliianii kureniia na orga-nizm cheloveka," *Vrach* 1 (1887): 5.

122. A. E. Sharbaka, "K vopros o vliianii nikotina i kureniia tabaku na nervnye tsenty," *Vrach* 5 (1887): 161–63; chart of pupil effects in continuation, *Vrach* 8 (1887): 189–93.

123. Poliakov, *Ne kuri,* 10.

124. Robert Jutte, *A History of the Senses: From Antiquity to Cyberspace* trans by James Lynn (Cambridge: Polity, 2005), 184–85.

125. Bussiron, *O vlianii tabaku*, 9–10.

126. *Tabak*, 10.

127. Nikol'skii, *O tabake*, 7.

128. Popov, *Deti!*, 7.

129. Zolotarev, *O preduprezhdenii*, 40–44.

130. Botkin, *Vrednye posledstviia*, 6; seen also in Grinevskii, *Bros'te,* 5.

131. Proctor, *Golden,* 27.

132. Bartolomeo, *Demon*, 66.

133. Bek, *Kurenie*, 35.

134. Grinevskii, *Bros'te,* 5.

135. Preis, *Tabak—vrag*, 10.

136. Krymskii, *Vred*, 12; Grinevskii, *Bros'te,* 5; Khmelevskii, *O stoikosti,* 14–17.

137. Popov, *Nachnite bor'bu*, 11.

138. Il'inski, *Polezno,* 30.

139. Ibid., 32.

140. Mikhailovskii, *Tabak,* 20.

141. Il'inskii, *Tri iada,* 30–31.

142. Popov, *Nachnite bor'bu*, 12.

143. Il'inskii, *Tri iada*, 30; Khmelevskii, *O stoikosti,* 22.

144. Nikol'skii, *O tabake*, 8.

145. Mount Athos, *Bros'te kurit*, 5.

146. M-ov', *Neskol'ko slov*, 8.

147. As translated earlier in relation to Mendel'son, "K voprosu," 583; Mikhailovskii, *Tabak*, 10–11.

148. Tate, *Cigarette Wars,* 26–27.

149. Laura Goering, "'Russian Nervousness': Neurasthenia and National Identity in Nineteenth-Century Russia," *Medical History* 47 (2003): 26.

150. Goering, "Russian Nervousness," 24–26; Beer, *Renovating Russia,* 37–44; Pawley, "Revo-lution in Health," 191–96

151. Beer, *Renovating Russia,* 31–32; Pawley, "Revolution in Health," 201.

152. Goering, "Russian Nervousness," 649.

153. Susan K. Morrissey, "The Economy of Nerves: Health, Commercial Culture, and the Self in Late Imperial Russia," *Slavic Review* 3 (Fall 2010): 649; Pawley, "Revolution in Health," 201.

154. Students of Grammatchikov, "K voprosu," 6.

155. Goering, "Russian Nervousness," 37; Beer, *Renovating Russia,* 55.

156. Irina Sirotkina, *Diagnosing Literary Genius: A Cultural History of Psychiatry in Russia, 1880–1930.* (Baltimore, MD: Johns Hopkins University Press, 2002), 97; Julie Vail Brown, "Psy-chiatrists and the State in Tsarist Russia," in *Social Control and the State* ed. Stanley Cohen and Andrew Scull (New York: St. Martin's Press, 1983), 267–87; Christine D. Worobec, *Possessed: Women, Witches, and Demons in Imperial Russia* (DeKalb: Northern Illinois University Press, 2007), 148–87.

157. Il'inskii, *Tri iada,* 24–25.

158. Daniel Pick, *Faces of Degeneration: A European Disorder, c. 1848–c. 1918* (New York: Cambridge University Press, 1989), 2–17.

159. Goering, "Russian Nervousness," 31–34.

160. Laura Briggs, "The Race of Hysteria: 'Overcivilization' and the 'Savage' Woman in Late Nineteenth-Century Obstetrics and Gynecology," *American Quarterly* 52, no. 2 (June 2000): 255.

161. Goering, "Russian Nervousness," 35.

162. Pick, *Faces of Degeneration,* 43.

163. Courtwright, *Forces,* 181.

164. Beliakov, *Tabak,* 43.

165. Ibid., 42–43.

166. Appolov, *Perestanem kurit'!,* 37–38.

167. Beliakov, *Tabak,* 43.

168. Ignatiev, "Kurenie," 74.

169. Many of these issues are now recognized as having some link to tobacco use. See Proctor, *Golden,* 19–20; Nikol'skii, *O tabake,* 6–7; Students of Grammatchikov, "K voprosu," 5–7.

170. Il'inskii,*Tri iada,* 19; also quoted in Preis, *Tabak i vino,* 42.

171. Popov, *Nachnite bor'bu,* 8.

172. Il'inskii, *Tri iada,* 44.

173. Il'inski, *Polezno,* 28. See also, E. Meier, *Tabak—Iad'* (Riga: Traktatnoe Obshchestvo v. Rossii, 1911) [repr in 1915 as *Dobryi sovet kuriashchim* (Petrograd: Ernst Biul'fing', 1915)]; Il'inski, *Tri iada,* 31.

174. Grinevskii, *Bros'te,* 14.

175. Proctor, *Golden,* 18, 149–53, 155–69.

176. Krymskii, *Vred,* 15

177. S. S. Gruzdeva, "Opyt' pogolovnago izsledovaniia mokroty na chatotochnyia aplochki u detei shkol'nago vozrasta," *Vrach* 40 (1889): 881–83.

178. Herlihy, *The Alcoholic Empire,* 92–97.

179. Jordan Goodman, "Webs of Drug Dependence: Towards a Political History of Smoking and Health," in *Ashes to Ashes: The History of Smoking and Health,* ed. S. Lock, L. A. Reynolds, and E. M. Tansey (Amsterdam: Rodopi, 1998), 16.

180. John Welshman, "Images of Youth: The Issue of Juvenile Smoking, 1880–1914," *Addiction* 91:, no. 9 (1996): 1380.

181. Petrone, *Tobacco,* 225–29; Matthew Hilton, "'Tabs', 'Fags' and the 'Boy Labour Problem' in Late Victorian and Edwardian Britain," *Journal of Social History* 28, no. 3 (1995): 587–607; Welshman, "Images of Youth," 1379–86.

182. Tate, *Cigarette Wars,* 20–21.

183. Preis, *Tabak—vrag,* 28.

184. Mount Athos, *Kakoi vred,* 9.

185. Priklonskii, *Upotreblenie,* 17–19.

186. Bek, *Kurenie,* 24.

187. Buial'skii, *O vrede,* 1–2; Zolotarev, *O preduprezhdenii,* 38.

188. Zolotarev, *O preduprezhdenii,* 38.

189. Students of Grammatchikov, "K voprosu," 5.

190. *Tabak,* 8.

191. Mikhailovskii, *Tabak,* 16–17.

192. Popov, *Deti!,* 7.

193. Steinberg, *Petersburg,* 252.

194. Popov, *Nachnite bor'bu,* 1887.

195. M-ov', *Neskol'ko slov,* 6.

196. Preis, *Tabak—vrag,* 32.

197. M-ov', *Neskol'ko slov,* 4.

198. Ibid., 6

199. Nikol'skii, *O tabake,* 9.

200. Udintsev, *O vrede,* 9.

201. Priklonskii, *Upotreblenie*, 28.
202. Beer, *Renovating Russia,* 12–14.
203. Preis, *Tabak—vrag,*
204. Zolotarev, *O preduprezhdenii*, 35.
205. Ibid., 30–31.
206. Popov, *Deti!* 7.
207. Botkin, *Vrednye posledstviia*, 13.
208. Ignatiev, "Kurenie," 9.
209. Ibid., 8.
210. Botkin, *Vrednye posledstviia*, 12.
211. Zolotarev, *O preduprezhdenii*, 39
212. Ibid., 39
213. Arsenii, *Bros'te kurit' tabak'*, 2.
214. Priklonskii, *Upotreblenie*, 36–37.
215. Popov, *Deti!* 11–12.
216. Zolotarev, *O preduprezhdenii*, 252.
217. Nikol'skii, *O kurenii tabaka*, 3.
218. Ibid., 6–7.
219. Grinevskii, *Bros'te,* 14; see also *P'ianstvo i kurenie tabaku*, 14.
220. Popov, *Deti!*, 10.
221. Preis, *Tabak—vrag*, 17.
222. Virenius, *Kurenie tabaka*, 3–5.
223. Preis, *Tabak—vrag,*
224. *P'ianstvo i kurenie tabaku*, 45.
225. Krymskii, *Vred*, 18–19
226. Ibid., 17.
227. Arsenii, *Bros'te kurit' tabak'*, 5.
228. Rudy, *Freedom*, 14; Becalossi Chiara, "The Origin of Italian Sexological Studies: Female Sexual Inversion, ca. 1870–1900," *Journal of the History of Sexuality,* 18: 1 (January 2009), 109.
229. Dogel, *Tabak,* 48.
230. Preis, *Tabak—vrag*, 16.
231. Ignatiev, "Kurenie," 74; Popov, *Nachnite bor'bu*, 8; Vvedenskii, *O kurenii tabaku,* 12
232. *P'ianstvo i kurenie tabaku*, 46.
233. Grinevskii, *Bros'te,* 16.
234. Arsenii, *Bros'te kurit' tabak'*, 3.
235. Students of Grammatchikov, "K voprosu," 5. On masturbation, see Thomas W. Laqueur, *Solitary Sex: A Cultural History of Masturbation* (New York: Zone Books, 2004); A. A. Mendel'son, *Onanizm i bor'ba s nim,* Biblioteka zhurnala *Gigiena i zdorov'e rabochei i krest'ianskoi sem'i* (Leningrad: tov. Zinov'eva, n.d).
236. Beliakov, *Tabak,* 41,
237. Vvedenskii, *O kurenii tabaku*, 12; see also Udintsev, *O vrede*, 6
238. Priklonskii, *Upotreblenie*, 14.
239. Appolov, *Perestanem kurit'!*, 34–35.
240. Komisarenko, *Pagubnoe*, 3.
241. Popov, *Nachnite bor'bu*, 7.
242. This charge was also made against Chinese cigar-labor in San Francisco. Nancy Tomes, *The Gospel of Germs: Men, Women, and the Microbe in American Life* (Cambridge, MA: Harvard University Press, 1998), 107, 210.
243. Engelstein, *Keys,* 195.
244. Meier, *Tabak*, 5–6.
245. Students of Grammatchikov, "K voprosu," 5; Morrissey, "The Economy of Nerves," 655.

246. Appolov, *Perestanem kurit'!*, 4.

247. Popov, *Deti!*, 3; Beliakov, *Tabak,* 8.

248. Zybin, *Tabak,* 3; Mikhailovskii, *Tabak,* 10–11; M-ov', *Neskol'ko slov,* 15; V. P. *Shto takoe—dymnaia privychka? O tabakokurenii* (Saint Petersburg: M. I. Fomina, 1914), 6; Arsenii, *Bros'te kurit' tabak'*, 5.

249. Vvedenskii, *O kurenii tabaku*, 4–5.

250. Popov, *Deti!* 8.

251. Botkin, *Vrednye posledstviia*, 18–19.

252. Herlihy, *The Alcoholic Empire,* 69.

253. M-ov', *Neskol'ko slov*, 9.

254. Rokau, *Interesnaia,* 115; Arsenii, *Bros'te kurit' tabak'*, 6.

255. Vvedenskii, *O kurenii tabaku*, 3.

256. Isidor Cherniaev, *Brashiura* (Moscow: E. I. Pogodika, 1882), 2–5; P. M. Sukhov, M. K. Vasil'ev, P. Aleksandrov, I. S. Bedrinskii, "K legendam i poveri'am o tabake," *Etnograficheskoe obozrenie: izdanie etnograficheskago otdela Imperatorskago Obshchestva Liubitelei estestvoznaniia, antropologii i etnografii cocosianiago pri Moskovskom Universitet* 1 (1898): 156; Aleksei Remizov, *O proiskhozhdenie moei khigi o tabake—Shto est' tabak* (Paris: Tchijoff, 1983), 53–68.

257. Roy R. Robson, "Old Believers in Imperial Russia: A Legend on the Appearance of Tobacco," in *The Human Tradition in Modern Russia,* ed. William B. Husband (Wilmington, DE: Scholarly Resources, 2000), 20–27.

258. Sukhov et al. "K legendam," 156–58.

259. Steinberg, *Petersburg,* 215.

260. Robson, "Old Believers; *Kurit' li mne ili net'?* (Rostov-na-Don: A. Pavlov, 1906).

261. Vvedenskii, *O kurenii tabaku,* 20; Popov, *Nachnite bor'bu,* 21; Mikhailovskii, *Tabak,* 23–25.

262. Vvedenskii, *O kurenii tabaku*, 24.

263. Nadieszda Kizenko, *A Prodigal Saint: Father John of Kronstadt and the Russian People* (University Park: Pennsylvania State University Press, 2000), 1–9. Quotation taken from V. P., *Shto takoe,* 1; see also Steinberg, *Petersburg,* 215–16.

264. As quoted in V. P., *Shto takoe,* 1.

265. As quoted in ibid., 2.

266. V. P., *Shto takoe,* 2.

267. Il'inskii, *Polezno*, 6.

268. Tregubov, *Normal'nyi sposob,* 10.

269. Bussiron, *O vlianii tabaku,* 17–18.

270. Bussiron, *O vlianii tabaku,* 20.

271. Ponomarev, *Stikhi,* 16; Priklonskii, *Upotreblenie,* 17; Zybin, *Tabak,* 11; Vvedenskii, *O kurenii tabaku,* 16–20; Botkin, *Vrednye posledstviia,* 10; Zolotarev, *O preduprezhdenii,* 47.

272. Preis, *Tabak—vrag,* 19–20.

273. Meier, *Tabak,* 1.

274. Arsenii, *Bros'te kurit' tabak'*, 7.

275. Popov, *Nachnite bor'bu,* 27–28; Mount Athos, *Kurenia tabaku,* 49–51; Blindovskii, *Kak brosit,* 4.

276. Zolotarev, *O preduprezhdenii,* 44–51

277. Nikol'skii, *O tabake,* 8.

278. *P'ianstvo i kurenie tabaku,* 45.

279. Popov, *Nachnite bor'bu,* 3–4.

280. Mikhailovskii, *Tabak,* 4; Dedelin, *Kak uchit'sia,* 5; Krymskii, *Vred,* 27; Bek, *Kurenie,* 41.

281. Preis, *Tabak—vrag,* 13.

282. Mikhailovskii, *Tabak,* 15.

283. Preis, *Tabak—vrag,* 13.

284. Nikol'skii, *O kurenii tabaka.* 12.

5. CONTESTED

1. V. V., *Kurite skol'ko khotite*, 20–22.

2. He attributed the theory to Leroy and Audiffrent, though there appeared to be no equivalent philosophers or psychologists in the period. Ibid., 26–31, quotation page 31. The general fascination with melancholy in the period is explored in Steinberg, *Petersburg*, 234–67.

3. V. V., *Kurite skol'ko khotite*, 28–36, quotations page 32 and 35.

4. Ibid., 57.

5. Ibid., 60–61, quotation page 60.

6. Ibid., 37–38, quotation page 37.

7. Ibid., 61.

8. V. Portugalov, "Tabak—gibel' molodezhi," *Vestnik vospitaniia: Nauchno-populiarnyi zhurnal' dlia roditelei i vospitatelei* (1891), 78–99, quotations pages 80, 87, and 95.

9. Claire Shaw, "Deafness and the Politics of Hearing," in *Russian History through the Senses: From 1700 to the Present*, ed. Matthew P. Romaniello and Tricia Starks (London: Bloomsbury, 2016), 193–218.

10. Mount Athos, *Kurenia tabaku*, 20.

11. Students of Grammatchikov and Ossendovskii, "K voprosu o vliianii kureniia na organizm cheloveka," *Vrach* 1 (1887): 4.

12. S. D. Vladychko, *Vlianie tabachnogo dyma na nervnuiu sistemu i organizum' voobshche* (St. Petersburg: Prakticheskaia meditsina, 1906), 58.

13. Vigié and Vigié, *L'herbe*, 25–50.

14. Courtwright, *Forces*, 70.

15. Nikolaos A. Chrissidis, "Sex, Drink, and Drugs: Tobacco in Seventeenth-Century Russia," Eve Levin, "Tobacco and Health in Early Modern Russia," and Erika Monahan, "Regulating Virtue and Vice: Controlling Commodities in Early Modern Siberia," in *Tobacco in Russian History and Culture: From the Seventeenth Century to the Present*, ed. Matthew P. Romaniello and Tricia Starks (New York: Routledge, 2009), 26–43, 44–60, and 61–82.

16. Bek, *Kurenie*, 7.

17. V. V., *Kurite skol'ko khotite*, 58.

18. Beliakov, *Tabak*, 23.

19. L. S. Minor, *Nauchnyia osnovy bor'by s kureniem tabaka* (Moscow: Tovarishchestva, 1914), 8–9.

20. Grinevskii, *Bros'te*, 19.

21. Botkin, *Vrednye posledstviia*, 11.

22. Poliakov, *Ne kuri*, 14.

23. I. I. Pontaga, *Izsledovanie russkago tabaka i papirosnago dyma* (Iu'ev: K. Mattisen, 1902).

24. A. A. Fal'kenberg, *Tabak i bakterii. iz. Vracha* No. 51 (St. Petersburg: Ia. Treia, 1892), 4.

25. Udintsev, *O vrede*, 6.

26. P. P. Orlov, *Vrednyia privychki i sposoby izbavit'sia ot nikh* (St. Petersburg: Knizhnyi sklad "Russkoe chtenie," n.d.), 46.

27. M. Valitskaia, *O vrede kureniia tabaku (Doklad, chitannyi v Pedagogicheskom musee Solianago gorodka v S.-Pb-ge). Iz No. 7 i 8 Zemskago vracha za 1890* (Kiev: Chernigovskoe gubernskoe upravleniie, 1890).

28. Minor, *Nauchnyia osnovy*, 8.

29. Ibid., 12, 16–17.

30. Rokau, *Interesnaia*, 75–76.

31. Il'inskii, *Tri iada*, 20; Mikhailovskii, *Tabak*, 10; Mount Athos, *Kakoi vred*, 12; Il'inskii, *Polezno*, 12.

32. Mikhailovskii, *Tabak*, 4.

33. Peter Bartrip, "Pushing the Weed: The Editorializing and Advertising of Tobacco in the *Lancet* and the *British Medical Journal*, 1880–1958" in *Ashes to Ashes: The History of Smoking*

and Health, ed. S. Lock, L. A. Reynolds, and E. M. Tansey (Amsterdam: Rodopi, 1998), 106–12; Hilton, *Smoking*, 63–65.

34. Tate, *Cigarette Wars*, 53–54

35. Hilton, *Smoking*, 66; Petrone, *Tobacco*, 240–53.

36. Rudy, *Freedom*, 22–25.

37. Galina Kichigina, *The Imperial Laboratory: Experimental Physiology and Clinical Medicine in Post-Crimean Russia* (Amsterdam: Rodopi, 2009), 9–10.

38. Buial'skii, *O vrede*.

39. Mount Athos, *Bros'te kurit!*, 10.

40. Dogel, *Tabak*, 74.

41. Grinevskii, *Bros'te*, 11.

42. Minor, *Nauchnyia osnovy*, 9.

43. Preis, *Tabak—Vrag*, 5.

44. Herlihy, *The Alcoholic Empire*, 29–30.

45. Keibel, *Kak nam' sleduet'*, 26–39.

46. Krymskii, *Vred*, 5.

47. Bek, *Kurenie*, 47.

48. Keibel, *Kak nam' sleduet'*, 28.

49. Ignatiev, "Kurenie," 72.

50. *O razvedenii i fabrikatsii tabaka*, 49.

51. Current measurements show a similar hierarchy, with Maryland, Turkish, Burley, and *rustica* having the lowest to highest nicotine contents. Jack E. Henningfield, Emma Calvento, and Sakire Pogun, *Nicotine Psychopharmacology* (Bethesda, MD: Springer, 2009), 62–63. Nicotine percentages hovered around 6% for makhorka versus 2% for American varieties according to Bartolomeo (*Demon*, 64). A similar case was made in Khmelevskii, *O stoikosti*, 7–9. Quotation from Beliakov, *Tabak*, 22.

52. *Ne po nosu tabak: Russkaia skazka*. 2nd ed. (Moscow: F. Iogansont, 1882).

53. Keibel, *Kak nam sleduet*, 33–34.

54. Mount Athos, *Bros'te kurit*, 11–12.

55. *O razvedenii i fabrikatsii tabaka*, 56.

56. Khmelevskii, *O stoikosti*, 23; 47; Beliakov, *Tabak*, 36.

57. Bek, *Kurenie*, 24, 47–48; see also Beliakov, *Tabak*, 36.

58. Dogel, *Tabak*, 39.

59. Il'inskii, *Tri iada*, 35.

60. Ibid., 34.

61. Minor, *Nauchnyia osnovy*, 20–21. Nicotine free cigarettes were also marketed in the United States in the 1880s and 1890s. Tate, *Cigarette Wars*, 19.

62. Udintsev, *O vrede*, 10.

63. A. L. Mendel'son, "K vorposu o vliianii kureniia na zdorov'e: Doklad II sektsii Obshchestva okhraneniia narodnago zdraviia, *Zhurnal Russkago obshchestva okhraneniia narodnago zdraviia: Dopushchen uchenym komitetom Ministerstva Narodnago Prosveshcheniia dlia fundamental'nykh bibliotek srednikh uchebnykh zavedenii, muzhskikh i zhenskikh* 9 (September 1897): 593.

64. Sebelius, *SGR*, 16–17.

65. Advertisement, "Tobacco in Russia: An Historico-Poetic Investigation by Uncle Misha," *Restorannoe delo* 2 (1912): 3.

66. "Mir papirosy," *Novyi Krai*, April 10, 1911, 5.

67. "A. Lopat and Son," *Novyi Krai*, March 24, 1911, 4.

68. "Kuria," *Novyi Krai*, January 5, 1908, 4.

69. Proctor, *Golden*, 365.

70. A. L. V. Khofman, *Regulirovanie kureniia i kreposti tabaka: Patentovano* (Samara: A. A. Lebson, 1913), 3–7, quotations from page 5, 6, and 7, testimonials starting page 14.

71. Since neither dependency nor addiction was understood at the time, nor did these terms correspond to language then used, fine distinctions do not hold. Eugene Raikhel, "From the Brain Disease *Model* to Ecologies of Addiction," in *Revisioning Psychiatry: Cultural Phenomenology, Critical Neuroscience, and Global Mental Health* eds. Laurence Kirmayer, Robert Lemelson, and Constance Cummings (Cambridge: Cambridge University Press, 2015), 343–74; William Garriott and Eugene Raikhel, "Addiction in the Making," *Annual Review of Anthropology* 44 (2015): 477–91.

72. David F. Mustov, "Drug Abuse Research in Historical Perspective," in *Pathways of Addiction: Opportunities in Drug Abuse Research*, ed. Committee on Opportunity in Drug Abuse Research (Washington, DC: National Academy Press, 1996), 284–94.

73. Harry Gene Levine, "The Discovery of Addiction: Changing Conceptions of Habitual Drunkenness in America," *Journal of Studies on Alcohol* 19, no. 1 (1978): 144, 151.

74. Peter Ferentzy, "From Sin to Disease: Differences and Similarities between Past and Current Conceptions of Chronic Drunkenness," *Contemporary Drug Problems* 26 (2001): 363–65; J. Warner, "Resolv'd to Drink No More: Addiction as a Preindustrial Construct," *Journal of the Study of Alcohol* 55 (1994): 685–91.

75. Petrone, *Tobacco*, 14; Courtwright, *Forces*, 174.

76. Arnold Jaffe, *Addiction Reform in the Progressive Age: Scientific and Social Responses to Drug Dependence in the United States, 1870–1930* (New York: Arno Press, 1981), passim; Courtwright, *Forces*, 141–42; Levine, "The Discovery of Addiction," 151.

77. David Joravsky, *Russian Psychology: A Critical History* (Oxford: Basil Blackwell, 1989), 17–19, 29–52.

78. Mariana Valverde, *Diseases of the Will: Alcohol and the Dilemmas of Freedom* (Cambridge: Cambridge University Press, 1998), 41; Marc J. Miresco, and Laurence J. Kirmayer, "The Persistence of Mind-Brain Dualism in Psychiatric Reasoning about Clinical Scenarios," *American Journal of Psychiatry* 163 (May 2006): 914; Laurence J. Kirmayer, "Mind and Body as Metaphors: Hidden Values in Biomedicine," *Biomedicine Explained* 13 (1988): 57–93; Levine, "The Discovery of Addiction," 143–74; William L. White, *Slaying the Dragon: The History of Addiction Treatment and Recovery in America* (Bloomington, IL: Chestnut Health Systems/Lighthouse Institute, 1998), 3; Richard J. Bonnie, "Responsibility for Addiction," *Journal of the American Academy of Psychiatry and the Law* 30 (2002): 405–13.

79. Courtwright, *Forces*, 180.

80. Sirotkina, *Diagnosing Literary Genius*, 11–12.

81. Ibid., 45–116; Julie Vail Brown, "Psychiatrists and the State in Tsarist Russia," in *Social Control and the State*, ed. Stanley Cohen and Andrew Scull (New York: St. Martin's Press, 1983), 269–70.

82. See for example the 1904 Ninth Pirogov Congress, which opened as one of the first public attacks on the tsarist state. Frieden, *Russian Physicians*, 231; Joravsky, *Russian Psychology*, 53–91.

83. Herlihy, *The Alcoholic Empire*, 38.

84. "Strashnaia bolezn'," *Trezvaia zhizn'* no. 2 (1905): 31–34.

85. Herlihy, *The Alcoholic Empire*, 37.

86. Ibid., 69.

87. Vvedenskii, *O kurenii tabaku*, 28–30; see also Grinevskii, *Bros'te*, 4.

88. Popov, *Nachnite bor'bu*, 22.

89. V. P., *Shto takoe*, 5.

90. Botkin, *Vrednye posledstviia*, 4.

91. Sirotkina, *Diagnosing Literary Genius*, 4.

92. Levine, "The Discovery of Addiction," 153–55.

93. Mount Athos, *Kurenia tabaku*, 14–15.

94. Tate, *Cigarette Wars*, 25–27.

95. Dr. Preis, as quoted in Blindovskii, *Kak brosit'*, 7.

96. Il'inskii, *Polezno*, 9–10; *Tabak*, 8–9.

97. Grinevskii, *Bros'te*, 20–21.

98. Priklonskii, *Upotreblenie*, 6–8.

99. Khmelevskii, *O stoikosti*, 20–21.

100. *P'ianstvo i kurenie tabaku*, 42.

101. Herlihy, *The Alcoholic Empire*, 9, 123.

102. In the Russian State Library catalog there were six editions of Dogel's *Tabak*.

103. Herlihy, *The Alcoholic Empire*, 39.

104. Dogel, *Tabak*, 46–51.

105. Nikol'skii, *O Tabake*, 2.

106. Herlihy, *The Alcoholic Empire*, 36–37.

107. Ibid., 36.

108. Nikol'skii, *O Tabake*, 11.

109. Ibid., 11.

110. Popov, *Nachnite bor'bu*, 4.

111. Bek, *Kurenie*, 3–4.

112. Priklonskii, *Upotreblenie*, 23.

113. Herlihy, *The Alcoholic Empire*, 37–39. Current studies show that only 5 percent of cessation attempts find initial success. Sebelius, *SGR*, 105.

114. Tormazov, *Zagadka kureniia*, 306, quotations 5 and 6.

115. Ibid., 9.

116. Ibid., 8, 16–28, 30–38.

117. Ibid., 35–42.

118. Tregubov, *Normal'nyi sposob*, 14

119. Keibel, *Kak nam sleduet*, 26.

120. Priklonskii, *Upotreblenie*, 41.

121. "Referati," *Pedagogicheskii sbornik izdavaemyi pri glavnom upravlenii voenno-uchebykh zavedenii*, Tom. 368 (September 1897): 505.

122. Nikol'skii, *O kurenii tabaka*, 13.

123. Ibid., 13–14.

124. Appollov, *Perestanem kurit'!* 51.

125. Buial'skii, *O vrede*.

126. Trakhtenberg, *Kak oni brosili kurit'*, passim.

127. Ibid., 15.

128. Zasidatel-Krzheminskii, *Tabachnoe otravlenie*, 26.

129. Grinevskii, *Bros'te*, 23.

130. Krymskii, *Vred*, 34.

131. Komisarenko, *Pagubnoe*, 6–7.

132. Tregubov, *Normal'nyi sposob*, 15.

133. Ibid., 16–18.

134. E. V. Korsun and M. A. Avkhukova, "Vklad S. P Botkina v razvitie otechestvennoi fitoterapii," *Klinicheskaia meditsina* 9 (2012): 22–23.

135. Tregubov, *Normal'nyi sposob*, 18.

136. Valverde, *Diseases of the Will*, 59–64.

137. Levine, "The Discovery of Addiction," 156.

138. Ibid., 158.

139. Ibid., 164.

140. Valverde, *Diseases of the Will*, 45, 51.

141. Beer, *Renovating Russia*, 116–24.

142. M. Menstrov, "Liudi bez voli," *Trezvaia zhizn'*, November 1905, 89–93.

143. For example, see Khofman, *Regulirovaniia*, 5; Nikol'skii, *O kurenii*, 13–14; A. A. Guliaev, *Zabytyi faktor khristianskogo vospitaniia voli* (Ufa: Elektricheskaia gubernskaia tipografiia, 1910), passim

144. Valverde, *Diseases of the Will*, 34.

145. Blindovskii, *Kak brosit'*, 15–16.

146. Arsenii, *Bros'te kurit' tabak'*, 7–8.

147. Mount Athos, *Kakoi vred*, 15–16.

148. *P'ianstvo i kurenie tabaku*, 42.

149. Herlihy, *The Alcoholic Empire*, 74–76.

150. Guliaev, *Zabytyi faktor*, 3.

151. Virenius, *Kurenie tabaka*, 6.

152. Catriona Kelly, "The Education of the Will: Advice Literature, *Zakal*, and Manliness in Early Twentieth-Century Russia," in *Russian Masculinities in History and Culture*, ed. Barbara Evans Clements, Rebecca Friedman, and Dan Healey (New York: Palgrave, 2002), 131–51.

153. Keibel, *Kak nam sleduet*, 37–39.

154. Anita Clair Fellman and Michael Fellman, *Making Sense of Self: Medical Advice Literature in Late Nineteenth-Century America* (Philadelphia: University of Pennsylvania Press, 1981), 29–38; Simon Pawley, "Revolution in Health: Nervous Weakness and Visions of Health in Revolutionary Russia, c. 1900–31," *Historical Research* 90 (2017): 191–94.

155. Sirotkina, *Diagnosing Literary Genius*, 125–42. Herlihy, *The Alcoholic, Empire*, 9; Susan K. Morrissey, "The Economy of Nerves: Health, Commercial Culture, and the Self in Late Imperial Russia," *Slavic Review* 3 (Fall 2010): 654; Goering, "Russian Nervousness," 45.

156. Brooks, *When Russia Learned to Read*, 260–61; N. Davydov, *Chuzhaia volia (Gipnoz): Original'naia drama v 4-x deistviiakh* (Dvink; I. A. Katsenelenbogen, 1905).

157. F. E. Rybaokov, "O primenenii gipnoza pri nekotorykh nervnykh razstroistvakh I patologicheskikh privychkakh," *Klinicheskii zhurnal* (December 1901): 571–88. A vast trove of pamphlets advocated hypnosis for healing illnesses, especially of the nerves. See also V. M. Bekhterev, *Gipnoz, vnushenie, telepatiia* (Moscow: Mysl', 1994); A. V. Gerber, *K ucheniiu o gipnoze v vnushenii i o primenenii ikh v lechenii nervnykh boleznei* (St. Petersburg: S. M. Propper, 1914); Grasse, *Gipnoz i vnushenie (Lechenie boleznei)*, trans. S. Ershova, 3rd ed. (St. Petersburg: V. I. Gubinskii, 1910); E. P. Radin, *Emotsional'nyia storony gipnoza i psikhoterapiia alkogolizma iz ambuliatorii dlia lecheniia gipnozom alkogolikov pri klinike dushevnykh i nervnykh boleznei v V.—Meditsinskoi Akademii akad. V. M. Bekhtereva*. Otd. ottisk iz "Russkago Vracha" No. 10–11-go. (St. Petersburg: Ia. Trei, 1905); F. E. Rybakov, *O lechenii p'ianstva gipnozom Iz psikhiatricheskoi kliniki Moskovskogo universiteta*. Otd. ottisk iz "Vracha" No. 18-go (St. Petersburg: Ia. Trei, 1898); A. Shiltov, *Sluchai zastrelago zapora, izlechennago gipnoterapiei v odin seans, i sedalishchnoi nevralgii u togo zhe bol'nago, ustupivshei semi seansam. Perepechatano iz gazety "Meditsina"* (St. Petersburg: Spb. gubernskaia tipografiia, 1891); V. V. Sreznevskii, *Gipnoz i volia: Rech, proiznesennaia v torzhestvennom zasedanii nauchnikh sobranii klinki dushevnykh i nervnykh boleznei 18 Ianvaria 1907 goda*. (St. Petersburg: N. N. Klobunov, 1907).

158. M. I. Bereznitskii, *Lechenie gipnozom morfinistov, alkogolikov i kuril'shchikov*, no. 7 ottisk iz "Russkii vrach" (St. Petersburg: Russkii Vrach, 1905), 1–3, 37.

159. Vladychko, *Vlianie tabachnogo dyma*, 59.

160. Herlihy, *The Alcoholic, Empire*, 8.

161. Transchel, *Under the Influence*, 69

162. "Anti-Cigarette League," *New York Times*, July 12, 1901, 5.

163. Bek, *Kurenie*, 45–47; Priklonskii, *Upotreblenie*, 39–41; Popov, *Nachnite bor'bu*, 29–30; Udintsev, *O vrede*, 12; Appolov, *Perestanem kurit'!*, 47.

164. Hilton, *Smoking*, 63.

165. Ian Tyrell, *Woman's World/Woman's Empire: The Woman's Christian Temperance Union in International Perspective, 1880–1930.* (Chapel Hill: University of North Carolina Press, 1991), 63; for the WCTU in Japan, Rumi Yasutake, "Men, Women, and Temperance in Meiji Japan: Engendering WCTU Activism from a Transnational Perspective," *The Japanese Journal of American Studies* 17 (2006): 91–111; Manako Ogawa, "The 'White Ribbon League of Nations' Meets Japan: The Trans-Pacific Activism of the Woman's Christian Temperance Union, 1906–1930," *Diplomatic History* 31, no. 1 (January 2007): 21–50; in Canada, Rudy, *Freedom*, 90–105

166. A. I. Tomilina, "Vospominaniia o kongresse 1903 goda Vsemirnago khristianskago soi-uza trezvosti zhenshchin," *Russkaia starina: Ezhemesiachnoe istoriecheskoe izdanie* (March 1916): 460–75; Report of the Eighth Convention of the World's Woman's Christian Temperance Union (n.p., 1910), 59, 166.

167. Virginia Berridge, *Demons: Our Changing Attitudes to Alcohol, Tobacco, and Drugs,* (Oxford: Oxford University Press, 2013), 1–13.

168. Kiernan, *Tobacco,* 43.

169. Statisticheskoe otdelenie (Glavnoe upravlenie neokladnykh sborov i kazennoi prodzhi pitei), *Popechitel'stva narodnoi trezvosti v 1904 godu* (St. Petersburg: B. O. Kirshbaum, 1907), 22. For more on the guardianship see Herlihy, *The Alcoholic Empire,* 14–35.

170. George E. Snow, "Alcoholism in the Russian Military: The Public Sphere and the Temperance Discourse, 1883–1917," *Jahrbücher für Geschichte Osteuropas* 45 (1997): 426.

171. N. A. Liubimov, *Dnevnik uchastnika pervogo vserossiskogo s"ezda po bor'be s narodnym p'ianstvom s. Peterburg 28 Dekabria 1909 g–6 Ianvaria 1910 g.* (Moscow: A. I Snegirevoi, 1911), 14–19.

172. Herlihy, *The Alcoholic Empire,* 97.

173. Grinevskii, *Bros'te,* 28.

174. Bek, *Kurenie,* 46.

175. John Welshman, "Images of Youth: The Issue of Juvenile Smoking, 1880–1914," *Addiction* 91, no. 9 (1996): 1379–81.

176. Burnham, *Bad Habits,* 91; Petrone, *Tobacco,* 112; Tate, *Cigarette Wars,* 5, 13, 30.

177. Welshman, "Images of Youth," 1383.

178. Matthew Hilton and Simon Nightingale, "'A Microbe of the Devil's Own Make': Religion and Science in the British Anti-Tobacco Movement, 1853–1908," in *Ashes to Ashes: The History of Smoking and Health,* ed. S. Lock, L. A. Reynolds, and E. M. Tansey (Amsterdam: Rodopi, 1998), 58; Hilton, *Smoking,* 72–76.

179. L. A. Zolotarev comp. *O preduprezhdenii kureniia tabaku v detskom vozrast: Populiarno-nauchnyi ocherk dlia roditelei i vospitatelei.* 2nd ed. (Moscow: I. N. Kushnerev, 1914).

180. *Tabak,* 17–18.

181. "Bor'ba s kureniem," *Pravda,* July 28, 1912, 9.

182. W. T. Stead, *Truth About Russia* (London: Cassell and Co. Ltd., 1888), 175–76.

183. The only reference to legal measures came from Dogel, *Tabak,* 60.

184. Priklonskii, *Upotreblenie,* 31.

185. Khmelevskii, *O stoikosti,* 133.

186. Bek, *Kurenie,* 45; Krymskii, *Vred,* 27–29; Priklonskii, *Upotreblenie,* 15, Botkin, *Vrednye posledstviia,* 20; Nikol'skii, *O kurenii tabaka,* 16.

187. Priklonskii, *Upotreblenie,* 39; Appolov, *Perestanem" kurit'!,* 47.

188. Birshtein, *K psikhologii,* 5.

189. Appolov, *Perestanem kurit'!,* 47, Bek, *Kurenie,* 40–41, 45; Priklonskii, *Upotreblenie,* 41; Udintsev, *O vrede,* 12; "K voprosu o vliianii kureniia na organizm" cheloveka," *Vrach* 1, no. 1 (January 1887): 4; Popov, *Nachnite bor'bu,* 23–24.

190. Grace G. Stewart, "A History of the Medicinal Use of Tobacco, 1492–1860," *Medical History* 11, no. 3 (July 1967): 228–68; Anne Charlton, "Medicinal Uses of Tobacco in History," *Journal of the Royal Society of Medicine* 97 (2004): 292–96.

191. Julie V. Brown, "Revolution and Psychosis: The Mixing of Science and Politics in Russian Psychiatric Medicine, 1905–13," *The Russian Review* 46 (1987): 283–302; Frieden, *Russian Physicians,* 231; Joravsky, *Russian Psychology,* 53–91.

192. Transchel, *Under the Influence,* 2, 41; Snow, "Alcoholism in the Russian Military," 417–19; Herlihy, *The Alcoholic Empire,* 129–45.

193. Transchel, *Under the Influence,* 34–36. Schrad, *Vodka Politics.*

194. Olga Novikoff, "The Temperance Movement in Russia," *Nineteenth Century* (September 1882): 439–59.

195. W. Arthur McKee, "Sobering Up the Soul of the People: The Politics of Popular Temperance in Late Imperial Russia," *The Russian Review* 58 (April 1999): 226.

196. Transchel, *Under the Influence,* 47.

197. Sally West, "Constructing Consumer Culture: Advertising in Imperial Russia to 1914" (PhD diss., University of Illinois Urbana-Champaign, 1995), 235.

198. Walker, *Under Fire,* 34–44.

199. Hilton, *Smoking,* 61–62.

200. The quotation has appeared in numerous forms but largely conforms to "Chelovek, kotoryi ne kurit i ne p'et ponevole vyzyvaet vopros—a ne svoloch li on?" Though it is popularly attributed to Chekhov, it is not clear from what work it might have come.

201. Geoffrey Borny, *Interpreting Chekhov* (Canberra, Australia: ANU E Press, 2006), 95. The piece was revived in 2010 and played for laughs by the comedian Steve Coogan.

202. Herlihy, *The Alcoholic Empire,* 14–30.

203. Translation by Ronald Hingley. Anton Chekhov, *The Oxford Chekhov* vol. 1, (London: Oxford University Press, 1968), quotations 155; text 151–58; 189–200. Alternatively, see Anton Chekhov "On the Harmfulness of Tobacco," trans. Michael R. Katz, *New England Review* 19, no. 4 (Fall 1998), 5–8; A. Chekhov, *O vrede tabaka: Tsena monolog v odnom deistvii* (Moscow: Litografii Moskovskoi teatral'noi bibliotek E. N. Ravsokhinoi, 1889), 1–12.

204. This from the 1889 version as presented in *The Oxford Chekhov,* 193.

205. Translation by Marian Fell in the collection Anton Chekhov, *Stories of Russian Life by Anton Tchekoff* (New York: Charles Scribner's Sons, 1916), 27.

206. Chekhov, *Stories of Russian Life,* 33.

207. "Plakaty dlia bor'by s kuren'em tabaku i alkogolizmom (glavnym obrazom v shkolakh)," *Obshchestvennyi vrach* (April 1912): 34.

208. Hilton, *Smoking,* 61–62.

209. Hilton and Nightingale, "Microbe," 52.

210. As quoted by West in "Constructing Consumer Culture," 223.

211. Morrissey, "The Economy of Nerves," 645.

212. Ibid., 663–69.

213. West, "Constructing Consumer Culture," 225, 235,

214. Ibid., 283.

215. Ibid., 236, 273.

216. "A Pleasant Pastime," *Restorannoe Delo* 2 (1912): 1.

217. Levine, "The Discovery of Addiction," 158–59.

218. "Papirosy—pamiati L. N. Tolstogo," *Novyi Krai,* March 24, 1911, 4.

EPILOGUE

1. Herlihy, *The Alcoholic Empire,* 146–51; Transchel, *Under the Influence,* 69–75.

2. Proctor, *Golden,* 44; Tate, *Cigarette Wars,* 65–92.

3. *Russkoi armii—Artisty Moskvy—Avtografy Moskovskikh artistov, sobrannye Komitetakh artistov Moskvy po sboru tabaku dlia armii v 1915 g.* (Moscow: Levinson, 1915).

4. Helen Rappaport, *Caught in the Revolution: Petrograd, Russia, 1917—A World on the Edge* (New York: St. Martin's Press, 2017), 101.

5. Neuberger, *Balkan Smoke,* 73–74.

6. Korno and Kitainer, *Balkanskaia zvezda,* 114–15.

7. Iu. P. Bokarev, "Tobacco Production in Russia: The Transition to Communism," in *Tobacco in Russian History and Culture,* ed. Matthew P. Romaniello and Tricia Starks (New York: Routledge, 2009), 151.

8. S. B Narkir'er, *Proizvodstvo tabachnykh i makhorochnykh fabric RSFSR v 1920 I 1921 gg.: Statisticheskii obzor* (Moscow: n.p., 1922), 27.

9. "Bratanie soldat," *Pravda*, October 3, 1917, 12.

10. Iu. P. Bokarev, "Tobacco in Russia," unpublished manuscript, last modified May 20, 2008.

11. Shortages also featured in memoirs from the British. French soldiers rioted over tobacco supply problems. Courtwright, *Forces,* 141.

12. Kafengauz, *Evoliutsiia*, 156, 198, 265.

13. Novikova and Shchemelev, *Nasha marka*, 62–63.

14. E. N. Burdzhalov, *The February 1917 Uprising in Petrograd*, trans. Donald J. Raleigh (Bloomington: Indiana University Press, 1987), 122–23.

15. Ruthchild, *Equality and Revolution*, 4–10.

16. Sheila Fitzpatrick, *The Russian Revolution: New Edition* (Oxford: Oxford University Press, 2008), 44, 53; Alexander Rabinowitch, *Prelude to Revolution: The Petrograd Bolsheviks and the July 1917 Uprising* (Bloomington, IN: Indiana University Press, 1968), 25.

17. "Tabachniki," *Pravda* June 21, 1917, p. 8. One worker recalled the activities of women throughout 1917 including working with injured revolutionaries; Chukaeva, "Ran'she i teper'," *Tabak* 4–5 (1937): 4.

18. Marina Romanova, "Tabachnyi kapitan," *Pravda*, December 3, 2001, http://www.pravda.ru/society/03-12-2001/836632-0/; Korno and Kitainer, *Balkanskaia Zvezda*, 119. For October at Dukat see N. Kh. Bargamov, "Oktiabr na 'Dukate'" *Tabak* 4–5 (1937): 3.

19. "Telegramma komanduiushchego voiskami Petrogradskogo voennogo okruga Avrova predsedateliu revvoensoveta Trotskomu," in *Kronshtadt 1921*, comp. V. P. Naumov and A. A. Kosakovskii (Moskva: Demokratia, 1997), no. 6, 49. See also Vladimir N. Brovkin, *Behind the Front Lines of the Civil War: Political Parties and Social Movements in Russia, 1918–1922* (Princeton, NJ: Princeton Legacy Library, 1994), 392; Ronald I. Kowalski, *The Russian Revolution, 1917–1921* (London: Routledge, 1997), 219; Paul Avrich, *Kronstadt, 1921* (Princeton, NJ: Princeton University Press, 2014), 38.

20. "Iz operativno-shifroval'noi svodki sekretno-operativnogo upravleniia VChK Leninu i Stalinu," cited in Avrich, *Kronshtadt 1921,* 191.

21. Bolshevik ambivalence and antipathy to women's issues had deep roots. Elizabeth Wood, *The Baba and the Comrade: Gender and Politics in Revolutionary Russia* (Bloomington: Indiana University Press, 2001), 30–33, 35–39, 43–48.

22. Hutchinson, *Politics and Public Health*, 191–95; Michael Kaser, *Health Care in the Soviet Union and Eastern Europe* (Boulder, CO: Westview Press, 1976); Henry Sigerist, *Medicine and Health in the Soviet Union* (New York: The Citadel Press, 1947), 29; Susan Gross Solomon and John F. Hutchinson, eds., *Health and Society in Revolutionary Russia* (Bloomington: Indiana University Press, 1990), 175–77, 181–83, 189–93.

23. N. A. Semashko, *Puti sovetskoi fizkul'tury* (Moscow: Vysshii sovet fizicheskoi kul'tury, 1926), 31; N. A. Semashko, *Nezabyvaemyi obraz*, 2nd ed. (Moscow: Politizdat, 1968), 15; B. S. Sigal *Vrednaia privychka (Kuren'e tabaka)* (Moscow: Gosmedizdat, 1929), 16

24. Tricia Starks, "Red Star/Black Lungs: Anti-Tobacco Campaigns in Twentieth-Century Russia," *Journal of the Social History of Alcohol and Drugs* 21, no. 1 (Fall 2006): 50–68.

25. John Reed, *Ten Days that Shook the World* (New York: Vintage Books, 1960), 123.

26. Kifiuriak and Kokoulin, *Tabachnaia fabrika "Iava,"* 4.

27. Elizabeth Waters, "Child-care Posters and the Modernization of Motherhood," *Sbornik-Study Group on the Russian Revolution* 13 (1987): 65; and her "Teaching Mothercraft in Post-Revolutionary Russia," *Australian Slavonic and East European Studies* 1 (July 1987): 29–56.

28. Courtwright, *Forces,* 191–93. Starks, "Red Star/Black Lungs," 50–68.

29. The article by demographer B. Urlanis started a firestorm of controversy in the late 1960s. See "Beregite muzhchin!," *Literaturnaia gazeta* 30 (1968): 12; "Krizis maskulinnosti v pozdnesovetskom diskurse," in *O muzhe(n)stvennosti*, ed. S. Oushakine (Moscow: Novoe literaturnoe obozrenie, 2002), 432–51.

Bibliography

ARCHIVES

Gosudarstvennyi arkhiv rossisskii federatsii (GARF)

JOURNALS AND NEWSPAPERS

Damskii mir
Klinicheskii zhurnal
Krest'ianin
Modnyi svet
Moskovskii listok
Narodnoe zdravie
Novyi Krai
Obshchestvennyi vrach
Otechestvennyia zapiski
Put' pravdy
Rabochii put

Rabotnitsa
Restorannoe delo
Russkii vestnik
Sanitarnoe delo
Trezvaia zhizn'
Vrach
Zdorov'e
Zemskii vrach
Zhenskoe dielo
Zhizn' tabachnika

BOOKS

Abramowich, Hirsz. *Profiles of a Lost World: Memoirs of East European Jewish Life before World War II*. Detroit: Wayne State University Press, 1999.

Ackerman, Diane. *A Natural History of the Senses*. New York: Random House, 1990.

Akimov, Vladimir. *On the Dilemmas of Russian Marxism, 1895–1903: The Second Congress of the Russian Social Democratic Labour Party; A Short History of the Social Democratic Movement in Russia*. CUP Archive, 1969.

Aleksandr. *Shto takoe—dymnaia privychka? Tabakokurenie*. St. Petersburg: M. I. Fomina, 1914.

Appolov, A. comp. *Perestanem kurit'! Shto takoe tabak i kakoi vred ot nego byvaet*. No. 148. Moscow: I. D. Sytin, 1904.

Arsenii. *Bros'te kurit' tabak'*. Moscow: A. I. Cnegireva, 1907.
——. (Nastoiatelia voskresenskago monastyria). *O poroke tabkokureniia*. St. Petersberg: A. S. Suvorina, 1905.
Atkinson, Dorothy, Alexander Dallin, and Gail Washofsky Lapidus, eds. *Women in Russia*. Stanford: Stanford University Press, 1977.
Avrich, Paul. *Kronstadt, 1921*. Princeton, NJ: Princeton University Press, 2014.
Avrutin, Eugene M., et al., eds. *Photographing the Jewish Nation: Pictures from S. An-sky's Ethnographic Expeditions*. Lebanon, NH: Brandeis University Press, 2009.
B., S. *Torzhestvo tabaku fiziologiia tabaku, trubki, sigar, papiros, pakhitos i tabakerki*. Translated from the French. St. Petersburg: Vnutr. strazhi, 1863.
Baburina, Nina, and Svetlana Artamonova, ed. *Russkii reklamnyi plakat*. Moscow: Kontakt-kul'tura, 2001.
Bain, John. *Cigarettes in Fact and Fancy*. Boston: H. M. Caldwell Co, 1906.
Balzer, Harley D., ed. *Russia's Missing Middle Class: The Professions in Russian History*. Armonk, NY: M. E. Sharpe, 1996.
Bardovskaia, L. *Sekret dvortsovoi tabakerki*. St. Petersburg: Tsarskoe selo, 2002.
Barnes, David S. *The Great Stink of Paris and the Nineteenth-Century Struggle against Filth and Germs*. Baltimore, MD: Johns Hopkins Press, 2006.
Bartolomeo, Iulius. *Demon v vodke i v tabake ili tabak i vino, to i drugoe, kak medlennyi iad, razrushaiushchii zdorov'e, sily, i sokrashchaiushchi zhizn' chelveka*. Moscow: I. E. Shiuman, 1871.
Beaver, Patrick. *The Match Makers: The Story of Bryant and May*. London: Henry Melland Limited, 1985.
Beer, Daniel. *Renovating Russia: The Human Sciences and the Fate of Liberal Modernity, 1880–1930*. Ithaca, NY: Cornell University Press, 2008.
Bek. *Kurenie: V obshchedostupnom izlozhenii*. Bezplatnoe prilozhenie k zhurnalu "Narodnoe zdravie," no. 25. St. Petersburg: Sankt Peterburgskaia elektropechatnia, 1902.
Bekhterev, V. M. *Gipnoz, vnushenie, telepatiia*. Moscow: Mysl', 1994.
Beliakov, S. A. *Tabak i vliianie kureniia ego na zdorov'e cheloveka*. Samara: Zemskaia tipografiia, 1904.
Benedict, Carol. *Golden-Silk Smoke: A History of Tobacco in China, 1550–2010*. Berkeley: University of California Press, 2011.
Berdov, P. N. *Pushkin: Vremennik Pushkinskoi komissii/AN SSSR. In-t literatury*. Moscow: Izd-vo AN SSSR, 1937.
Bereznitskii, M. I. *Lechenie gipnozom morfinistov, alkogolikov i kuril'shchikov*. No. 7 ottisk iz "Russkii vrach." St. Petersburg: Russkii vrach, 1905.
Bernstein, Laurie. *Sonia's Daughters: Prostitutes and Their Regulation in Imperial Russia*. Berkeley: University of California Press, 1995.
Berridge, Virginia. *Demons: Our Changing Attitudes to Alcohol, Tobacco, and Drugs*. Oxford: Oxford University Press, 2013.
Birshtein, I. A. *K psikhologii kureniia*. Moscow: Moskovskii voennyi okrug, 1913.
Blindovskii, A. *Kak brosit' kurit'*. Kiev: A. O. Shterenzon, 1912.
Bogdanov, Igor. *Dym otechestva, ili kratkaia istoriia tabakokureniia*. Moscow: Novoe literaturnoe obozrenie, 2007.
Bonnell, Victoria E. *Roots of Rebellion: Workers' Politics and Organizations in St. Petersburg and Moscow, 1900–1914*. Berkeley: University of California Press, 1983.
——, ed. *The Russian Worker: Life and Labor under the Tsarist Regime*. Berkeley: University of California Press, 1983.

Borny, Geoffrey. *Interpreting Chekhov*. Canberra, Australia: ANU E Press, 2006.

Botkin, S. P. *Vrednye posledstviia ot kureniia tabaku*. Moscow: P. V. Bel'tsov, 1914.

Bowlt, John E., and Matthew Drutt, eds. *Amazons of the Avant-Garde: Alexandra Exter, Natalia Goncharova, Liubov Popova, Olga Rozanova, Varvara Stepanova, and Nadezhda Udaltsova*. New York: Guggenheim Museum Publications, 2000.

Bradley, Joseph. *Muzhik and Muscovite: Urbanization in Late Imperial Russia*. Berkeley: University of California Press, 1985.

Brandt, Allan M. *The Cigarette Century: The Rise, Fall, and Deadly Persistence of the Product That Defined America*. New York: Basic Books, 2007.

Braudel, Fernand. *Civilization and Capitalism: 15th–18th Century*. Vol. 1. *The Structures of Everyday Life: The Limits of the Possible*. Berkeley: University of California Press, 1992.

Brennan, W. A., *Tobacco Leaves: Being a Book of Facts for Smokers*. Menasha, WI: Index Office, Inc., 1915.

Broadberry, Stephen, and Mark Harrison, eds. *The Economics of World War I*. Cambridge: Cambridge University Press, 2005.

Brokgauz, F. A., and I. A. Efron, *Entsiklopedicheskii slovar XXXII*. St. Petersburg: I. A. Efron, 1901.

Brooks, Jeffrey. *When Russia Learned to Read: Literacy and Popular Literature, 1861-1917*. Evanston, IL: Northwestern University Press, 2003.

Brovkin, Vladimir N. *Behind the Front Lines of the Civil War: Political Parties and Social Movements in Russia, 1918–1922*. Princeton, NJ: Princeton Legacy Library, 1994.

Buial'skii, I. *O vrede ot izlishchnego kureniia tabaka*. No. 170. *Sanktpetersburg Vedomostei*. St. Petersburg: Imperatorskii akademii nauk, 1859.

Bunker, Steven B. *Creating Mexican Consumer Culture in the Age of Porfirio Diaz*. Albuquerque: University of New Mexico Press, 2012.

Burdzhalov, E. N. *The February 1917 Uprising in Petrograd*. Translated by Donald J. Raleigh. Bloomington: Indiana University Press, 1987.

Burnham, John C. *Bad Habits: Drinking, Smoking, Taking Drugs, Gambling, Sexual Misbehavior, and Swearing in American History*. New York: New York University Press, 1993.

Bussiron. *O vlianii tabaku kuritel'nogo, niukhal'nogo i tsigar, na zdorov'e, nravstvennost' i um' cheloveka*. St. Petersburg: K. Zhernakov, 1845.

Chekhov, Anton. *O vrede tabaka: Tsena monolog v odnom deistvii*. Moscow: Litografii Moskovskoi teatral'noi bibliotek E. N. Ravsokhinoi, 1889.

———. *The Oxford Chekhov*. Vol. 1. Translated by Ronald Hungley. London: Oxford University Press, 1968.

———. *P'esy. 1895–1904* vol. 13. *Polnoe sobranie sochinenii i pisem: V 30 t. Cochineniia: V 18 t*. Moscow: Nauka, 1974–82.

———. *Stories of Russian Life by Anton Tchekoff*. Translated by Marian Fell. New York: Charles Scribner's Sons, 1916.

———. *Zagodochnaia natura*. Bibliotechka zhurnala Krasnoarmeets. Moscow: Pravda, 1944.

Chernevich, Elena, ed. *Russkii graficheskii dizain, 1880–1917*. Moscow: Vneshsigma, 1997.

Cherniaev, Isidor. *Brashiura*. Moscow: E. I. Pogodika, 1882.

Christian, David. *"Living Water": Vodka and Russian Society on the Eve of Emancipation*. Oxford: Clarendon Press, 1990.

Chulkhov, M. *Istoriia zakonodatel'stva: Tabachnoi promyshlennosti v Rossii do Ekateriny II*. Kazan: Ivan Dubrovin, 1855.

Classen, Constance, David Howes, and Anthony Synnott. *Aroma: The Cultural History of Smell*. London: Routledge, 1994.

Clements, Barbara Evans. *Bolshevik Women*. Cambridge: Cambridge University Press, 1997.

Clements, Barbara Evans, Rebecca Friedman, and Dan Healey, eds. *Russian Masculinities in History and Culture*. London: Palgrave, 2002.

Clowes, Edith W., Samuel D. Kassow, and James L. West, eds. *Between Tsar and People: Educated Society and the Quest for Public Identity in Late Imperial Russia*. Princeton, NJ: Princeton University Press, 1991.

Cohen, Stanley, and Andrew Scull, eds. *Social Control and the State*. New York: St. Martin's Press, 1983.

Committee on Opportunity in Drug Abuse Research, ed. *Pathways of Addiction: Opportunities in Drug Abuse Research*. Washington, DC: National Academy Press, 1996.

Cooper, Patricia A. *Once a Cigar Maker: Men, Women, and Work Culture in American Cigar Factories, 1900–1919*. Urbana: University of Illinois Press, 1987.

Corbin, Alain. *The Foul and the Fragrant: Odor and the French Social Imagination*. Cambridge, MA: Harvard University Press, 1986.

Courtwright, David T. *Forces of Habit: Drugs and the Making of the Modern World*. Cambridge, MA: Harvard University Press, 2001.

Cox, Howard. *The Global Cigarette: Origins and Evolution of British American Tobacco, 1880–1945*. New York: Oxford University Press, 2000.

Crawford, John Martin, ed. *The Industries of Russia: Manufactures and Trade with a General Industrial Map*. St. Petersburg: Department of Trade and Manufacture of the Imperial Ministry of Finance, 1893.

Dal', V. I. *Tolkovyi slovar' zhivago velikoruskago iazyka*. Moscow: Lazarevskii institute vostochnykh iazykov, 1863.

Davydov, N. *Chuzhaia volia (Gipnoz): Original'naia drama v 4-x deistviiakh*. Dvink: I. A. Katsenelenbogen, 1905.

Dedelin, O. *Kak uchit'sia ot' kureniia*. Translated from the German. Moscow: Izdaniia, 1909.

Demin, A. K., ed. *Kurenie ili zdorov'e v Rossii*. Moscow: Fond Zdorov'e i okruzhaiushchaia sreda, 1996.

———. *Rossia: Delo Tabak, rassledovanie massovogo ubiistva*. Moscow: Rossiiskaia assotsiatsiia obshchestvennogo zdorov'ia, 2012.

De Vries, Jan, *The Industrious Revolution: Consumer Behavior and the Household Economy, 1650 to the Present*. Cambridge: Cambridge University Press, 2008.

Dmitriev, K. *Kak vosdelyvat' tabak i podgotovliat' ego v prodazhu*. Moscow: I. S. Gabai, 1894.

Dobryi sovet kuriashchim. Petrograd: Ernst Biul'fing', 1915.

Dogel, I. M. *Tabak kak prikhot' i neschastie cheloveka: Rech', chitannaia na godichnom akte Kazanskago universiteta, 1884*. 3rd ed. Kazan: Imperatorskii universitet, 1886.

Douglas, Mary. *Purity and Danger: An Analysis of Concepts of Pollution and Taboo*. Reprint, London: Routledge, 2002.

———. *The World of Goods*. New York: Basic Books, 1979.

Druzhinin, N. M. *Okhrana zhenskogo i detskogo truda v fabrichnoi promyshlennosti Rossia: Diplomnoe sochinenie*. Moscow: ZAO, 2005.

Dvadtsatipiatiletie tabachnoi fabriki V. I. Asmolova v Rostov na Donu. (Kratkii istoricheskii ocherk fabriki) izdanie v pamiat iubileinago goda. Moscow: A. Gatnukh, 1882.

Dzhervis, M. V. *Russkaia tabachnaia fabrika v XVIII i XIX vekakh.* Leningrad: Akademii nauk SSSR, 1933.

Dziuvett, F. *Beregite vashe zdorov'e: Shto nado delat' shtoby byt' zdorovym, Azbuka gigieny dlia detei v shkole i sem'e (So svedeniiami o vrede alkogolia i tabaka).* Perevod s angliiskago P. Khlebnikova. Biblioteka I. Gorbunova-Posadova dlia detei i dlia iunoshestva, no 197. Moscow: I. N. Kushnerev i ko., 1912.

Edwards, Henry Sutherland. *The Russians at Home: Unpolitical Sketches.* 2nd ed. London: Wm. H. Allen and Co, 1861.

Egiz, S. A., ed. *Sbornik statei i materialov po tabachnomu delu.* St. Petersburg: V. F Kirshbaum, 1913.

Eklof, Ben, Josh Bushnell, and Larissa Zakharova, eds. *Russia's Great Reforms, 1855-1881.* Bloomington: Indiana University Press, 1994.

Emsley, John. *The Shocking History of Phosphorus: A Biography of the Devil's Element.* Basingstoke: Macmillan Publishing, 2000.

Engel, Barbara Alpern. *Between the Fields and the City: Women, Work and Family in Russia, 1861–1914.* Cambridge: Cambridge University Press, 1996.

——. *Breaking the Ties that Bound: The Politics of Marital Strife in Late Imperial Russia,* Ithaca, NY: Cornell University Press, 2011.

——. *Mothers and Daughters: Women of the Intelligentsia in Nineteenth-Century Russia.* Cambridge: Cambridge University Press, 1983.

Engelstein, Laura. *The Keys to Happiness: Sex and the Search for Modernity in Fin-de-Siècle Russia.* Ithaca, NY: Cornell University Press, 1992.

——. *Moscow, 1905: Working-Class Organization and Political Conflict.* Stanford: Stanford University Press, 1982.

Entsiklopedicheskie slovar'. St. Petersburg: Izdatel'skoe delo, 1901.

Episkop, Evlogii, *Tabak i ego vrednoe vliianie na cheloveka.* Saratov: A. F. Vinkler, 1914.

Fairbank, John King, Katherine Frost Bruner, and Elizabeth MacLeod Matheson, eds. *The I. G. in Peking: Letters of Robert Hart, Chinese Maritime Customs, 1868–1907.* Vol. 1. Cambridge, MA: The Belknap Press of Harvard University Press, 1975.

Fal'kenberg, A. A. *Tabak i bakterii.* iz. *Vracha* no. 51. St. Petersburg: Ia. Treia, 1892.

Federenko, L. N. *Kurenie v Rossii.* Rossiiskaia akademiia obrazovaniia iuzhnoe otdelenie. Slaviansk-na-kubain: Slavianskii filial Armavirskogo gosudarstvennogo pedagogicheskogo instituta, 2002.

Fellman, Anita Clair, and Michael Fellman. *Making Sense of Self: Medical Advice Literature in Late Nineteenth-Century America.* Philadelphia: University of Pennsylvania Press, 1981.

Ferrence, Roberta G. *Deadly Fashion: The Rise and Fall of Cigarette Smoking in North America.* New York: Garland Publishing, 1989.

Fesenko, E. I. *Bros'te kurit'.* Odessa: P. V. Bel'tsov, 1914.

Filtzer, Donald A. *A Dream Deferred: New Studies in Russian and Soviet Labour History.* Bern: Peter Lang, 2008.

Fishzon, Anna. *Fandom, Authenticity, and Opera: Mad Acts and Letter Scenes in Fin-de-Siècle Russia.* New York: Palgrave Macmillan, 2013.

Fitzpatrick, Sheila. *The Russian Revolution: New Edition.* Oxford: Oxford University Press, 2008.

Fitzpatrick, Sheila, and Yuri Slezkine, eds. *In the Shadow of Revolution: Life Stories of Russian Women from 1917 to the Second World War.* Princeton, NJ: Princeton University Press, 2000.

Frieden, Nancy Mandelker. *Russian Physicians in an Era of Reform and Revolution, 1856–1905*. Princeton, NJ: Princeton University Press, 1981.

Frierson, Cathy A. *All Russia is Burning! A Cultural History of Fire and Arson in Late Imperial Russia*. Seattle: University of Washington Press, 2002.

Galkin, R. A., V. N. Mal'tsev, N. P. Lopukhov, and O. L. Nikitin, eds. *Tabak ili zhizn': Aktual'nye problemy profilaktiki kureniia*. Samara: Perspektiva, 2000.

Gamalei, A. F. *Ob upotreblenii spiritnykh napitkov i kurenii tabaku* iz. zhurnala "Ogni." N.p.: A. M. Ponomareva, n.d.—voennyi tsensor.

Gately, Iain. *Tobacco: The Story of How Tobacco Seduced the World*. New York: Grove Press, 2001.

Gerber, A. V. *K ucheniiu o gipnoze v vnushenii i o primenenii ikh v lechenii nervnykh boleznei*. St. Petersburg: S. M. Propper, 1914.

Gerritsen, Anne, and Giorgio Riello, eds. *The Global Lives of Things: Materiality, Material Culture and Commodities in the First Global Age*. London: Routledge, 2015.

Gilman, Sander L. *Jewish Frontiers: Essays on Bodies, Histories, and Identities*. New York: Palgrave Macmillan, 2004.

Gilman, Sander, and Zhou Xun, eds. *Smoke: A Global History of Smoking*. London: Reaktion Books, 2004.

Glants, Musya, and Joyce Toomre, eds. *Food in Russian History and Culture*. Bloomington: Indiana University Press, 1997.

Glickman, Rose L. *Russian Factory Women: Workplace and Society, 1880–1914*. Berkeley: University of California Press, 1984.

Gompers, Samuel. *Seventy Years of Life and Labor: An Autobiography*. Edited by Nick Salvatore. Ithaca, NY: Cornell University Press, 1984.

Goodman, Jordan. *Tobacco in History: The Cultures of Dependence*. London: Routledge, 1993.

Gorshkov, Boris B. *Russia's Factory Children: State, Society, and Law, 1800–1917*. Pittsburgh: University of Pittsburgh Press, 2009.

Grasse. *Gipnoz i vnushenie (Lechenie boleznei)*. Translated by S. Ershova. 3rd ed. St. Petersburg: V. I. Gubinskii, 1910.

Greene, F. V. *Sketches of Army Life in Russia*. New York: Charles Scribner's Sons, 1880.

Grigorovich, D. V. *Polnoe sobranie sochineneii D. V. Grigorovicha v 12 tomakh*, tom. 11. St. Petersburg: A. F. Marksa, 1896.

Grinevskii, Adolf Fedorovich, *Bros'te kurit'! O vrede kureniia tabaku dlia zdorov'ia*. 2nd ed. Moscow: I. Efimov, 1905, 1889.

Guliaev, A. A. *Zabytyi faktor khristianskogo vospitaniia voli*. Ufa: Elektricheskaia gubernskaia tipografiia, 1910.

Hahn, Barbara. *Making Tobacco Bright: Creating an American Commodity, 1617–1937*. Baltimore, MD: Johns Hopkins University Press, 2011.

Hamm, Michael F., ed. *The City in Late Imperial Russia*. Bloomington: Indiana University Press, 1986.

Hartley, Janet M. *Siberia: A History of the People*. New Haven, CT: Yale University Press, 2014.

Healey, Dan. *Homosexual Desire in Revolutionary Russia: The Regulation of Sexual and Gender Dissent*. Chicago: University of Chicago Press, 2001.

Henningfield, Jack E., Emma Calvento, and Sakire Pogun. *Nicotine Psychopharmacology*. Bethesda, MD: Springer, 2009.

Herlihy, Patricia. *The Alcoholic Empire: Vodka and Politics in Late Imperial Russia*. Oxford: Oxford University Press, 2002.

———. *Odessa: A History, 1794–1914*. Cambridge, MA: Harvard University Press, 1986.

Hillyar, Anna, and Jane McDermid. *Revolutionary Women in Russia, 1870–1917: A Study in Collective Biography*. Manchester: Manchester University Press, 2000.

Hilton, Marjorie L. *Selling to the Masses: Retailing in Russia, 1880–1930*. Pittsburgh: University of Pittsburgh Press, 2011.

Hilton, Matthew. *Smoking in British Popular Culture, 1800–2000*. Manchester: Manchester University Press, 2000.

Howes, David, ed. *Empire of the Senses: The Sensual Culture Reader*. 2004. Reprint, London: Bloomsbury, 2014.

Howes, David, and Constance Classen. *Ways of Sensing: Understanding the Senses in Society*. London: Routledge, 2014.

Husband, William B., ed. *The Human Tradition in Modern Russia*. Wilmington, DE: Scholarly Resources, 2000.

Hutchinson, John F. *Politics and Public Health in Revolutionary Russia, 1890–1918*. Baltimore, MD: Johns Hopkins University Press, 1990.

I., E. *Shto vy delaete?* Nizhnii-Novgorod: I. A. Shelemet'eva, 1915.

Iakovlev, V., ed. *Revoliutsionnaia zhurnalistika 70-kh godov*. Paris, 1905.

Il'inskii, A. I., comp. *Polezno, ili vredno kurit', niukhat' i zhevat' tabak'*. Moscow: I. D. Sytin, 1888.

———. *Tri iada: Tabak, alkogol' (vodka), i sifilis (O vliianii ikh na byt' i zdorov'e cheloveka i ego potomstva i o tom—kak predokhranit sebia ot prichiniamago imi vreda)*. 2nd ed. Moscow: Kh. Barkhudarian, 1898.

Ipatov, A. D., comp. *Bylye gody: Vospominaniia starykh rabochikh tabachnykh fabrik g. Saratova*. Saratov: Saratovskoe oblastnoe izdatelstvo, 1937.

Iushkov, N. F. *Fabrikant luchshikh patentovannykh mundshtukov dlia sigar i papiros: Dramaticheskaia kartinka, v 1 deistvii*. Kazan: I. S. Perov, 1907.

Ivankin, Feodorva Fedotovich, and Leonid Dmitrii Romanovich. *Tabak i spichki v Rossii, 1875–1920 gg*. Moscow: Staraia basmannaia, 2009.

Ivanova, E. A., comp. *Rumiantsevskie chteniia—2015*. Moscow: Pashkov dome, 2015.

Jaffe, Arnold. *Addiction Reform in the Progressive Age: Scientific and Social Responses to Drug Dependence in the United States, 1870–1930*. New York: Arno Press, 1981.

Joravsky, David. *Russian Psychology: A Critical History*. Oxford: Basil Blackwell, 1989.

Judge, Edward H. *Plehve: Repression and Reform in Imperial Russia, 1902–1904*. Syracuse, NY: Syracuse University Press, 1983.

Jutte, Robert. *A History of the Senses: From Antiquity to Cyberspace*. Translated by James Lynn. Cambridge: Polity, 2005.

Kafengauz, Lev Borisovich, *Evoliutsiia promyshlennogo proizvodstva Rossii (posledniaia tret' XIX v.–30–e gody XX v.)*. Moscow: Epifaniia, 1994.

Kahan, Arcadius. *Russian Economic History: The Nineteenth Century*. Chicago: University of Chicago Press, 1989.

Karafa-Korbut, K. I. *Ustavy ob aktsiznykh sborakh*. Tom. iii. St. Petersburg: I. I Zubkova, 1914.

Karas, N. M. *Uvlekatel'nyi mir Moskovskoi reklamy XIX-nachala XX veka*. Moscow: Muzei istorii goroda Moskvy, 1996.

Kasatkin, A. K. *O vrede kureniia tabaka*. St. Petersburg, 1910.

Kaser, Michael. *Health Care in the Soviet Union and Eastern Europe.* Boulder, CO: Westview Press, 1976.

Kazanskii obshchestvo trezvosti. *O tabake: Sredstvo izbavit'sia ot mnogikh boleznei.* Kazan: Imperatorskii universitet, 1910.

Kaznakov, S. N. *Paketovyia tabekerki imperatorskogo farforovogo zaboda.* St. Petersburg: Sirius, 1913.

Kechedzhi-Shapovalov, Mikhail Vasil'evich. *Tabakovodstvo v Rossi.* St. Petersburg: Ulei, 1912.

Keibel. *Kak nam' sleduet' kurit' shtoby umen'shit' vred tabaka dlia zdorov'ia.* St. Petersburg: V. Bezobraz, 1890.

Kelly, Catriona. *Refining Russia: Advice Literature, Polite Culture, and Gender from Catherine to Yeltsin.* Oxford: Oxford University Press, 2001.

Kelly, Catriona, and David Shepherd, eds. *Constructing Russian Culture in the Age of Revolution: 1881–1940.* Oxford: Oxford University Press, 1998.

Khmelevskii, Vitol'd. *O stoikosti i kolichestvennom opredelenii nikotina v trupakh zhivotnykh, otravelennykh' etim' alkoloidom': Dissertatsiia na stepen doktora meditsiny.* St. Petersburg: Russkaia skoropechantia I. S. Pakhimova, 1876.

Khofman, A. L. V. *Regulirovanie kureniia i kreposti tabaka: Patentovano.* Samara: A. A. Lebenson, 1913.

Kichigina, Galina. *The Imperial Laboratory: Experimental Physiology and Clinical Medicine in Post-Crimean Russia.* Amsterdam: Rodopi, 2009.

Kiernan, V. G. *Tobacco: A History.* London: Hutchinson Radius, 1991.

Kifuriak, S. V., and O. I. Kokoulin. *Tabachnaia fabrika "Iava."* Moscow: Pishchevaia promyshlennost, 1978.

Kirmayer, Laurence, Robert Lemelson, and Constance Cummings, eds. *Revisioning Psychiatry: Cultural Phenomenology, Critical Neuroscience, and Global Mental Health.* Cambridge: Cambridge University Press, 2015.

Kivelson, Valerie A., and Joan Neuberger, eds. *Picturing Russia: Explorations in Visual Culture.* New Haven, CT: Yale University Press, 2008.

Kizenko, Nadieszda. *A Prodigal Saint: Father John of Kronstadt and the Russian People.* University Park: Pennsylvania State University Press, 2000.

Klein, Richard, *Cigarettes Are Sublime.* Durham, NC: Duke University Press, 1993.

Klimova, Ekaterina, and Irina Zolotinkina, comps. Anastasiia Rudakova, ed. *Reklamnyi plakat v Rossii, 1900–1920-e.* St. Petersburg: Palace Editions, 2010.

Kluger, Richard. *Ashes to Ashes: America's Hundred-Year Cigarette War, the Public Health, and the Unabashed Triumph of Philip Morris.* New York: Vintage Books, 1997.

Komisarenko, P. K. *Pagubnaia privychka.* 9th ed. Moscow: A. I. Momontov, 1913.

Korablev, Iu. I. ed. *Rabochee dvizhenie v Petrograde v 1912–1917: Dokumenty i materialy* Leningrad: Lenizdat, 1958.

Kornblatt, Judith Deutsch. *The Cossack Hero in Russian Literature: A Study in Cultural Mythology.* Madison: The University of Wisconsin Press, 1992.

Korno, V. I., and M. G. Kitainer. *Balkanskaia zvezda: Stranitsy istorii.* Iaroslavl: Niuans, 2000.

Korsmeyer, Carolyn. *Making Sense of Taste: Food and Philosophy.* Ithaca, NY: Cornell University Press, 1999.

Kotel'nikov, V. G. *Vozdelyvane prostogo tabaka-makhorki.* 2nd ed. St. Petersburg: Izd. A. F. Devriena, 1899.

Kowalski, Ronald I. *The Russian Revolution, 1917–1921*. London: Routledge, 1997.

Kozharinov, Veniamin. *Russkaia parfiumeriia: Illiustrirovannaia istoriia*. Moscow: Neisvestnaia Rossiia Chastnaia Kollektsiia, 2005.

Kozlowski, Lynn T., Jack E. Henningfield, and Janet Brigham. *Cigarettes, Nicotine, and Health: A Biobehavioral Approach*. Thousand Oaks, CA: Sage, 2001.

Kratkii ocherk deiatelnosti tabachnoi fabrik "Brat'ev Kogen'." Kiev: I. I. Chokolov, 1897.

Kratkii ocherk tabakokureniia v Rossii, v minuvshem 19-m stoletii: Za period vremeni s 1810 po 1906 god. Kiev: Petr Barskii, 1906.

Krementsov, Nikolai. *The Cure: The Story of Cancer and Politics from the Annals of the Cold War*. Chicago: University of Chicago Press, 2002.

Krylov, A. *Tabak: Prakticheskoe rukovodstvo k vozdelyvaniiu tabaka*. Moscow: N. Ris', 1869.

Krymskii, E. S. *Vred dlia zdorov'ia ot kureniia i niukhaniia tabaku i sredstva perestat' kurit'*. Zvenigorodka: E. S. Krysmkii, 1889.

Kudelli, P. F., comp. *Rabotnitsa v 1905 g. v S.-Peterburge: Sbornik statei i vospominanie*. Leningrad: Priboi, 1926.

Kurit' li mne ili net'? Rostov-na-Donu: A. Pavlov, 1906.

Laqueur, Thomas W. *Solitary Sex: A Cultural History of Masturbation*. New York: Zone Books, 2004.

Lenin, V. I. *Collected Works*. 4th ed. Moscow: Progress Publishers, 1964.

———. *Polnoe sobranie sochinenii*, vol. 3. Moscow: Gosizdat, 1958.

Leonov, A. I., ed. *Russkoe iskusstvo: Ocherki o zhizni i tvorchestve khudozhnikov, Pervaia polovina deviatnadtsatogo veka*. Moscow: Gosizdat Isskustvo, 1954.

Liubimenko, V. N. *Tabachnaia promyshlennost' v Rossii*. Petrograd: Komis. po izuch. Estest. Proizvoditel'nykh sil Rossii, 1916.

———. *Tabak*. Petrograd: M. S. Sabashnikovy, 1922.

Liubimov, N. A. *Dnevnik uchastnika pervogo vserossiskogo s"ezda po bor'be s narodnym p'ianstvom S. Peterburg 28 Dekabria 1909 g–6 Ianvaria 1910 g*. Moscow: A. I. Snegirevoi, 1911.

Lock, S., L. A. Reynolds, and E. M. Tansey, eds. *Ashes to Ashes: The History of Smoking and Health*. Amsterdam: Rodopi, 1998.

Lowth, G. T. *Around the Kremlin; or, Pictures of Life in Moscow*. London: Hurst and Blackett, 1868.

MacKay, John. *True Songs of Freedom: Uncle Tom's Cabin in Russian Culture and Society*. Madison: University of Wisconsin Press, 2013.

Maiorova, Olga. *From the Shadow of Empire: Defining the Russian Nation through Cultural Mythology, 1855–1870*. Madison: University of Wisconsin Press, 2010.

Malinin, A. V. *O chem umolchal MINZDRAV*. Moscow: Russkii tabak, 2003.

———. *Tabachnaia istoriia Rossii*. Moscow: Russkii Tabak, 2006.

Marchand, Roland. *Advertising the American Dream: Making Way for Modernity, 1920–1940*. Berkeley: University of California Press, 1985.

Markovich, K. *Otchet: po sboru papiros, tabaku i kuritel'nykh prinadlezhnostei, proizvedennomu v g. Rostove n/D. i po nekotorym stantsiiam Vladinavnazskoi zheleznoi dorogi*. Rostov na Don: Pechantia S. P. Iakovleva, 1904.

Martin, Alexander M. *Enlightened Metropolis: Constructing Imperial Moscow, 1762–1855*. Oxford: Oxford University Press, 2013.

McDermid, Jane, and Anna Hillyar. *Midwives of the Revolution: Female Bolsheviks and Women Workers in 1917*. Athens: Ohio University Press, 1999.

McReynolds, Louise. *Russia at Play: Leisure Activities at the End of the Tsarist Era*. Ithaca, NY: Cornell University Press, 2003.

Meaken, Annette M. B. *Woman in Transition*. London: Methuen and Co., 1907.

Meier, E. *Tabak—Iad'*. Riga: Traktatnoe obshchestvo v Rossii, 1911.

——. *Dobryi sovet kuriashchim* (Petrograd: Ernst Biul'fing', 1915).

Mendel'son, A. A. *Onanizm i bor'ba s nim*. Biblioteka zhurnala *Gigiena i zdorov'e rabochei i krest'ianskoi sem'i*. Leningrad: tov. Zinov'eva, n.d.

Menning, Bruce W. *Bayonets before Bullets: The Imperial Russian Army, 1861–1914*. Bloomington: Indiana University Press, 2000.

Mezhov, V. I. *Iadovityia svoistva tabaka i gibel'noe vliianie ikh na chelovecheskii organizm*. St. Petersburg: V. Bezobrazov i comp., 1871.

Mikhailovskii, V. *Tabak i vrednoe vliianie ego na cheloveka*. 5th ed. St. Petersburg: E. A. Pozdniakov, 1894.

Miller, Daniel. *Stuff*. Cambridge: Polity, 2010.

Minor, L. S. *Nauchnyia osnovy bor'by s kureniem tabaka*. Moscow: Tovarishchestva, 1914.

Morozov, S. D., and V. B. Zhiromska, eds. *Istoriia rossiiskoi povsednevnosti: Materialy dvadtsat' shestoi vserossiiskoi zaochnoi nauchnoi konferentsii*. St. Petersburg: Nestor, 2013.

Morrissey, Susan K. *Suicide and the Body Politic in Imperial Russia*. Cambridge: Cambridge University Press, 2006.

Mount Athos Skete of St. Il'inskii. *Kureniia tabaku, kak odna iz neprostitel'nykh prikhotei cheloveka*. 2nd ed. # 62. Odessa: D. Pliushchev, 1896.

Mount Athos St. Panteleimon Monastery. *Bros'te kurit'! O vrede kureniia tabake dlia zdorov'ia*. 6th ed. Moscow: I. Efimov, 1905.

——. *Kakoi vred prinosit cheloveku tabak?* Odessa: E. I. Fesenko, 1896.

——. *P'ianstvo i kurenie tabaku i ikh vrednaia posledstviia*. 2nd ed. Moscow: Efimov, 1904.

——. *O p'ianstve i drugikh bogoprotivnykh privychkakh kurenii tabaka, skvernoslovii, penii mirskikh pesen, igrishchakh, kataniiakh, sueverii i bozhbe. S ukazaniem dvukh dobrodetelei, kotoryia legko dovodiat do istinnago schastiia*. Moscow: I. Efimov, 1901.

M-ov', Vl. *Neskol'ko slov o tabake i ego upotreblenii (Otdel'nyi ottisk iz shurnala "Staroobriadets" no. 5 za 1906 g)*. Nizhnyi Novgorod: I. M. Mashistov, 1906.

Narkir'er, S. *Proizvodstvo tabachnykh fabric RSFSR v 1919 godu (v tsifrakh)*. Moscow: Vyschii sovet narodnogo khoziastva, 1921.

Naumov, V. P., and A. A. Kosakovskii, comps. *Kronshtadt 1921*. Moscow: Demokratia, 1997.

Nead, Lynda. *Victorian Babylon: People, Streets and Images in Nineteenth-Century London*. New Haven, CT: Yale University Press, 2000.

Ne po nosu tabak Russkaia skazka. 2nd ed. Moscow: F. Iogansont, 1882.

Neuberger, Mary C. *Balkan Smoke: Tobacco and the Making of Modern Bulgaria*. Ithaca, NY: Cornell University Press, 2013.

Nikol'skii, D. P. *O kurenii tabaka sredi uchashchikhsia*. no. 42. St. Petersburg: Russkago vracha, 1902.

——. *O tabake i vrede ego kureniia*. St. Petersburg: Ministerstva vnutrennikh del, 1894.

Norris, Stephen M. *A War of Images: Russian Popular Prints, Wartime Culture, and National Identity, 1812–1945*. DeKalb: Northern Illinois University Press, 2006.

Norton, Barbara T., and Jehanne M. Gheith, eds. *An Improper Profession: Women, Gender, and Journalism in Late Imperial Russia*. Durham, NC: Duke University Press, 2001.

Nove, Alec. *An Economic History of the U.S.S.R.* London: The Penguin Press, 1969.

Novikova, V. G., and N. N. Shchemelev. *Nasha marka: Ocherki istorii Donskoi gosudarst-vennoi tabachnoi fabriki*. Rostov: Rostovskoi knizhnoe izd., 1968.

Novoderevenskii, P. I. *Iskusstvo krasivo odevat'sia: Prakticheskiia ukapaniia dlia muzh-chin, kak odevat'sia deshevo i iziashchno, ne podvergaia sebia ekspluatatsii portnykh.* Narva: R. Peder, 1903.

Nye, Robert A. *Crime, Madness, and Politics in Modern France: The Medical Concept of National Decline.* Princeton, NJ: Princeton University Press, 1984.

Ocherk 25-letnei deiatel'nosti tabachnoi fabriki A. N. Shaposhnikova v S.-Peterburge 2 Ianvaria 1873–1898. St. Petersburg: Eduarda Goppe, 1897.

Olearius, Adam. *The Travels of Olearius in Seventeenth-Century Russia.* Translated by Samuel H. Baron. Stanford: Stanford University Press, 1967.

O razvedenii i fabrikatsii tabaka. Moscow: Aleksandr Semen, 1852.

Orlov, P. P. *Vrednyia privychki i sposoby izbavit'sia ot nikh.* 2nd ed. St. Petersburg: Knizhnyi sklad "Russkoe chtenie," n.d.

O tabake. Moscow: I. D. Sytkin i ko.,1890.

O tabake i vrede ego kureniia. Prerevolutionary pocket book with no author, publisher, or date.

Otchet tovarishchestva Rostovsko-Donskoi tabachnoi fabriki za 1903 god. Rostov: tip F.A. Polubatko, 1904.

Otchet tovarishchestva tabachnoi fabriki "A. N. Shaposhnikov' i Ko." v S.-Peterburge za 1912 god: Vtoroi operatsionnyi god. St. Petersburg: N. I. Evstif'ev, 1913.

Otto, Robert. *Publishing for the People: The Firm Posrednik, 1885–1905.* New York: Garland Publishing, 1987.

Oushakine, S., ed. *O muzhe(n)stvennosti.* Moscow: Novoe literaturnoe obozrenie, 2002.

P., V. *Shto takoe—dymnaia privychka? O tabakokurenii.* St. Petersburg: M. I. Fomina, 1914.

Paltusova, I. N. *Torgovaia reklama i upakovka v Rossii, XIX–XX vv.* Moscow: GIM, 1993.

Pankratova, A. M., ed. *Rabochee dvizhenie v Rossii v XIX veke: Sbornik dokumentov i materialov.* Tom 1–4. Moscow: Gosizdat, 1950.

Parant. *O tabake.* Translated from the French. St. Petersburg: Smirnov, n.d. prerevolutionary.

Pennock, Pamela E. *Advertising Sin and Sickness: The Politics of Alcohol and Tobacco Marketing, 1950–1990.* DeKalb: Northern Illinois University Press, 2007.

Perrot, Philippe. *Fashioning the Bourgeoisie: A History of Clothing in the Nineteenth Century.* Translated by Richard Bienvenu. Princeton, NJ: Princeton University Press, 1994.

Petrone, Gerard S. *Tobacco Advertising: The Great Seduction.* Atglen, PA: Schiffer Publishing, 1996.

P'ianstvo i kurenie tabaku i ikh vrednye posledstviia. 2nd ed. Moscow: I. Efimov, 1904.

Pick, Daniel. *Faces of Degeneration: A European Disorder, c. 1848–c. 1918.* New York: Cambridge University Press, 1989.

Podrobnyi ukazatl' po otdelam vserossiiskoi promyshlennoi i khudozhestvennoi vystavki 1896 g. v Nizhnem-Novgorode: Otdel IX Proizvodstva fabrichno-remeslennyia. Moscow: Russkago t-va pechatnago i izdatel'skago dela, 1896.

Poliakov, Petr Iv. *Ne kuri, ne niukhai i ne zhui tabaku (Pis'mo uchenogo i opytnogo vracha)* Graivoron: I. S. Banin, 1891.

Polianskii, A., comp. *Deistvie tabachnago dyma na zhivotnykh i cheloveka (Stoit'-li kurit'? Kak rekomenduetsia kurit'?).* Novonikslaevsk: Soiuz-Bank, 1919.

Polunov, Alexander. *Russia in the Nineteenth Century: Autocracy, Reform, and Social Change, 1814–1914*. London: M. E. Sharpe, 2005.

Pomerantsev, N. P. *O tabake i vrede ego kureniia: Beseda s uchenikami v–viii klassov Shelaputinskoi gimnazii gimnazicheskago vracha*. Moscow: M. M. Tarchigin, 1908.

Pomeranz, Kenneth. *The Great Divergence: China, Europe, and the Making of the Modern World Economy*. Princeton, NJ: Princeton University Press, 2000.

Ponomarev, I. V. *Stikhi o kurenii tabaka: Na pol'zu blizhnemu*. Kamyshin: Lebedeva i Fadeev, 1904.

Pontaga, I. I. *Izsledovanie russkago tabaka i papirosnago dyma*. Iu'ev: K. Mattisen, 1902.

Popov, Evgenii. *Deti! Nikogda ne nachinaite kurit tabak*. Perm: P. F. Kamenskii, 1884.

———. *Nachnite bor'bu so strast'iu k tabaku*. 3rd ed. Perm: Gubernskoe pravlenie, 1887.

Popov, Mikh. *Makhorkha*. Sofiia: Zemsnab, 1948.

Porter, Roy, ed. *Rewriting the Self: Histories from the Renaissance to the Present*. London: Routledge, 1997.

Preis, Nik. Pav. *Tabak i vino—vragi chelovechestva*. 5th ed. Khar'khov: Pechatnoe delo, 1902.

———. *Tabak—vrag chelovechestva (avto-kompiliativnyi sbornik)*. Khark'kov': Pechatnoe delo, 1902.

Priklonskii, Ivan Ivanovich. *Upotreblenie tabaka i ego vrednoe na organizm cheloveka vliianie*. Moscow: K. Tikhomirov, 1909.

Proctor, Robert N. *Golden Holocaust: Origins of the Cigarette Catastrophe and the Case for Abolition*. Berkeley: University of California Press, 2011.

———. *The Nazi War on Cancer*. Princeton, NJ: Princeton University Press, 1999.

Prozhogin N. P. *Vremennik Pushkinskoi komissii, 1978* AN SSSR. OLIA. Pushkin. komis. Leningrad: Nauka. Leningr. otd-nie, 1981.

Pushkareva, I. M. *Rabochee dvizhenie v Rossii v period reaktsii, 1907–1910 gg*. Moscow: Nauka, 1989.

Pushkareva, I. M., et al., eds. *Rabochee dvizhenie v Rossii: 1895–Febral' 1917 g., Khrnoika* vyp. 1 1895. Moscow: Pervaia obraztsovaia tipografiia, 1992.

Pushkareva, I. M., K. I. Borodkin, S. V. Glazunov, A. V. Novikov, S. I. Potolov, and I. V. Shil'nikova. *Trudovye konflikty i rabochee dvizhenie v Rossii na rubezhe 19–20 vv*. St. Petersburg: Aleteiia, 2011.

Rabinowitch, Alexander. *Prelude to Revolution: The Petrograd Bolsheviks and the July 1917 Uprising*. Bloomington, IN: Indiana University Press, 1968.

Radin, E. P. *Emotsional'nyia storony gipnoza i psikhoterapiia alkogolizma iz ambuliatorii dlia lecheniia gipnozom alkogolikov pri klinike dushevnykh i nervnykh boleznei v V.— Meditsinskoi Akademii akad. V. M. Bekhtereva*. Otd. ottisk iz "Russkago Vracha" No. 10–11-go. St. Petersburg: Ia. Trei, 1905.

Ragozin, Evgenii. *Istoriia tabaka i sistemy naloga na nego v Evrope i Amerike*. St. Petersburg: A. Benke, 1871.

Rappaport, Helen. *Caught in the Revolution: Petrograd, Russia, 1917—A World on the Edge*. New York: St. Martin's Press, 2017.

Reed, John. *Ten Days that Shook the World*. New York: Vintage Books, 1960.

Remizov, Aleksei. *O proiskhozhdenie moei khigi o tabake – Shto est' tabak*. Paris: Tchijoff, 1983.

Reynolds, Patrick, and Tom Shachtman. *The Gilded Leaf: Triumph, Tragedy, and Tobacco, Three Generations of the R. J. Reynolds Family and Fortune*. Boston: Little, Brown and Company, 1989.

Rindisbacher, Hans J. *The Smell of Books: A Cultural-Historical Study of Olfactory Perception in Literature*. Ann Arbor: University of Michigan Press, 1992.

Rokau. *Interesnaia i liubopytnaia istoriia kurivshikh', niuchavshikh' i zhevashikh' tabak': S legendarnymi pravdivym skazaniem o ego pagubnom' vlianii na zdorov'e cheloveka* Moscow: A. V. Kudriavtseva, 1885/6.

Romaniello, Matthew P., and Tricia Starks, eds. *Russian History through the Senses: From 1700 to the Present*. London: Bloomsbury, 2016.

——, eds. *Tobacco in Russian History and Culture: From the Seventeenth Century to the Present*. New York: Routledge, 2009.

Ruane, Christine. *The Empire's New Clothes: A History of the Russian Fashion Industry, 1700–1917*. New Haven, CT: Yale University Press, 2009.

Ruckman, Jo Ann. *The Moscow Business Elite: A Social and Cultural Portrait of Two Generations, 1840–1905*. DeKalb: Northern Illinois University Press, 1984.

Rudy, Jarrett. *The Freedom to Smoke: Tobacco Consumption and Identity*. Montreal: McGill-Queen's University Press, 2005.

Russkoi armii—Artisty Moskvy—Avtografy Moskovskikh artistov, sobrannye Komitetakh artistov Moskvy po sboru tabaku dlia armii v 1915 g. Moscow: Levinson, 1915.

Ruthchild, Rochelle Goldberg. *Equality and Revolution: Women's Rights in the Russian Empire, 1905–1917*. Pittsburgh: University of Pittsburgh Press, 2010.

Rybokov, F. E. *O lechenii p'ianstva gipnozom. Iz psikhiatricheskoi kliniki Moskovskogo universiteta*. Otd. ottisk iz "Vracha" No. 18-go. St. Petersburg: Ia. Trei, 1898.

Sahadeo, Jeff. *Russian Colonial Society in Tashkent, 1865–1923*. Bloomington: Indiana University Press, 2007.

Schrad, Mark Lawrence. *Vodka Politics: Alcohol, Autocracy, and the Secret History of the Russian State*. Oxford: Oxford University Press, 2014.

Schudson, Michael. *Advertising, the Uneasy Persuasion: Its Dubious Impact on American Society*. New York: Routledge, 1984.

Sebelius, Kathleen. *How Tobacco Smoke Causes Disease: The Biology and Behavioral Basis for Smoking-Attributable Disease; A Report of the Surgeon General*. Rockville, MD: U.S. Department of Health and Human Services, 2010.

Semashko, N. A. *Nezabyvaemyi obraz*. Moscow: Gosizdat, 1959.

——. *Puti sovetskoi fizkul'tury*. Moscow: Vyshii sovet fizicheskoi kul'tury, 1926.

Shapovalov, Andrei Valer'evich. *Ocherki istorii i kul'tury potrebleniia tabak v Sibiri: XVII-pervaia polovina XX vv*. Novosibirsk: Progress-servis, 2002.

Shiltov, A. *Sluchai zastrelago zapora, izlechennago gipnoterapiei v odin seans, i sedalishchnoi nevralgii u togo zhe bol'nago, ustupivshei semi seansam*. Perepechatano iz gazety "Meditsina." St. Petersburg: Spb. gubernskaia tipografiia, 1891.

Sigal, B. S. *Vrednaia privychka (Kuren'e tabaka)*. Moscow: Gosmedizdat, 1929.

Sigerist, Henry. *Medicine and Health in the Soviet Union*. New York: The Citadel Press, 1947.

Sirotkina, Irina. *Diagnosing Literary Genius: A Cultural History of Psychiatry in Russia, 1880–1930*. Baltimore, MD: Johns Hopkins University Press, 2002.

Sivulka, Juliann. *Soap, Sex, and Cigarettes: A Cultural History of American Advertising*. Belmont, CA: Wadsworth Publishing Company, 1998.

Slezkine, Yuri. *The Jewish Century*. Princeton, NJ: Princeton University Press, 2004.

Smith, Alison K. *For the Common Good and Their Own Well-Being: Social Estates in Imperial Russia*. Oxford: Oxford University Press, 2014.

——. *Recipes for Russia: Food and Nationhood under the Tsars*. DeKalb: Northern Illinois University Press, 2008.

Smith, Mark M. *Sensing the Past: Seeing, Hearing, Smelling, Tasting, and Touching in History*. Berkeley: University of California Press, 2007.

Snopkov, Aleksandr, Pavel Snopkov, and Aleksandr Shkliaruk. *Reklama v plakate: Russkii torgovo-promyshlennyi plakat za 100 let/Advertising Art in Russia*. Moscow: Kontakt Kul'tura, 2007.

Sobel, Richard. *They Satisfy: The Cigarette in American Life*. Garden City, NY: Anchor Press/Doubleday, 1978.

Solomon, Susan Gross, and John F. Hutchinson, eds. *Health and Society in Revolutionary Russia*. Bloomington: Indiana University Press, 1990.

Spacks, Patricia Meyer. *Boredom: The Literary History of a State of Mind*. Chicago: University of Chicago Press, 1995.

Sreznevskii, V. V. *Gipnoz i volia: Rech, proiznesennaia v torzhestvennom zasedanii nauchnikh sobranii kliniki dushevnykh i nervnykh boleznei 18 Ianvaria 1907 goda*. St. Petersburg: N. N. Klobunov, 1907.

Stal'skii, I., comp. *Donskaia gosudarstvennaia tabachnaia fabrika: Ocherk po materialam starykh kadrovikov DGTF A. K. Vasil'eva, E. I. Riabininoi, O. P. Ogarenko, i V. I. Shcherbakova*. Moscow: Gosizdat, 1938.

Starks, Tricia. *The Body Soviet: Propaganda, Hygiene, and the Revolutionary State*. Madison: University of Wisconsin Press, 2008.

Statisticheskoe otdelenie (Glavnoe upravlenie neokladnykh sborov i kazennoi prodazhi pitei). *Popechitel'stva narodnoi trezvosti v 1904 godu*. St. Petersburg: V. O. Kirshbaum, 1907.

Stead, W. T. *Truth about Russia*. London: Cassell and Co. Ltd., 1888.

Steinberg, Mark D. *Petersburg Fin de Siècle*. New Haven, CT: Yale University Press, 2011.

——. *Proletarian Imagination: Self, Modernity, and the Sacred in Russia, 1910–1925*, Ithaca, NY: Cornell University Press, 2002.

Stites, Richard. *The Women's Liberation Movement in Russia: Feminism, Nihilism, and Bolshevism, 1860–1930*. Princeton, NJ: Princeton University Press, 1978.

Stranichka iz istorii promyshlennosti iugo-vostochnoi Rossii: Tabachnaia fabrika F. K. Shtaf v Saratove Saratov: F. M. Kimmel', 1896.

Sviatlovskii, V. V. *Materialy dlia otsenki zdorov'ia rabochikh na sveklosakharnykh zavodakh i na tabachnykh fabrikakh*. izdanie zhurnala *Zemskii Vrach*. Chernigov: Gubernskaia pravleniia, 1889.

Tabak: Sredstvo izbavit'sia ot mnogikh boleznei. Kazan: Imperatorskago Universiteta, 1888.

Tate, Cassandra. *Cigarette Wars: The Triumph of "The Little White Slaver."* New York: Oxford University Press, 1999.

Tilley, Nannie M. *The R. J. Reynolds Tobacco Company*. Chapel Hill: University of North Carolina Press, 1985.

Tolstoi, L. N. *Polnoe sobranie sochinenii*, vol. 25 and 27. Moscow: Gosizdat, 1937.

——. *What Shall We Do Then? On the Moscow Census. Collected Articles*. Translated by Leo Weiner. Boston: Dana Estes and Company, 1904

——. *Why Do Men Stupefy Themselves? And Other Writings*. Translated by Aylmer Maude Blauvelt, NY: Strength Books, 1975.

Tomes, Nancy. *The Gospel of Germs: Men, Women, and the Microbe in American Life.* Cambridge, MA: Harvard University Press, 1998.

Tormazov, S. *Zagadka kureniia.* St. Petersburg: M. O. Vol'f', 1907.

Trakhtenberg, Vl. O. *"Kak oni brosili kurit'" Basnia-sharzh v 2-kh kartinakh.* St. Petersburg: Trud, 1904.

Transchel, Kate. *Under the Influence: Working-Class Drinking, Temperance, and Cultural Revolution in Russia, 1895–1932.* Pittsburgh: University of Pittsburgh Press, 2006.

Tregubov, I. *Normal'nyi sposob brosit' kurit'.* Batum: D. L. Kapelia, 1912.

Troinitskii, S. *Farforovyia tabakerki imperatorskago ermitazha.* Petrograd: Starye gody, 915.

Troyat, Henri. *Daily Life in Russia under the Last Tsar.* Translated by Malcolm Barnes. Stanford: Stanford University Press, 1961.

Tugendgol'd', Aleksandr. *Fiziologicheskiia izseldovaniia o deistvii nikotina.* Moscow: V. Grachev, 1864.

Tursi, Frank V., Susan E. White, and Steve McQuilken. *Lost Empire: The Fall of R. J. Reynolds Tobacco Company.* Rochester, WA: Gorham Printing, 2000.

Turchinskii, L. M., comp. *Russkie poety XX veka: Materialy dlia bibliografii.* Moscow: Znak, 2007.

Tyrell, Ian. *Woman's World/Woman's Empire: The Woman's Christian Temperance Union in International Perspective, 1880–1930.* Chapel Hill: University of North Carolina Press, 1991.

Udintsev, F. A. *O vrede kureniia (Nauchno-populiarnyi ocherk).* Kiev: Imperatorskii universitet sv. Vladimira, 1913.

Ukhanov, I. N. *Kuritel'nyi trubki: xviii-nachalo xx veka fantaziia i kur'ez v melkoi plastike.* St. Petersburg: Gosudarstvennyi ermitzah, 2009.

Ustav bol'nichnoi kassy pri tabachnoi fabrike Ottoman, t-va Laferm', nakhodiashcheisia v S. Peterburge, Kolokol'naia ul., no. 8. St. Petersburg: Br. V. I. Linnik, 1913.

Ustav tovarishchestva fabrik tabachnikh izdelii pod firmoiu "Laferm": Vysochaishe utverzhdennyi vo 2-i den' Ianvaria 1870 goda. St. Petersburg: Brat'i Shumakher, 1883.

Ustav tovarishchestva tabachnoi fabriki "Brat'ia Shapshal"" St. Petersburg: Rumanov, 1905.

Ustav tovarishchestva tabachnoi fabriki "Dukat"" v Moskve. Moscow: Russkoe tovarishchestvo, 1910.

V., A. *Shto govoriat' uchenye liudi o kurenii tabaka.* St. Petersburg: Aleks-Nevsk. O-va trezvosti, 1914.

V., V. *Kurite skol'ko khotite: Istoriia upotrebleniia tabaka, psikhologicheskiia osnovy etoi privychki, bezvrednost' i ee vashneishie gigienicheskiia pravila kureniia.* St. Petersburg: Gosudarstvennaia tipografiia, 1890.

Valitskaia, Mariia Konstantinovna. *Izsledovanie zdorov'ia rabochikh' na tabachnykh' fabrikakh': Nabliudeniia proizvedeny na 12 tabachnykh' fabrikakh' iuga Rossii s 3-mia risunkami i 1-i diagrammoi.* St. Petersburg: Tovarishchestvo Paravoi Skoropechatni Iblonskii i Perott, 1889.

——. *O vrede kureniia tabaku (Doklad, chitannyi v Pedagogicheskom musee Solianago gorodka v S.-Pb-ge).* Iz No. 7 i 8 *Zemskago vracha* za 1890. Kiev: Chernigovskoe gubernskoe upravleniie, 1890.

Valverde, Mariana. *Diseases of the Will: Alcohol and the Dilemmas of Freedom*. Cambridge: Cambridge University Press, 1998.

Vashik, Klaus, and Nina Baburina. *Real'nost' utopii: Isskusstvo Russkogo plakata XX veka*. Moscow: Progress-Traditsiia, 2003.

Vigié, Marc, and Muriel Vigié. *L'herbe à Nicot: Amateurs de tabac, fermiers généraux et contrebandiers sous l'Ancien Régime*. Paris: Fayard, 1989.

Violin, Ia. A. *Tabak i ego vred dlia zdorov'ia*. Kazan: Shtaba zapasnoi armii, 1920.

Virenius, A. *Kurenie tabaka*. St. Petersburg: N. V. Gaevskii, 1907.

Vladimir, Allan M. *On the Dilemmas of Russian Marxism, 1895–1903: The Second Congress of the Russian Social Democratic Labour Party: A Short History of the Social Democratic Movement in Russia*. CUP Archive, 1969.

Vladychko, S. D. *Vlianie tabachnogo dyma na nervnuiu sistemu i organizm' Voobshche*. St. Petersburg: Prakticheskaia meditsina, 1906.

Vvedenskii (Sviashchennik). *O kurenii tabaku*. Otdela rasprostraneniia dukhovno-nravstv. knig. pri Mosk. Obshchestve Liubit. Dukhovn. Prosveshcheniia. 5th ed. Moscow: T. Dortmam, 1915.

Walker, Robin. *Under Fire: A History of Tobacco Smoking in Australia*. Carlton, Victoria: Melbourne University Press, 1984.

Walton, Stuart. *Out of It: A Cultural History of Intoxication*. New York: Harmony Books, 2001.

West, James L., and Iurii A. Petrov. *Merchant Moscow: Images of Russia's Vanished Bourgeoisie*. Princeton, NJ: Princeton University Press, 1998.

West, Sally. *I Shop in Moscow: Advertising and the Creation of Consumer Culture in Late Tsarist Russia*. Dekalb: Northern Illinois University Press, 2011.

White, William L. *Slaying the Dragon: The History of Addiction Treatment and Recovery in America*. Bloomington, IL: Chestnut Health Systems/Lighthouse Institute, 1998.

Wilkins, Mira, and Harm Schröter, eds. *The Free-Standing Company in the World Economy, 1830–1996*. Oxford: Oxford University Press, 1998

Winter, Joseph C., ed. *Tobacco Use by Native North Americans: Sacred Smoke and Silent Killer*. Norman: University of Oklahoma Press, 2000.

Wood, Elizabeth. *The Baba and the Comrade: Gender and Politics in Revolutionary Russia*. Bloomington: Indiana University Press, 2001.

World Health Organization. *European Tobacco Control Status Report 2013*. Geneva, Switzerland: World Health Organization, 2013

——. *WHO Report on the Global Tobacco Epidemic, 2013*. Geneva, Switzerland: World Health Organization, 2013.

Worobec, Christine D., ed. *The Human Tradition in Imperial Russia*. Lanham, MD: Rowman and Littlefield, 2010.

——. *Possessed: Women, Witches, and Demons in Imperial Russia*. DeKalb: Northern Illinois University Press, 2007.

Zasidatel'-Krzheminskii, V. I. *Tabachnoe otravlenie: V sviazi s ucheniem ob angionevrozakh i bolezn'iu Raynand*. St. Petersburg: Prakticheskaia meditsina, 1911.

Zelnick, Reginald E. *Labor and Society in Tsarist Russia: The Factory Workers of St. Petersburg, 1855–1870*. Stanford: Stanford University Press, 1971.

——, ed. *Worker and Intelligentsia in Late Imperial Russia: Realities, Representations, Reflections*. Berkeley: University of California, 1999.

Zhurnal: Sostoiavshagosia 24 Febralia–8 Marta 1914 g. pri Glavnom upravlenii neokladnykh sborov i kazennoi prodazhi pitei soveshchaniia po voprosu o vliianii tabachnago ustava na tabakovodstvo i fabrikatsiiu tabaka. St. Petersburg: Ministerstva Finansov, 1914.

Zolotarev, L. A., comp. *O preduprezhdenii kureniia tabaku v detskom vozraste: Populiarno-nauchnyi ocherk dlia roditelei i vospitatelei.* 2nd ed. Moscow: I. N. Kushnerev, 1914.

Zybin, Aleksandr, comp. *Tabak, kak pagubnaia strast', i ego vrednoe vliianie na dukhovnuiu i telesnuiu zhizn' cheloveka.* Kungur': M. Letunov, 1907.

Index

Page numbers in italics refer to figures, maps, and tables.

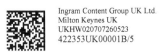

Ingram Content Group UK Ltd.
Milton Keynes UK
UKHW020707260523
422353UK00001B/5

9 781501 722059